Antifungal Agents
Advances and Problems

Special Topic

Progress in
Drug Research

Edited by Ernst Jucker, Basel

Advisor
Annemarie Polak

Authors
Johannes Müller and Annemarie Polak
Reinhard Kappe and Dagmar Rimek
Annemarie Polak
Michael Seibold and Kathrin Tintelnot

Birkhäuser Verlag
Basel · Boston · Berlin

Editor

Dr. E. Jucker
Steinweg 28
CH-4107 Ettingen
Switzerland
e-mail: jucker.pdr@bluewin.ch

A CIP catalogue record for this book is available from the Library of Congress, Washington D.C., USA

Bibliographic information published by Die Deutsche Bibliothek.
Die Deutsche Bibliothek lists this publication in the Deutsche Nationalbibliografie; detailed bibliographic data is available in the Internet at <http://dnb.ddb.de>.

ISBN 3-7643-6926-4 Birkhäuser Verlag, Basel – Boston – Berlin

Member of the BertelsmannSpringer Publishing Group
Printed on acid-free paper produced from chlorine-free pulp. TCF ∞
Cover design and layout: Gröflin Graphic Design, Basel

ISBN 3-7643-6926-4
9 8 7 6 5 4 3 2 1

www.birkhauser.ch

Contents

Foreword by the Editor

In the early 1990s Annemarie Polak and P.G. Hartmann expressed some hope that the battle for an effective therapy in dermatology as well as in deep mycoses could be won (PDR *37*, 181 (1991)). Five years later (PDR *49*, 219 (1996)), in an update of the above review and in summarising the then prevailing situation, A. Polak came to the conclusion that the search for new antifungals was an everlasting battle: despite the fact that important new antifungals were discovered and introduced into therapy, the breakthrough was still far away. This battle is still going on, and this volume *Antifungal Agents – Advances and Problems* aims at providing the reader with a concise overview of the situation, but might also give an impulse to further research in this important field of human disorders.

Antifungal Agents – Advances and Problems contains five chapters, each representing an up-to-date review covering the major problems of medical mycology. Physicians confronted with the various forms and problems of fungal diseases will welcome this monograph as a useful tool in their daily work and as a source of relevant original literature. Advanced students will benefit from the concise form of the presentation covering all major aspects of antifungals and their therapeutic application.

The main emphasis of the book is on antifungal therapy (chapter 4), covering the present state of art of chemotherapy for dermatomycoses, subcutaneous and invasive mycoses and also thoroughly dealing with open questions and unsolved problems.

In addition to this status quo review, an outlook into the future, to new biochemical and/or genetic targets, as well as to the new approaches interfering with the host defence or the virulence of fungi, which will become more important in the future, is provided. The author of this chapter, Annemarie Polak, not only shared her extended knowledge and experience but she also acted as Advisor for the entire monograph. The Editor is especially indebted to her.

The first chapter deals with various growth forms of the pathogenic fungi and classifies these fungi based on characteristics of their sexual life cycle and on their RNA/DNA pattern.

The second chapter describes the clinical manifestations of the complete set of human fungal infections known today. In addition to the clinical symptoms, on which the main emphasis lies, data on prevalence, overall importance and epidemiology are provided.

The third chapter deals with the various laboratory methods in the field of diagnosis of fungal infections which are necessary and suitable for a timely and accurate diagnosis. The identification techniques are described according to the fungal group involved, i.e. techniques for yeast and filamentous fungi are separate.

The last chapter deals with the field of susceptibility testing. On one hand the most relevant standard methods and their intrinsic problems related to media, fungi or drugs are presented; on the other hand, the usefulness of susceptibility data in connection with epidemiology and guidance of therapy is discussed. A special part of this last chapter is dedicated to the question whether a correlation exists between *in vitro* and *in vivo* data.

The Editor is grateful to the authors for their comprehensively written articles which in a very concise form cover all aspects of the current situation in the field of fungal diseases and therapeutic possibilities. My sincere thanks also go the members of Birkhäuser Publishing who participated in the production of this monograph. Thus, I am indebted to Beatrice Menz and Gabriele Fertöszögi for their great help as members of the Editorial Department. H.-P. Ebneter, Eduard Mazenauer and Gregor Messmer did contribute – as in the past decades – their vast knowledge, experience and innovative skill in the production of this book: for all their efforts and, especially, for the harmonious cooperation, I cannot thank all of them enough.

My very special thanks go to Hans-Peter Thür, Birkhäuser Publishing CEO. For a number of decades, Hans-Peter Thür participated directly in the efforts linked with the PDR series, and it was he who initiated this new series of monographs dealing with specific topics of drug research. My gratitude to Hans-Peter is linked with sadness that due to my advanced age and my wish for fewer responsibilities, this harmonious cooperation and our team-work come to an end with this PDR Special Topic volume.

Basel, February 2003 Dr. E. Jucker

Antifungal Agents – Advances and Problems (E. Jucker, Ed.)

Classification and taxonomy of fungi pathogenic for warm-blooded hosts

By Johannes Müller[1] and Annemarie Polak[2]

[1]Brandelweg 24, D-79312 Emmendingen-Maleck, Germany
[2]Spitzenrainweg 45, CH-4147 Aesch, Switzerland

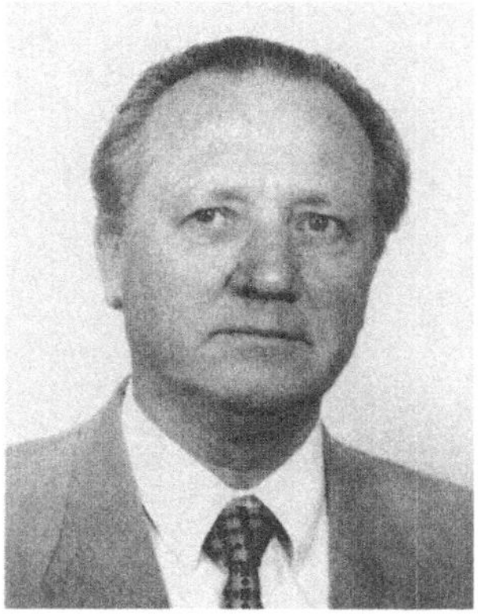

Johannes Müller

received the Doctor rerum naturalium *from the University of Munich in 1956. In 1960, he joined the Institute of Hygiene and Microbiology at Freiburg i. Br. At this time there was a department for extensive medical and microbiological diagnostics in bacteriology, virology, parasitology, and serology. Johannes Müller created a diagnostic and research unit for medical mycology. His main interest was electron microscopy. In 1973, Johannes Müller was awarded the title "Medizinischer Fachmikrobiologe DHGM"; in 1978, he received the "Habilitation" for medical microbiology and hygiene at the medical faculty of the University Freiburg and became professor in 1984. From 1975 to 1986 he was head of the division of parasitology and mycology at the institute of hygiene, and from 1986–1992 he was head of the mycology unit. Johannes Müller was mainly interested in host-parasite relationships in mycology, ultrastructure, pathogenesis, and immunology and development of new diagnostic methods. He was active member of various international research societies and later became an honorary member of several of these societies.*

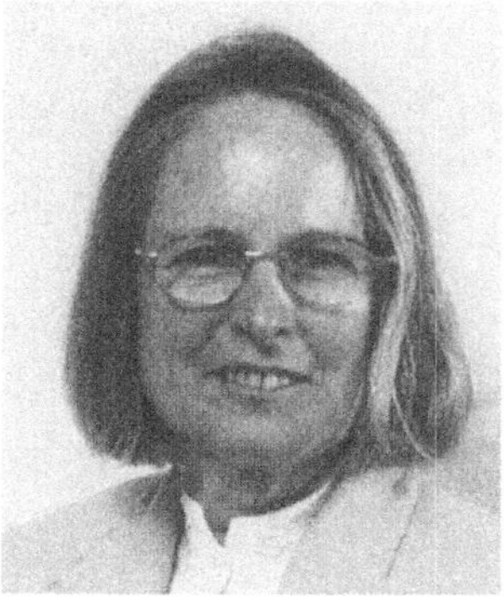

Annemarie Polak

received her Ph.D. in microbiology from the Eidgenössische Technische Hochschule (ETH), Zürich, Switzerland, in 1969. In the same year, she joined Hoffmann LaRoche as a microbiologist in the tropical medicine group. Her research interest included mode of action studies and detecting new antifungals. She became a specialist in the field of research on antifungals and was later promoted to Scientific Expert, a cadre position at Roche. In 1989, A. Polak did her "Habilitation" at the Institute of Microbiology and Hygiene in the Medical Faculty of the University Freiburg i. Br. (Germany) and received a professorship for medical mycology in 1995.

Summary

The kingdom of fungi is described with emphasis on fungi pathogenic for warm-blooded hosts. The various growth forms of the most frequent causative agents of fungal infections are described and their classification based on characteristics of their sexual life cycle and on their DNA/RNA pattern is summarized in various tables.

Contents

Keywords
Taxonomy, pathogenic fungi, *Zygomycota, Ascomycota, Basidiomycota.*

1 Introduction

Fungi are regarded as a separate kingdom of eukariotic organisms apart from plants and animals. They are heterotrophic, i.e., lacking chlorophyll, and are dependent on organic carbon compounds for their nutrition. They feed by excretion of enzymes into the colonized substrate and subsequent uptake of digested compounds through the cell wall and cytoplasmic membrane.

2 Morphology

Like human cells, fungi are eukariotic cells, in contrast to bacteria. The genome is organized in a nucleus surrounded by a membrane, which is continuous with the endoplasmatic reticulum. Cellular division is accompanied by meiosis or mitosis. Cell organelles such as mitochondria, ribosomes, vacuoles, lipid bodies, and other storage inclusions are also present. The only fungus-specific target for antifungal chemotherapy is the cell wall, which

Table 1.
Causative agents of zygomycosis; Division: *Zygomycota*

Order	Family	Genus	Species
Mucorales	*Mucoraceae*	*Absidia*	*A. corymbifera*
		Apophysomyces	*A. elegans*
		Mucor	*M. circinelloides*
			M. racemosus
		Rhizomucor	*R. miehei*
			R. pusillus
			R. variabilis
		Rhizopus	*R. microsporus*
			R. oryzae
	Cunninghamellaceae	*Cunninghamella*	*C. bertholletiae*
	Syncephalastraceae	*Syncephalastrum*	*S. racemosum*
	Saksenaeaceae	*Saksenaea*	*S. vasiformis*
Mortierellales	*Mortierellaceae*	*Mortierella*	*M. wolfii*
Entomophthorales	*Basidiobolaceae*	*Basidiobolus*	*B. ranarum*
	Ancylistaceae	*Conidiobolus*	*C. coronatus*
			C. incongruus

consists mainly (90%) of the carbohydrates glucan, mannan, and chitin, the latter two being absent in mammalian cells.

Pathogenic fungi grow in two different morphologic shapes. The main elements are apically growing hyphae. These filamentous fungi invade the substrate by single hyphae. The entire thallus is called mycelium. Unicellular fungi grow in the yeast form characterized by propagating in forming buds.

Suppression of hyphal growth due to environmental factors, e.g., nutritional conditions, temperature, host defense etc., often leads to deformation of the fungal thallus. This phenomenon is called dimorphism and must be regarded in diagnostic procedures. Dimorphism is conspicuous for *Histoplasma capsulatum*, *Blastomyces dermatitidis*, *Paracoccidioides brasiliensis*, and *Penicillium marneffei*, the hyphal form being saprophytic and the parasitic one being yeast-like in shape. *Candida albicans* also shows dimorphism; however, both phases of this species are responsible for pathogenicity.

The majority of fungi pass sexual life cycles (teleomorph) with formation of sexual propagules. The sexual life cycle is the basis of ranging the fungi in a natural classification system with regard to biological relationship. The teleomorph life cycle of fungi pathogenic for warm-blooded hosts, however,

Table 2.
Opportunistic causative agents of candidosis and geotrichosis. Division: *Ascomycota*; Class: *Hemiascomycetes*; Order: *Saccharomycetales*

Familiy	Genus	Species: teleomorph name	Species: anamorph name
Candidosis			
Saccharomycetaceae	*Issatchenkia*	*I. orientalis*	*Candida krusei*
Endomycetaceae	*Stephanoascus*	*S. ciferrii*	*Candida ciferrii*
	Pichia	*P. guilliermondii*	*Candida guilliermondii*
Metschnikowiaceae	*Clavispora*	*C. lusitaniae*	*Candida lusitaniae*
Unclassified opportunistic agents of candidosis			
			Candida albicans
			C. dubliniensis
			C. glabrata
			C. parapsilosis
			C. tropicalis
			C. zeylanoides
Geotrichosis:			
Dipodascaceae	*Dipodascus*	*D. capitatus*	*Geotrichum capitatum*
		–	*Geotrichum clavatum*

is mostly realized only under specific ecological conditions that are rarely to be observed in the laboratory. The asexual life cycle (anamorph) is the most commonly observed life phase. Without exception only the anamorph phase is found to be responsible in the situation of infection. Many filamentous fungi propagate readily under laboratory conditions by asexual sporulation in a broad variety of spore configurations, which is helpful for identification. Yeasts readily propagate asexually by budding. Formation of filamentous elements apart from the spherical or elipsoidical yeast cells are called pseudohyphae and pseudomycelium, respectively. The lack of morphological characteristics in yeasts necessitates the use of biochemical characters in their identification.

The classification of fungi is generally based on characteristics of their sexual life cycle, on their DNA/RNA pattern, on morphological characteristics of their asexual life cycle, and on biochemical properties. Teleomorphs and anamorphs each are listed under their own names in the classification of fungi.

For a considerable number of fungi, a teleomorph is not known. These fungi are classified in artificial taxa summarized as Fungi imperfecti or *Deuteromycetes*.

Table 3.
Keratinophilic fungi, causative agents of dermatophytosis. Divison: *Ascomycota*; Class: *Euascomycetes*

Familiy	Genus	Species: teleomorph name	Species: anamorph name
Order: *Onygales*			
Arthrodermataceae	*Arthroderma*	–	*Epidermophyton floccosum*
		–	*Microsporum audouinii*
		A. otae	*Microsporum canis*
		A. gypseum	*Microsporum gypseum*
		A. incurvatum	*Microsporum gypseum*
		–	*Trichophyton mentagrophytes*
		A. vanbreuseghemii	*Trichophyton interdigitale*
		–	*Trichophyton rubrum*
		–	*Trichophyton schoenleinii*
		–	*Trichophyton tonsurans*
		–	*Trichophyton verrucosum*
		–	*Trichophyton violaceum*
Often present in close relationship with a dermatophytic infection:			
Order: *Microascales*			
Microascaceae	*Microascus*	*M. brevicaulis*	*Scopulariopsis brevicaulis*

3 Classification

Out of the more than 100,000 described species of fungi, about 100 are known to be regularly involved in fungal infections of humans or animals, called mycoses; only a dozen of these cause more than 90% of fungal infections in humans. They are widely classified together with non-pathogenic fungi in the same taxa.

The clinically significant fungi are scattered in several locations of the fungal kingdom. Pathogenicity is a multifactorial complex, and fungi have acquired capacities to infect warm-blooded organisms more than once in the course of evolution. However, orders containing primarily pathogenic fungi are phylogenetically closely interrelated, suggesting that pathogenicity is an evolutionarily rare phenomenon.

On the other hand, the spectrum of clinically relevant fungi is expanding steadily, particularly in patients with severe immunodeficiency. In recent decades, several hundred fungi were described as emerging pathogens in patients of risk with compromized immunological defense capacity. However, the number of fungi capable of invading warm-blooded hosts remains a very

Table 4.
Primary causative agents of systemic mycoses. Division: *Ascomycota*; Class: *Euascomycetes*

Familiy	Genus	Species: teleomorph name	Species: anamorph name
Order: *Onygenales*			
Onygenaceae	*Ajellomyces*	*A. dermatitidis*	*Blastomyces dermatitidis*
		–	*Coccidioides immitis*
		A. crescens	*Emmonsia crescens*
		A. capsulatus	*Histoplasma capsulatum*
		–	*Histoplasma duboisii*
		–	*Paracoccidioides brasiliensis*
Order: *Ophiostomatales*			
Ophiostomataceae		–	*Sporothrix schenckii*

small proportion in the total number of fungal species. The elucidation of pathogenetic pathways in fungal infections concerns equally pathogenic properties of the fungal pathogen as well as deficiencies in the host´s defense.

Taxonomical classification, and therefore nomenclature as well, is a science open for steadily increasing insights into the phylogenetic relationships of organisms. Therefore, changes of names are relatively frequent because of increasing knowledge of sexual life cyles of pathogenic fungi and because of molecular genetic exploration. These historical facts, combined with the laboratory experience that fungi in the expression of their morphological characteristics are widely dependent on the biochemical composition of culture media, are the reason that a considerable number of fungi changed their names in the past, and the existence of a great variety of synonyma makes the handling of the taxonomy of fungi rather difficult.

4 Nomenclature

The kingdom *Eumycota* is subdivided in a hierarchical manner, each rank being named with, and recognizable by, a particular ending:

Division:	-mycota
Class:	-mycetes
Order:	-ales
Family:	-aceae

Table 5.
Opportunistic causative agents of hyalohyphomycosis. Division: *Ascomycota*; Class: *Euascomycetes*

Familiy	Genus	Species: teleomorph name	Species: anamorph name
Order: *Eurotiales*			
Trichocomaceae		–	*Aspergillus flavus*
		–	*Aspergillus fumigatus*
	Emericella	*E. nidulans*	*Aspergillus nidulans*
		–	*Aspergillus niger*
		–	*Aspergillus terreus*
		–	*Paecilomyces variotii*
		–	*Penicillium marneffei*
Order: *Hypocreales*			
Hypocreaceae		–	*Acremonium falciforme*
		–	*Acremonium kiliense*
		–	*Acremonium recifei*
		–	*Fusarium oxysporum*
	Nectria	*N. haematococca v. breviconia*	*Fusarium solani*
	Gibberella	*G. moniliformis*	*Fusarium verticillioides*
	Hypocrea	*H. pseudokoningii*	*Trichoderma pseudokoningii*
		H. rufa	*Trichoderma viride*

A family is composed of genera (singular: genus), and these contain species. A species name is binomial, consisting of the genus name with the species-specific epitheton.

5 Taxonomy

The taxonomy given in the following chapters for the most frequent causative agents of fungal infections is similar to the phylogeny-based classification of fungi. The use of the traditional artificial system of *Deuteromycetes* (Fungi imperfecti) is avoided; however, locating the causative agents of fungal infections in the phylogeny-based classification system often remains doubtful and must be open for possible future revision.

A complete survey of all fungi presently known as clinically relevant for humans is given in the monograph by G.S. de Hoog and colleagues [1]. This handbook presents the newest state of classification and nomenclature of these fungi, including a description of each species hereby enabling its identification.

Table 6.
Causative agents of phaeohyphomycosis and chromomycosis; infections caused by dematiaceous fungi. Division: *Ascomycota*; Class: *Euascomycetes*

Familiy	Genus	Species: teleomorph name	Species: anamorph name
Order: *Chaetothyriales*			
Herpotrichiellaceae		–	*Cladophialophora arxii*
		–	*Cladophialophora bantiana*
		–	*Cladiophialophora carrionii*
		–	*Exophiala berberi*
		–	*Fonsecaea compacta*
		–	*Fonsecaea pedrosoi*
		–	*Fonsecaea dermatitidis*
	Capronia	*C. semiimmersa*	*Phialophora americana*
		–	*Phialophora richardsiae*
		–	*Phialophora verrucosa*
Order: *Microascales*			
Microascaceae		–	*Scedosporium prolificans*
	Pseudallescheria	*P. boydii*	*Scedosporium apiospermum*
		P. boydii	*Graphium eumorphum*
Order: *Dothideales*			
Dothioraceae	*Discosphaerina*	*D. fulvida*	*Aureobasidium pullulans*
Mycosphaerellaceae		–	*Cladosporium trichoides*
Order: *Pleosporales*			
Pleosporaceae		–	*Alternaria alternata*
		–	*Alternaria tenuis*
		–	*Drechslera sp.*
Order: *Leotiales*			
Leotiaceae		–	*Ochroconis constricta*

Members of the kingdom *Eumycota* are currently restricted to four divisions: *Chytridiomycota, Zygomycota, Ascomycota,* and *Basidiomycota*. This taxonomic overview covers those groups within the *Eumycota* that contain species having been isolated in relation to human or animal mycoses. No fungi with clinical significance belong to the division *Chytridiomycota*.

5.1 Zygomycota

The *Zygomycota*, class *Zygomycetes*, are regarded as organisms on a low developmental stage in an evolutionary sense. Their hyphae are irregular in shape, not septate, containing a multiplicity of nuclei. They propagate sexually by

Table 7.
Causative agents of mycetoma. Division: *Ascomycota*; Class: *Euascomycetes*

Familiy	Genus	Species: teleomorph name	Species: anamorph name
Order: *Dothideales*			
Lophiostomataceae		–	*Madurella grisea*
		–	*Madurella mycetomi*
		–	*Pyrenochaeta romoroi*
Herpotrichiellaceae?		–	*Phialophora jeanselmei*
Order: *Microascales*			
Microascaceae		*Pseudallescheria boydii*	*Scedosporium apiospermum*
Order: *Hypocreales*			
Hypocreaceae		–	*Acremonium kiliense*
		–	*Acremonium falciforme*
		–	*Acremonium recifei*
		–	*Acremonium granulomatosis*
Order: *Pleosporales*			
Leptosphaeriaceae	*Leptosphaeria*	*L. senegalensis*	–

isogamic reproduction; the fusion of gametes leads to the formation of zygospores being located in sporangia. Asexual reproduction forming numerous spores is common.

The causative agents of zygomycoses are summarized in Table 1.

5.2 Ascomycota

The thallus of the *Ascomycota* is a mycelium, regular in hyphal diameter and with septa, or is yeast-like in shape. During their sexual life cycle after karyogamy and meiosis, haploid ascospores, 4–8 in number, are produced in a closed ascus. The *Ascomycota* harbor the majority of fungi pathogenic for warm-blooded hosts in at least 15 orders.

The class *Archiascomycetes* with only one family, *Pneumocystidaceae*, is the taxon containing the pathogen *Pneumocystis carinii*, formerly regarded as a protozoon.

The causative agents of candidosis and geotrichosis are placed in the class *Hemiascomycetes* and are summarized in Table 2.

The causative agents of dermatophytosis are members of the *Arthrodermataceae*. These fungi are summarized in Table 3.

Table 8.
Basidiomycetous causative agents of mycoses.

Familiy	Genus	Species: teleomorph name	Species: anamorph name
a. Division: *Basidiomycota*; Class: *Urediniomycetes*, Order: *Sporidiales*			
Sporidiobolaceae	*Rhodosporium*	*R. diabovatum*	*Rhodotorula glutinis*
		R. sphaerocarpum	*Rhodotorula glutinis*
		–	*Rhodotorula minuta*
		–	*Rhodotorula mucilaginosa*
	Sporidiobolus	*S. johnsonii*	*Sporobolomyces salmonicolor*
b. Division: *Basidiomycota*; Class: *Hymenomycetes*, Order: *Tremellales*			
Filobasidiaceae		–	*Cryptococcus curvatus*
	Filobasidiella	*F. neoformans*	*Cryptococcus neoformans var. grubii*
		F. neoformans	*Cryptococcus neoformans var. neoformans*
		F. bacillispora	*Cryptococcus neoformans var. gattii*
		–	*Malassezia furfur*
		–	*Malassezia globosa*
		–	*Malassezia obtusa*
		–	*Malassezia pachydermatis*
		–	*Malassezia restricta*
		–	*Malassezia slooffiae*
		–	*Malassezia sympodialis*
		–	*Trichosporon asahii*
		–	*Trichosporon asteroides*
		–	*Trichosporon cutaneum*
		–	*Trichosporon inkin*
		–	*Trichosporon mucoides*
		–	*Trichosporon ovoides*

The primary causative agents of systemic mycoses, belonging to the same order *Onygenales* as the causative agents of dermatophytosis, are summarized in Table 4.

The opportunistic causative agents of hyalohyphomycosis are placed in the orders *Eurotiales* and *Hypocreales*. They are summarized in Table 5.

The causative agents of phaeohyphomycosis and chromomycosis, infections caused by dematiaceous fungi (black fungi containing melanin), are members of the orders *Chaetothyriales*, *Microascales*, *Dothideales*, and *Pleosporales*; they are summarized in Table 6.

Mycetomas are fungal infections with a homogeneous clinical picture but a broad divergence regarding the causative agents. These fungi are members of the orders *Dothideales, Microascales,* and *Hypocreales* (see Table 7).

5.3 Basidiomycota

A minority of causative agents of mycoses are basidiomycetous fungi, placed in the two classes *Urediniomycetes* and *Hymenomycetes;* they are summarized in Table 8.

References

1 G.S. de Hoog, J. Guarro, J.Gené and M.J. Figueras: Atlas of clinical fungi, 2nd ed., Centralbureau voor Schimmlecultures, Utrecht and University Rovira I Virgili 2000.

Antifungal Agents – Advances and Problems (E. Jucker, Ed.)

Fungal diseases

By Reinhard Kappe[1] and Dagmar Rimek[2]

[1]Institut für Medizinische Mikrobiologie und Hygiene am HELIOS Klinikum Erfurt, Nordhäuser Str. 74, D-99089 Erfurt, Germany
[2]Thüringer Landesamt für Lebensmittelsicherheit und Verbraucherschutz, Dezernat Medizinische Mikrobiologie, Nordhäuser Str. 74, D-99089 Erfurt, Germany

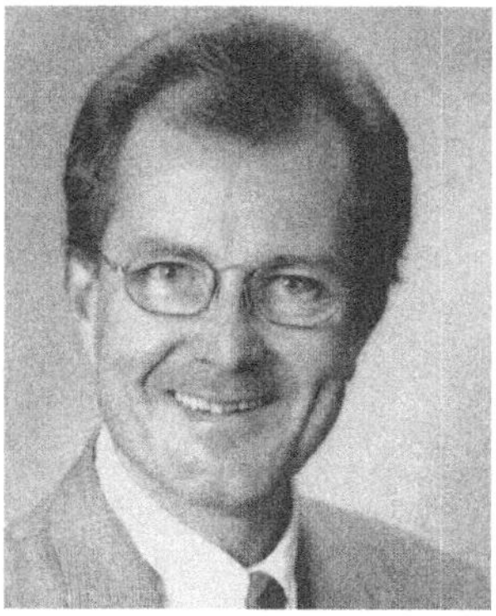

Reinhard Kappe

received his M.D. from the University of Freiburg i. Br., Germany, in 1983. Ever since, his scientific interests were focused on medical mycology. Postdoctoral positions included (1) research associate at the University of Freiburg i. Br., Germany, (2) research fellow of the German Research Foundation and adjunct professor at the Department of Microbiology and Immunology of the Southern Illinois University at Springfield, Illinois, USA, and (3) clinical microbiologist and senior research associate at the University of Heidelberg, Germany. He was board certified for medical microbiology and epidemiology of infectious diseases (1993) and for hygiene and environmental medicine (1999). Since 2000, Reinhard Kappe has been the head of the Institute of Medical Microbiology and Hygiene at the Helios Medical Center in Erfurt, Germany.

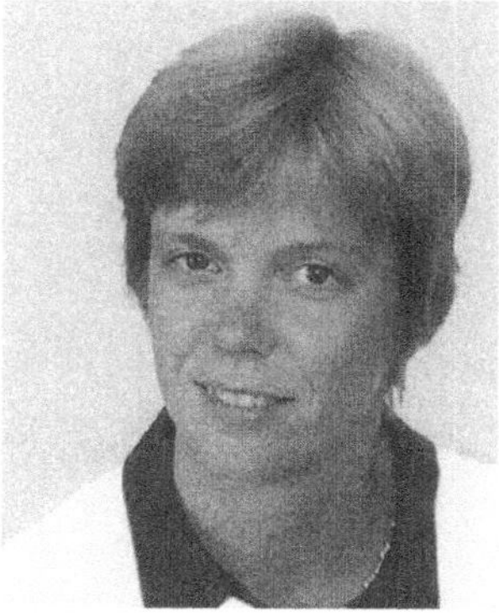

Dagmar Rimek

studied medicine and cell biology and received her M.D. from the University of Lübeck, Germany, in 1993. Postdoctoral positions included positions as clinical microbiologist and research associate at the Universities of Homburg/Saar, Heidelberg, and Rostock, Germany. She was board certified for medical microbiology and epidemiology of infectious diseases in 1998. Since 2002, Dagmar Rimek has been senior microbiologist at the Department of Medical Microbiology of the TLLV (Thüringisches Landesamt für Lebensmittelsicherheit und Verbraucherschutz), Erfurt, Germany.

Summary

In this chapter, we present concise reviews on the clinical manifestations of the complete set of human fungal infections known today. Emphasis is given to the clinical symptoms. The classification corresponds to the body sites affected, from systemic to superficial. Within the groups, the order of presentation follows the order of prevalence and overall importance of the fungal infections. Short paragraphs on the ecology of the causative fungi and the epidemiology of the corresponding diseases, including the mode of aquisition, the susceptible population, and the geographical distribution, precede each clinical entity.

Contents

Keywords
Candidosis, cryptococcosis, aspergillosis, zygomycosis, fusariosis, scedosporiosis, pseudallescheriosis, pneumocystosis, histoplasmosis, coccidioidomycosis, blastomycosis, paracoccidioidomycosis, penicilliosis, sporotrichosis, chromoblastomycosis, phaeohyphomycosis, eumycetoma, basidiobolomycosis, conidiobolomycosis, lobomycosis, dermatophytosis, pityriasis versicolor, tinea nigra, white piedra, black piedra, systemic, invasive, cutaneous, subcutaneous, superficial, fungal, mycotic.

Glossary of abbreviations
AIDS, aquired immune deficiency sydrome; HIV, human immune deficiency virus; IgE, immunoglobulin class E; ABPA, allergic bronchopulmonary aspergillosis; spp., species = more than one species.

1 Introduction

Three general types of human diseases may be caused by fungi [1, 2]:

(1) Allergies may follow sensitization to specific fungal antigens.
(2) Intoxications may be due to mycotoxins generated by fungi.
(3) Infections may be caused by fungi, which actively grow on or in a human host.

Fungal allergies and mycotoxicoses are not dealt with in this review. They are not treated with antimycotic drugs. The most common form of mycotic disease is infection – i.e., actual growth of a fungus on a human or animal host [3]. Mycosis refers to infection caused by a fungus. The names of many fungal infections are formed by coupling mycosis as a suffix with another word that designates the etiologic agent (e.g., coccidioidomycosis) or the site of involvement (e.g., otomycosis) [2, 4]. In general, the establishment of an infection depends on the host defenses, or the lack thereof, the route of exposure to the fungus, the size of the inoculum, and the virulence of the organism [2].

According to current taxonomic understanding, rhinosporidiosis, formerly a putative fungal infection caused by the non-culturable organism *Rhinosporidium seeberi*, has been omitted, because today it is believed to be a parasite rather than a fungus. On the other hand, pneumocystosis, formerly believed to be a protozoan infection by the non-culturable organism *Pneumocystis jiroveci*, is included, because recent genetic studies have proven its fungal nature [5].

This chapter provides a clinical classification followed by a concise coverage of the epidemiology and the clinical manifestations of systemic, subcutaneous, cutaneous, and superficial mycotic infections.

2 Clinical classification of fungal infections

The clinical classification of fungal infections is based on the body sites predominantly involved (Table 1, modified from [2]). For practical purposes including the laboratory diagnosis, this clinical classification has proven to be superior to a taxonomical classification, because there are many fungi from completely different taxa that cause almost identical clinical diseases [6–8]. For a taxonomical classification of the etiologic fungi, see Chapter 1 of this volume.

In general, systemic mycoses are life threatening. They are often difficult to diagnose and even more difficult to treat [9–11]. In contrast, subcutaneous, cutaneous, and superficial mycoses are restricted to body sites that are easily accessible for diagnostic sampling and local therapy. They are never life threatening and are relatively easy to diagnose and to treat.

3 Systemic mycoses with worldwide distribution

These infections – with the exception of cryptococcosis – have long been known as opportunistic mycoses [12]. The true opportunistic character of cryptococcosis was revealed by the AIDS pandemic. Virtually everybody is exposed to the causative fungi, which colonize the human environment or the human body itself. Immunosuppressed patients may develop life-threatening infections. Survival does not confer protective immunity. The etiologic agents are classified in biohazard group no. 2 on a scale of 4 [13].

3.1 Candidosis, deep (synonyms: invasive, disseminated, systemic, visceral)

3.1.1 Epidemiology

The natural habitat of *Candida albicans* is the oral cavity and the intestinal tract of warm-blooded animals including man. Other *Candida* spp. can be iso-

Table 1.
Clinical classification of fungal infections

Body sites involved	Mycosis	Etiology
Blood stream, disseminated, internal organs	*Worldwide occurrence*	
	Candidosis, deep	*Candida albicans, Candida* spp.
	Cryptococcosis	*Cryptococcus neoformans*
	Aspergillosis	*Aspergillus fumigatus*, other *Aspergillus* spp.
	Zygomycosis	Species of *Rhizopus, Absidia, Rhizomucor*, and others
	Fusariosis	*Fusarium* spp.
	Scedosporiosis (Pseudallescheriosis)	*Scedosporium apiospermum* (*Pseudallescheria boydii*)
	Pneumocystosis	*Pneumocystis jiroveci*
	Predominantly endemic occurrence	
	Coccidioidomycosis	*Coccidioides immitis*
	Histoplasmosis	*Histoplasma capsulatum*
	Blastomycosis	*Blastomyces dermatitidis*
	Paracoccidioidomycosis	*Paracoccidioides brasiliensis*
	Penicilliosis	*Penicillium marneffei*
Subcutis	Sporotrichosis	*Sporothrix schenckii*
	Chromoblastomycosis	*Phialophora verrucosa, Fonsecaea pedrosoi*, and others
	Phaeohyphomycosis	*Alternaria* spp., *Bipolaris* spp. and others
	Eumycetoma	*Madurella mycetomatis, Scedosporium* spp. and others
	Lobomycosis	*Lacazia loboi*
	Basidiobolomycosis	*Basidiobolus ranarum*
	Conidiobolomycosis	*Conidiobolus coronatus*
Cutis, hair, and nails	Dermatophytosis	*Trichophyton* spp., *Microsporum* spp., *Epidermophyton floccosum*
	Candidosis of skin, mucosa, or nails	*Candida albicans, Candida* spp.
Skin surface	Pityriasis versicolor	*Malassezia furfur*
	Tinea nigra	*Hortaea werneckii*
Hair shaft	Black piedra	*Piedraia hortae*
	White piedra	*Trichosporon* spp.

lated from environmental sources, such as soil, food, water, and plants [14, 15]. Invasive candidosis is the most prevalent deep-seated mycosis, estimated at a worldwide annual incidence of 500 cases per one million population (including self-limiting forms) [16]. It most commonly affects immunocompromised patients with neutropenia, postsurgical patients, burn patients, and neonates.

3.1.2 Clinical manifestations

According to the portal of entry and the pathogenesis, three types of deep, internal diseases caused by *Candida* spp. are observed:

(1) Candidemia may result from contamination of indwelling intravascular catheters, surgical procedures, or trauma to the skin, gastrointestinal, or respiratory tract. Initially, the patients have intermittent, prolonged, or persistent fever and are unresponsive to antibacterial chemotherapy. Numerous organ manifestations may rise from hematological dissemination: hepatosplenic candidosis, miliary nephritis and pneumonia, endophthalmitis, endocarditis, myocarditis, meningitis, arthritis, osteomyelitis, and macronodular skin lesions. Some of them may resolve spontaneously or heal *ad integrum* under antimycotic therapy; others may result in permanent defects, e.g., loss of vision after endophthalmitis.
(2) In immunocompromised and postsurgical patients, heavy *Candida* colonization of the gastrointestinal, respiratory, or urinary tract may lead to direct fungal invasion of the mucosa or serosa followed by penetration into adjacent deeper tissue, producing infections such as esophagitis, peritonitis, bronchitis, cystitis, or pyelonephritis.
(3) In small children, obstruction or failure of drainage in the urinary or gastrointestinal tract may lead to an accumulation of *Candida* biomass, which forms fungus balls in the renal pelvis, the stomach, or other natural body cavities. There is usually no invasion of the mucosa or deeper tissue. Surgical drainage and removal of the fungal mass resolves the problem.

3.2 Cryptococcosis

3.2.1 Epidemiology

Cryptococcus neoformans appears to be ubiquitous in the soil. It has been isolated from a variety of fruits, from the Australian red river gum tree, and from pigeon droppings, which provides a reservoir of organisms. Cryptococcosis is a sporadic infection with a worldwide distribution. The portal of entry is the lung after inhalation of yeast cells of *C. neoformans*. Impaired cellular immunity – as in patients with lymphoma or AIDS – is a prerequisite for clinical manifestation.

3.2.2 Clinical manifestations

The pulmonary infection remains only modestly symptomatic, with cough and chest pain, or asymptomatic. The heavily encapsulated blastospores of *C. neoformans* are neurotropic and disseminate to the central nervous system. Meningitis takes the form of chronic meningitis, with progressive headache, personality changes, dementia, and focal neurological findings related to cranial nerve involvement. The usual progression of symptoms is fever, headache, stiff neck, and disorientation. The cerebrospinal fluid is typically clear, with predominantly mononuclear cells, elevated protein, and normal or reduced glucose. Further dissemination may occur to the skin and internal organs [17, 18].

3.3 Aspergillosis

3.3.1 Epidemiology

Aspergillus fumigatus and other *Aspergillus* spp. grow on dead organic matter all over the world. Conidiospores are produced abundantly for aerial dissemination. Humans inhale the spores, and susceptible immunocompromised patients, such as patients with hematological malignancies and patients after organ transplantation, develop *A. fumigatus*-associated diseases [19, 20].

3.3.2 Clinical manifestations

Three distinct, well-characterized clinical types of aspergillosis are observed: (1) *Invasive aspergillosis*. Invasive aspergillosis may be localized in the lungs or generalized and disseminated. The course depends largely on the underlying illness. Virtually all cases of invasive pulmonary aspergillosis occur in patients with severe granulocyte dysfunction. These include patients with acute leukemia, immunosuppression after organ transplantation, and long-term, high-dose steroid treatment. The pulmonary pathology includes thrombosis, infarction, and hemorrhage. Dissemination from the lungs may result in generalized aspergillosis, involving the brain, heart, kidney, and many other sites.

(2) *Aspergilloma.* A fungus ball, consisting of *Aspergillus* hyphae, develops in a pulmonary cavity, caused originally by tuberculosis, bronchiectasis, carcinoma, or malformation. The radiographic appearance of an air space surrounding the cavity (air crescent) is highly characteristic. Many patients with aspergilloma are asymptomatic. Some have productive cough and hemoptysis. Dyspnea and pulmonary hemorrhage are serious complications. Aspergilloma of the paranasal sinuses may clinically appear as chronic sinusitis.

(3) *Allergic bronchopulmonary aspergillosis (ABPA).* Major diagnostic criteria include asthma, pulmonary infiltrates, eosinophilia (in blood), elevated serum IgE levels, and *Aspergillus* plugs with positive culture from sputum.

3.4 Zygomycosis (rhinocerebral, pulmonary)

3.4.1 Epidemiology

Mucorales are ubiquitous, thermotolerant saprophytes. Sporangiospores are produced in abundance. They are inhaled or ingested by humans. Patients with ketoacidosis from uncontrolled diabetes, leukemias, and immune deficiencies are at risk for zygomycosis [21, 22].

3.4.2 Clinical manifestations

(1) *Rhinocerebral zygomycosis.* In patients with ketoacidosis, invasion begins typically in the nasal region and progresses rapidly to involve the sinuses, palate, eye, and retroorbital area, with invasion of the brain and

cavernous sinus. Symptoms include facial and orbital pain, headache, and diplopia. There is characteristic edema of the involved facial areas, necrosis, and a black nasal discharge. Damage to the fifth and seventh cranial nerves, orbital cellulitis, and exophthalmia are frequent manifestations.

(2) *Pulmonary and disseminated zygomycosis.* After inhalation of sporangiospores by patients with leukemia, the lung is primarily involved. The pulmonary lesions may be focal or diffuse. The invasion of blood vessels is typical and results in profound destruction of lung parenchyma. The usual course is 1 to 4 weeks from onset to death. However, hematogenous dissemination appears to be a rare event.

(3) *Intestinal zygomycosis and other forms.* After ingestion of sporangiospores, the wall of the stomach may be the portal of entry for a particularly destructive form of zygomycosis. The fungus invades adjacent tissue without respecting anatomical borders.

3.5 Fusariosis

3.5.1 Epidemiology

Fusarium spp. are worldwide common saprophytes on dead organic matter. Several species are well known as plant pathogens. Small, one- or two-celled microconidia can be inhaled by humans.

3.5.2 Clinical manifestations

Invasive fusariosis resembles invasive aspergillosis in many respects [23, 24]. Almost exclusively, neutropenic patients with leukemia or patients who received a liver allograft are affected. Initial signs on chest radiography are often patchy, irregular infiltrates without clearly defined margins. Hematogenous dissemination almost invariably involves the skin, with typical deep reddish lesions that soon become hemorrhagic and necrotic. The overall natural course of invasive fusariosis is even more desastrous than invasive aspergillosis. If untreated, the patients invariably die within a few days to several weeks.

3.6 Scedosporiosis (Pseudallescheriosis)

3.6.1 Epidemiology

Scedosporium apiospermum (*Pseudallescheria boydii*) has been isolated worldwide from numerous natural substrates including soil, foul water, sewage, etc. Small children who have been saved from drowning may acquire cerebral scedosporiosis by uptake of contaminated water into the lungs and the sinuses, from where the fungus spreads to the brain [25, 26].

3.6.2 Clinical manifestations

(1) *Pulmonary and disseminated scedosporiosis.* This clinical syndrome resembles other forms of hyalohyphomycoses (fungal infections producing non-pigmented hyphae in the tissue). It occurs in patients with leukemia and may be underdiagnosed due to its clinical and histopathological similarity to aspergillosis and fusariosis.
(2) *Pneumonia with brain abscesses.* Typically, after a near-drowning, children with contaminated water remaining in the lungs and sinuses for several minutes may, after several days to weeks, develop frontotemporal, cerebral abscesses.
(3) *Chronic subcutaneous abscess.* In older literature, *S. apiospermum* has frequently been reported as an agent of white grain eumycetoma (see also Section 5, "Subcutaneous mycoses").

3.7 Pneumocystosis

3.7.1 Epidemiology

Pneumocystis jiroveci (formerly *Pneumocystis carinii* f. sp. *hominis*) has been proven to be a fungus rather than a protozoon by genetic analyses [5]. It lives as a saprophyte in the lower respiratory tract of man and animals such as rats, rabbits, dogs, goats, and sheep. A reservoir in the inanimate nature has not been found yet. The primary exposition is by inhalation of unknown infectious particles.

3.7.2 Clinical manifestations

(1) *Interstitial, plasma cellular pneumonia of premature infants.* Fever is usually absent and the onset is subtle, with mild tachypnea. After 1 week, respiratory distress becomes severe, with flaring of the nasal alae and cyanosis.
(2) *Pneumonia of immunosuppressed patients, mainly patients with AIDS.* Early symptoms include dyspnea, dry cough, and fever. On the chest radiograph, the infiltrates become apparent first in the perihilar area, spread peripherally, and produce a bilateral diffuse alveolar disease.

4 Predominantly endemic deep mycoses

Common features of the following five predominantly geographically restricted systemic mycoses include: (1) temperature-dependent morphological dimorphism of the etiologic organisms: at 20 °C they grow as moulds, and at 37 °C they grow as yeast (or spherules in the case of *Coccidioides*), the latter one being the parasitic form; (2) natural occurrence in the soil and/or in animals; (3) lungs as the portal of entry, while skin lesions are less common; (4) hematological dissemination to almost any organ possible; (5) etiologic agents classified in biohazard group no. 3 on a scale of 4 [13]; and (6) cell-mediated immunity most important for protection.

4.1 Histoplasmosis

4.1.1 Epidemiology

Histoplasma capsulatum grows in soil with a high nitrogen content. It is associated with bat and avian habitats. The main endemic area is the Ohio-Mississippi Valley in the northern U.S. However, some autochthonous cases have been reported in southern Mexico, Indonesia, the Philippines, and Turkey. Histoplasmosis is the most common pulmonary mycosis of humans and animals. In the U.S., 500,000 new infections occur every year, with 100,000 cases being symptomatic, 2000 requiring hospitalization, and 50 resulting in death [2]. Almost every single case observed in Europe is imported from an endemic area.

Histoplasma capsulatum var. *duboisii* causes a distinct form of predominantly subcutaneous histoplasmosis in central Africa.

4.1.2 Clinical manifestations

(1) *Acute pulmonary histoplasmosis.* Symptoms range from a mild flu-like illness that clears spontaneously to a moderate or severe disease, which develops 1–3 weeks after inhalation of airborne microconidia. The moderate form is characterized by cough, retrosternal or pleuritic chest pain, dyspnea, and hoarseness. In more severe cases, fever, chills, headache, myalgia, night sweats, loss of appetite, and weight loss also develop. Radiologic examination may reveal multiple small nodular infiltrates scattered throughout the lungs, with hilar lymphadenopathy usually present. Coin lesions and histoplasmomas (2 to 3 cm in diameter) may also be produced.

(2) *Disseminated histoplasmosis.* Progressive disseminated histoplasmosis occurs in about 1 in 2000 infections. The most common sites of involvement, after the lung, are the reticuloendothelial tissues of the spleen, liver, lymph nodes, and bone marrow. Disseminated histoplasmosis may be completely benign and inapparent or acute and progressive. Fever and weight loss are the most common symptoms. Shock, respiratory distress, hepatic and renal failure, and coagulopathy may complicate severe cases. This form of histoplasmosis is associated with compromised cell-mediated immunity such as in patients with AIDS.

(3) *African histoplasmosis.* The predominant sites affected are the skin and bones. The bone lesions are often painless. More widespread infections involve the liver, spleen, and other organs and may evolve into febrile wasting illnesses that are fatal within weeks or months if left untreated.

4.2 Coccidioidomycosis

4.2.1 Epidemiology

The endemic foci in the U.S., Mexico, Argentina, and other scattered areas of Central and South America are characterized by a semiarid climate and alkaline soil. Virtually everyone who inhales the arthroconidia of *Coccidioides immitis* becomes infected and acquires a positive delayed-type hypersensitivity response. Skin test surveys with coccidioidin confirmed the areas of endemicity defined by isolation of *C. immitis* from soil [2, 27].

4.2.2 Clinical manifestations

(1) *Primary coccidioidomycosis.* The primary form follows inhalation of arthroconidia, and in most individuals the infection is asymptomatic. After an incubation period of 10 to 16 days, others may have fever, chest pain, cough, or weight loss. Radiographic examination often reveals discrete nodules in the lower lobes, which usually resolve without complication in 3 weeks to 3 months. A small percentage of patients retain cavities, nodules, or calcifications, but endogenous reactivation of residual pulmonary lesions is rare.

(2) *Disseminated coccidioidomycosis.* Disseminated or secondary coccidioidomycosis develops within a few months as a complication of the primary form. The numerous forms of secondary coccidioidomycosis include chronic and progressive pulmonary disease, single or multiple extrapulmonary dissemination, or generalized systemic infection. Extrapulmonary lesions most frequently involve the meninges, skin, or bone. Draining sinus tracts may evolve from subcutaneous and osseous lesions.

4.3 Blastomycosis

4.3.1 Epidemiology

Blastomycosis is endemic in North and South America. *Blastomyces dermatitidis* was isolated from soil samples near river beds in connection with outbreaks involving 3 to 48 persons [2, 28].

4.3.2 Clinical manifestations

(1) *Cutaneous blastomycosis.* Initial skin lesions, consisting of one or more subcutaneous nodules, develop on exposed areas, such as face, hand, wrist, and lower leg. Spread may occur to the trunk. After weeks to months, the nodules may eventually ulcerate and develop into elevated granulomatous lesions with advancing borders.

(2) *Pulmonary blastomycosis.* Acute pulmonary blastomycosis produces two distinct patterns of illness. One is a systemic, influenza-like illness characterized by fever, chills, myalgias, arthralgias, photophobia, and headache. The second type consists of pleuritic chest pain of abrupt onset. Chest radiographs reveal segmental airspace disease, which varies from patchy, nodular opacities to extensive confluent densities.
(3) *Disseminated blastomycosis.* From the lungs, the yeasts disseminate throughout the body, with a characteristic predilection for the skin and bones. Other frequently involved extrapulmonary sites include the genitourinary tract, the central nervous system, and the spleen.

4.4 Paracoccidioidomycosis

4.4.1 Epidemiology

The infection is confined to Central and South America. Infections are presumed to follow exposure to the organisms from an exogenous source. The natural habitat of *Paracoccidioides brasiliensis* is unresolved.

4.4.2 Clinical manifestations

The initial episode of pulmonary paracoccidioidomycosis is inapparent. However, the organism may be reactivated after months to years. After reactivation, the pulmonary lesions are granulomatous nodules that cavitate, but rarely calcify. *P. brasiliensis* tends to spread to the skin and mucocutaneous tissue, particularly to the corners of the mouth, lips, gingiva, and tongue [7].

4.5 Penicilliosis

4.5.1 Epidemiology

Penicillium marneffei naturally occurs in bamboo rats and similar mammals in southeast Asia. Patients infected with HIV aquire penicilliosis by inhalation [29].

4.5.2 Clinical manifestations

The first lesions are pulmonary and often are clinically inapparent. Hematogenous dissemination occurs intracellularly in macrophages. The patients develop fever and weight loss. Skin lesions, cough, and generalized malaise are also often present. The organism is found in the bloodstream, in skin lesions, in organs of the reticuloendothelial system, such as bone marrow, or in enlarged thoracic and abdominal lymph nodes. When untreated, penicilliosis is mostly fatal.

5 Subcutaneous mycoses

The subcutaneous mycoses are local, traumatic, primary infections of the subcutis, provoking a leukocytic response and leading to cysts or granulomata. Most of these are chronic, sometimes disfiguring, infections that may last for decades.

5.1 Sporotrichosis

5.1.1 Epidemiology

Sporotrichosis is a chronic disease caused by a soil fungus, *Sporothrix schenckii*. It is a rare disease with worldwide occurence and affects persons with activities involving contact with plants or plant products, e.g., horticulture, farming, or berry picking [8, 28].

5.1.2 Clinical manifestations

(1) *Subcutaneous sporotrichosis*. At the site of traumatic implantation of the organism into the skin, typically the hand or fingers, a small, moveable, nontender nodule develops, which may eventually ulcerate. The primary lesion heals, and new ones develop nearby, classically along the lymph node stations of the arm.

(2) *Disseminated sporotrichosis*. Other forms of sporotrichosis include primary pulmonary sporotrichosis after inhalation of fungal spores. In patients with impaired cell-mediated immunity, *S. schenckii* may disseminate from cutaneous lesions to the bones and joints and other internal organs.

5.2 Chromoblastomycosis

5.2.1 Epidemiology

In chromoblastomycosis, the fungi occur as brownish to golden pigmented, muriform, blastospore-like cells in the tissue. The etiological agents of chromoblastomycosis are wide-spread in the environment, being found in soil, wood, and decomposing plant matter. Human infection follows inoculation of the fungus into the skin through cuts or wounds due to thorns or wood splinters. The disease is most prevalent in rural, arid parts of warmer climates, where individuals go barefoot. Most cases have been reported in Central and South America [7, 25, 26].

5.2.2 Clinical manifestations

Chromoblastomycosis is a verrucous dermatitis that occurs mostly on the extremities. It is characterized by localized, slowly expanding, grayish, dry, raised, and crusted lesions. Superficial warty to cauliflower-like tumors and deformations develop, due to hyperkeratosis and acanthosis.

5.3 Phaeohyphomycosis

5.3.1 Epidemiology

The term phaeohyphomycosis is applied to all infections characterized by the presence of darkly pigmented, melanized, septate hyphae in tissue. The numerous causative fungi have been collectively termed dematiaceous fungi. They occur in soil and plant debris.

5.3.2 Clinical manifestations

The painless, firm, and tender phaeomycotic cyst usually develops on the extremities and may enlarge to several centimeters. The affected area is surrounded by a fibrous, collagenous secretion of the host, and hence no inflammation occurs. Skin and tissue surrounding the cyst are relatively normal [12].

5.4 Eumycetoma

5.4.1 Epidemiology

A wide spectrum of saprophytic fungi may induce eumycetoma, which develops after traumatic inoculation with soil. The term eumycetoma is restricted to infections caused by fungi, but not to clinically similar mycetomata caused by bacteria (actinomycetes). The feet, lower extremities, hands, and other exposed areas are most often involved. The incidence is highest in tropical climates [7].

5.4.2 Clinical manifestations

The pathology is characterized by suppuration and abscess formation, granulomata, and the formation of draining sinuses containing granules of the fungi. A mycetoma, whether fungal or bacterial, always contains grains. The color and consistency of the grains are characteristic for individual causative agents.

5.5 Basidiobolomycosis

5.5.1 Epidemiology

Basidiobolus ranarum has been isolated worldwide from dead vegetation and from the intestinal tract of reptiles, fish, and amphibians. Patients are mainly boys below the age of ten. Over 100 cases have been reported in moist, tropical Africa and Asia [30].

5.5.2 Clinical manifestations

The infection begins on the limbs, buttocks, or perineum with a small, firm, moveable nodule in the subcutaneous tissue. The skin is generally intact, and the lesions are not painful. They persist for several months, spread slowly but relentlessly, and may form large masses that are attached to the skin.

5.6 Conidiobolomycosis

5.6.1 Epidemiology

Conidiobolus coronatus is a soil saprophyte and an insect parasite that has been isolated worldwide. Less than 100 cases, confined to tropical areas in Nigeria, India, and Southeast Asia, have been reported [30].

5.6.2 Clinical manifestations

The initial lesions are hard nodules in the nasal submucosa. Nasal symptoms include obstruction, rhinorrhoe, and epistaxis. The lesions may expand to form large, disfiguring tissue masses in the face, paranasal sinuses, and pharynx.

5.7 Lobomycosis

5.7.1 Epidemiology

Approximately 100 human cases have been reported in the Amazon river basin. Natural infection has been discovered in Atlantic bottle-nose dolphins. The causative agent, *Lacazia loboi,* may be a fungus, but thus far has not been cultured [26].

5.7.2 Clinical manifestations

The initial lesions are small, hard subcutaneous nodules usually appearing in the extremities, face, or ear and resembling keloids. Lymph nodes are not involved. The infection is chronic and progressive and does not resolve spontaneously.

6 Cutaneous mycoses

This category contains disorders in which living parts of the outermost skin layers (epidermis, stratum spinosum, stratum corneum), mucocutaneous membranes, genitalia, or external ears are affected. Adjacent dead skin or hairs may be involved.

6.1 Dermatophytosis

6.1.1 Epidemiology

Dermatophytes are classified as geophilic, zoophilic, or anthropophilic, depending on whether their usual habitat is soil, animals, or humans. According to current taxonomy [26], little more than 10 species of the 3 genera *Trichophyton, Microsporum,* and *Epidermophyton* are able to cause human infection.

6.1.2 Clinical manifestations

The clinical forms of dermatophytoses were termed ringworm or tinea because of the raised circular lesions. Tinea capitis appears as dull gray, circular patches of alopecia, scaling, and itching of the scalp. Tinea barbae, tinea corporis, tinea cruris, tinea pedis, and tinea manus are caused mostly by *Trichophyton rubrum* and less commonly by *Trichophyton interdigitale* or *Epidermophyton floccosum.* The lesions on glabrous skin are annular and scaly, and they may be embellished with erythema, vesicles, or allergic reactions. In tinea unguium, or onychomycosis, the nails initially show white, patchy, or pitted lesions on the surface, followed by hyphal invasion beneath the nail with discoloration and deformation of the nail [31].

6.2 Candidosis of skin, mucosa, or nails

6.2.1 Epidemiology

Candida spp. are members of the normal flora of the skin and mucous membranes of the oral cavity and the gastrointestinal tract, which are colonized during birth or shortly thereafter. Superficial candidosis occurs worldwide in newborns, elderly patients, and patients with severe underlying diseases. It is the most common fungal infection of mucous membranes [14].

6.2.2 Clinical manifestations

(1) *Thrush*. This is an abundant growth of *Candida* species, mostly *C. albicans*, in the oral cavity. A whitish, removable layer covers the reddish, eroded, easily bleeding mucosa. The infection may extend into the esophagus (see also deep candidosis, Section 3.1.2).

(2) *Vulvovaginitis*. Erythema or irritation occurs, mostly noted on the skin of the vulva. A whitish, dry and crumbling fluor is produced with a sweetish smell. *Candida* vaginitis most often affects pregnant women, diabetics, and women receiving antibacterial or hormonal treatment, including birth control pills. The corresponding infection of the glans penis is known as balanitis.

(3) *Intertrigo*. This is an infection of moist or occluded areas of the skin. The erythematous intertriginous lesions are papular, plaque-like, or confluent. Satellite lesions consisting of pustules or erythematous papules may surround these areas. A special form is perleche, an infection of the corner of the mouth, mostly in elderly or diabetic people. Often, co-infection with gram-positive bacteria, such as *Staphylococcus aureus*, is observed.

(4) *Paronychia*. *Candida* spp. are associated with chronic nail infections and may cause paronychia. Unlike dermatophytosis of the nail, the skin around the nail infection becomes swollen, erythematous, and painful.

(5) *Chronic mucocutaneous candidosis.* In patients with T-cell abnormalities, persistent or recurrent mucosal, cutaneous, or nail infections develop in infancy or early childhood.

7 Superficial mycoses

This category concerns fungi living on compounds, such as lipids, available on the human skin surface and on hairs, without provoking any immune response.

7.1 Pityriasis versicolor

7.1.1 Epidemiology

Yeasts of the genus *Malassezia* are common saprobes on the human skin in lipid excretions. The incidence of pityriasis versicolor increases where the climate is hot and humid and is highest in the tropics.

7.1.2 Clinical manifestations

The characteristic lesions consist of patches of fine brown scaling, particularly on the upper trunk, neck, and upper arms. In light-skinned subjects, the affected skin may appear darker than normal. In dark-skinned individuals, the affected skin loses color and becomes depigmented. The patients seek medical care for cosmetic reasons [2, 12].

7.2 Tinea nigra

7.2.1 Epidemiology

Hortaea werneckii, a ubiquitous saprophyte in nature, has a predilection for affecting females, persons under 20 years of age, and hyperhydrotic individuals. Tinea nigra is most frequently found in tropical areas and coastal regions.

7.2.2 Clinical manifestations

Brown or black superficial skin lesions, mostly on the palm of the hand, sometimes on the sole, are usually solitary, innocuous macules, with sharply defined margins. The brownish color is darkest at the advancing periphery [26].

7.3 Black piedra

7.3.1 Epidemiology

The disorder is caused by *Piedraia hortae*. It has been reported mostly in humid, tropical regions, particularly in South America in those populations where the hair is treated with oily substances. The infection is spread by common use of combs, hair brushes, or utensils used for washing the hair [12].

7.3.2 Clinical manifestations

Black piedra is a colonization of the hair shaft, characterized by the presence of adherent, hard, black nodules of 1 to 2 mm in diameter, leaving the hairs largely undamaged. When untreated, the disorder may remain for years.

7.4 White piedra

7.4.1 Epidemiology

This disorder occurs in the temperate regions of Asia and South America and infrequently in other countries. *Trichosporon* spp. have been isolated from soil, air, and human skin.

7.4.2 Clinical manifestations

In the case of white piedra, soft, white nodules are formed on the hair shaft, mostly of beard, axillary, or pubic hairs. It is caused by several *Trichosporon* spp., each of which has a characteristic localization, e.g., *Trichosporon ovoides* on capital hair and *Trichosporon inkin* on crural hair [26].

8 Conclusions

Most of the fungi are widespread in inanimate nature. Only rarely do they parasitize living plants and animals. Virtually all of the human fungal parasites, including the endemic species, are highly opportunistic. In general, only patients with severe underlying diseases and impaired cell-mediated immunity are at risk to acquire clinically apparent, deep fungal infections. Healthy individuals also become infected. However, their fungal infections are clinically inapparent, mild, or self-limiting. The clinical symptoms of fungal diseases of all body sites may resemble non-infectious diseases or infections due to other microorganisms. Therefore, the diagnosis of a mycosis usually relies on laboratory methods. Although associated with a high mortality, in principal even invasive, disseminated fungal infections can be cured by the timely application of specific antifungal drugs. Hence, the etiology of fungal diseases must be clarified as early as possible.

References

1 D.H. Howard (ed.): Fungi pathogenic for humans and animals. Marcel Dekker, New York 1983.
2 T.G. Mitchell, in: W.K. Joklik, H.P. Willett, D.B. Amos and C.M. Wilfert (eds.): Zinsser Microbiology, Appleton and Lange, Norwalk/San Mateo 1988, 879–947.
3 R.D. Baker, in: E. Uehlinger (ed.): Handbuch der speziellen pathologischen Anatomie und Histologie, Springer-Verlag, New York 1971, Band III/5.
4 F.C. Odds, T. Arai, A.F. DiSalvo, E.G.V. Evans, R.J. Hay, H.S. Randhawa, M.G. Rinaldi and T.J. Walsh: J. Med. Vet. Mycol. *30*, 1 (1992).
5 J.R. Stringer, J.C. Edman, M.T. Cushion, F.F. Richards and J. Watanabe: J. Med. Vet. Mycol. *30* (Suppl. 1), 271 (1993).
6 R.D.G.Ph. Simons (ed.): Medical Mycology, Elsevier, Amsterdam 1954.
7 K.J. Kwon-Chung and J.W. Bennett (eds.): Medical Mycology, Lea & Febiger, Philadelphia 1992.
8 G.L. Mandell, J.E. Bennett, R. Dolin (eds.): Mandell, Douglas, and Bennett's Principle and Practice of Infectious Diseases, Churchill Livingstone, Philadelphia, London 2000.
9 G. Bader (ed.): Die viszeralen Mykosen, Gustav Fischer Verlag, Jena 1965.
10 H. Gemeinhardt (ed.): Endomykosen, Gustav Fischer Verlag, Stuttgart, New York 1989.

11 S. Ascioglu, J.H. Rex, B. de Pauw, J.E. Bennett, J. Bille, F. Crokaert, D.W. Denning, J.P. Donnelly, J.E. Edwards, Z. Erjavec et al.: Clin. Infect. Dis. *34*, 7 (2002).

12 M.D. Richardson and D.W. Warnock (eds.): Fungal infection, Blackwell Scientific Publications, London 1993.

13 G.S. de Hoog: Mycoses *39*, 407 (1996).

14 F.C. Odds (ed.): *Candida* and candidosis, Baillière and Tindall, London 1988.

15 G.P. Bodey (ed.): Candidiasis, Raven Press, New York 1993.

16 J. Müller, R. Kappe, D. Kubitza, R. Feßler and I. Scheidecker: Mycoses *31* (Suppl. 1), 29 (1988).

17 M.L. Littmann and J.E. Walter (eds.): Cryptococcosis, Grune & Stratton, New York 1956.

18 T.G. Mitchell and J.R. Perfect: Clin. Microbiol. Rev. *8*, 515 (1995).

19 A.A. Brakhage, B. Jahn and A. Schmidt (eds.): *Aspergillus fumigatus*, Karger, Basel 1999.

20 J.P. Latgé: Clin. Microbiol. Rev. *12*, 310 (1999).

21 H.J. Scholer, E. Müller and M.A.A. Schipper, in: D.H. Howard (ed.): Fungi pathogenic for humans and animals, part A, Marcel Dekker, New York 1983, 9–59.

22 J.A. Ribes, C.L. Vanover-Sams and D.J. Baker: Clin. Microbiol. Rev. *13*, 236 (2000).

23 P.E. Nelson, M.C. Dignani and E.J. Anaissie: Clin. Microbiol. Rev. *7*, 479 (1994).

24 E.I. Boutati and E.J. Anaissie: Blood *90*, 999 (1997).

25 G. Darai, M. Handermann, E. Hinz and H.-G. Sonntag (eds.): Lexikon der Infektionskrankheiten des Menschen, Springer-Verlag, Berlin, Heidelberg, New York 1997.

26 G.S. de Hoog, J. Guarro, J. Gené and M.J. Figueras (eds.): Atlas of clinical fungi, Centraalbureau voor Schimmelcultures/Universitat Rovira i Virgili, Utrecht/Reus 2000.

27 D.A. Stevens (ed.): Coccidioidomycosis, Plenum Publishing Corporation, New York 1980.

28 J.W. Rippon (ed.): Medical Mycology, W.B. Saunders Company, Philadelphia 1982.

29 C.R. Cooper: ASM News, 64, 390 (1998).

30 E. Drouhet and P. Ravisse, in: M. Borgers, R. Hay and M.G. Rinaldi (eds.): Current topics in medical mycology, Prous Science Publications, Barcelona 1993, 215–245.

31 C. Seebacher and R. Blaschke-Hellmessen (eds.): Mykosen: Epidemiologie – Diagnostik – Therapie, Gustav Fischer Verlag, Jena 1990.

Antifungal Agents – Advances and Problems (E. Jucker, Ed.)

Diagnosis of fungal diseases

By Reinhard Kappe[1] and Dagmar Rimek[2]

[1]Institut für Medizinische Mikrobiologie und Hygiene am HELIOS Klinikum Erfurt, Nordhäuser Str. 74, D-99089 Erfurt, Germany
[2]Thüringer Landesamt für Lebensmittelsicherheit und Verbraucherschutz, Dezernat Medizinische Mikrobiologie, Nordhäuser Str. 74, D-99089 Erfurt, Germany

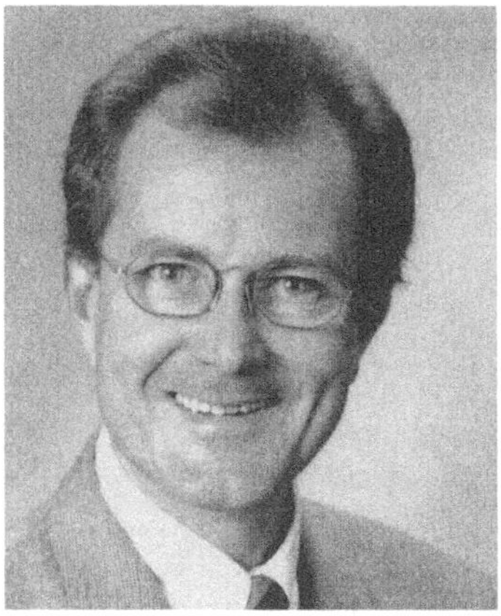

Reinhard Kappe

received his M.D. from the University of Freiburg i. Br., Germany, in 1983. Ever since, his scientific interests were focused on medical mycology. Postdoctoral positions included (1) research associate at the University of Freiburg i. Br., Germany, (2) research fellow of the German Research Foundation and adjunct professor at the Department of Microbiology and Immunology of the Southern Illinois University at Springfield, Illinois, USA, and (3) clinical microbiologist and senior research associate at the University of Heidelberg, Germany. He was board certified for medical microbiology and epidemiology of infectious diseases (1993) and for hygiene and environmental medicine (1999). Since 2000, Reinhard Kappe has been the head of the Institute of Medical Microbiology and Hygiene at the Helios Medical Center in Erfurt, Germany.

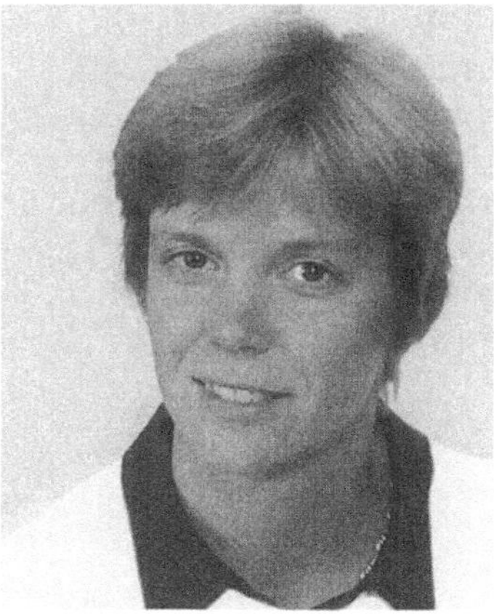

Dagmar Rimek

studied medicine and cell biology and received her M.D. from the University of Lübeck, Germany, in 1993. Postdoctoral positions included positions as clinical microbiologist and research associate at the Universities of Homburg/Saar, Heidelberg, and Rostock, Germany. She was board certified for medical microbiology and epidemiology of infectious diseases in 1998. Since 2002, Dagmar Rimek has been senior microbiologist at the Department of Medical Microbiology of the TLLV (Thüringisches Landesamt für Lebensmittelsicherheit und Verbraucherschutz), Erfurt, Germany.

Summary

In this chapter, we focus on diagnostic laboratory methods that are necessary and suitable for providing physicians with a timely and accurate diagnosis of fungal diseases. After discussing some pre-analytical aspects, the complete set of methods, i.e., microscopy, histopathology, culture, antigen detection, DNA detection, and antibody detection, is concisely described. Identification techniques depend on the fungal group involved. Therefore, separate paragraphs are dedicated to the identification of yeasts and filamentous fungi, which include moulds, dermatophytes, and dimorphic fungi.

Contents

Keywords
Calcofluor white, Grocott-Gomori, *Candida* mannan antigen, *Aspergillus* galactomannan, *Cryptococcus* glucuronoxylomannan, beta-glucan, real time PCR, mycoserology, PFGE, RAPD.

Glossary of abbreviations
DNA, desoxyribonucleic acid; EDTA, ethylene diamine tetra acetate; HIV, human immunodeficiency virus; rpm, rotations per minute; H&E, hematoxylin and eosine stain; PAS, periodic

acid Schiff's stain; GMS, Grocott-Gomori's methenamine silver stain; EIA, enzyme immunoassay; PCR, polymerase chain reaction; PFGE, pulsed field gel electrophoresis; RAPD, random amplified polymorphic DNA; CSF, cerebrospinal fluid; BAL, bronchoalveolar lavage fluid; KOH, potassium hydroxide.

1 Introduction

The diagnosis of fungal diseases needs to be timely and accurate, usually to the species level of the etiologic agent. The first steps of clinical and laboratory diagnostic procedures are non-specific and must be suitable for the complete spectrum of possible microorganisms. Therefore, pre- and post-analytical aspects and large parts of the laboratory analysis are procedures that allow the detection of both bacteria and fungi. The collection and processing of samples, the preparation of smears for microscopy, and even initial media for culture and isolation should be multi-purpose procedures and tools, designed for the detection of a wide range of etiologic agents. Specific mycological techniques, which require a separate laboratory, special equipment, and specially trained personnel, are necessary for the identification (see Sections 7.2 and 7.3 in this chapter) and the susceptibility testing of fungi (see Chapter 5 (Seibold and Tintelnot), this volume).

2 Principal approaches to the diagnosis of fungal diseases

From superficial, cutaneous, and subcutaneous lesions, specimens such as scales, scrapings, swabs, or biopsies are collected and examined microscopically and culturally or histopathologically, if this is clinically considered necessary.

Confirmation or exclusion of *deep* fungal disease in the clinical setting of patients at risk for such infections is much more complicated. The first clinical signs of systemic or deep fungal infection usually include fever that is unresponsive to antibiotics or new persistent, patchy, irregular infiltrates in chest radiography.

The clinical manifestations of fungal diseases of all body sites often resemble non-infectious diseases or infections due to microorganisms other than fungi. The results of clinical examination and radiological investigations are rarely diagnostic [1, 2]. Therefore, the diagnosis of mycoses usually relies on laboratory methods [3–18].

3 General guidelines for laboratory diagnosis

In the first approach, general procedures are applied that are suitable for the detection of a wide range of microorganisms, including bacteria and fungi. If only a small volume of a particular specimen is available for which numerous laboratory investigations are requested, a restriction of laboratory tests is required. Priority should then be given to culture rather than microscopy, because culture is generally more sensitive and enables species identification and susceptibility testing [19].

3.1 Indication for collection of samples

A few superficial or cutaneous mycoses, e.g., pityriasis versicolor, can be diagnosed clinically and managed without a laboratory diagnosis.

However, for the vast majority of fungal diseases, especially deep mycoses, the fungal etiology must be proven. Inappropriate collection, storage, or processing of specimens can result in a missed diagnosis. Therefore, the following sections are dedicated to these points.

3.2 Types of specimens

Many of the clinical specimens are collected in the same way as for the detection of bacteria. In fact, in many cases, one good sample is sufficient for both bacteriological and mycological studies. However, it is important to indicate on the laboratory request form that a mycological investigation should be performed, because of the potential need of additional culture media or prolonged incubation times. Table 1 is a comprehensive list of the types of clinical specimens from which the detection of fungi can be expected in the case of a fungal disease.

For the diagnosis of pulmonary fungal infections, sputum, induced sputum, and tracheal and bronchial secretions are less suitable than bronchoalveolar lavage fluid or transbronchial biopsies [20, 21].

Table 1.
List of types of clinical specimens for the laboratory diagnosis of fungal infection.

Investigation	Types of specimens
Microscopy and culture	Skin scrapings and scales, nail clippings, hair roots, swabs from lesions in the mouth or from vaginal discharge, scrapings of corneal ulcers, vitreous humor, blood, bone marrow, cerebrospinal fluid, urine samples from midstream, transurethral catheter, or suprapubic aspiration, fluids from sterile body compartments (such as pleura, peritoneal cavity, joint), sputum, tracheal and bronchial secretions, bronchoalveolar lavage fluid, tissue specimens, tips from central venous catheters, stool
Antigen detection	Serum, cerebrospinal fluid
DNA amplification (PCR)	EDTA-blood, serum, respiratory tract samples, biopsies, fluids from sterile body compartments
Antibody detection	Serum

3.3 Collection

In general, clinical specimens should be collected from body sites with pathological alterations *before* treatment is installed. Fluids, semiliquid samples, skin scrapings and scales, nail clippings, and hair roots are collected into clear, dry, sterile polystyrene vessels. Swabs go into tubes containing transport medium (some authors recommend avoiding medium for anaerobic bacteria [22]). For blood cultures, at least 10 ml of venous blood is injected into bottles with broth, which supports the growth of bacteria and fungi. Small tissue pieces are transferred into clear, sterile polystyrene tubes containing saline.

For skin scrapings and scales, nail clippings, and hair roots, it is important to clean cutaneous and scalp lesions with 70% ethanol prior to sampling, as this will reduce the likelihood of bacterial contamination of cultures.

3.4 Transport and storage

The specimens must be collected in tightly closed, break-proof tubes that are correctly labeled (patient data, type of specimen, collection date and time). A completed laboratory request form must be enclosed. The tubes for transportation must be packaged and labelled according to the guidelines laid down for the transport of biological materials by the relevant national and international authorities (no leakage, no breaking, correct labeling). The samples should be sent to the laboratory immediately, if possible within 2–4 hours after collection. If the transport and/or processing of the specimens is delayed, swabs, liquids, and tissue samples should be kept at 2–8 °C, and skin scrapings, nail clippings and hairs should be kept at room temperature. Blood culture bottles should be kept at room temperature or at 37 °C, depending on the recommendations of the manufacturer.

3.5 Processing

Visually clear, liquid samples of >0.5 ml volume are centrifuged at 3000 × g for 5 minutes to concentrate cells and microorganisms. The supernatant is transferred to a new sterile polystyrene tube and stored at 2–8 °C for use in assays for the detection of soluble antigens or DNA. The pellet is resuspended in the remaining approximately 200 µl of fluid and used for the preparation of smears and for cultures.

Large solid samples, such as tissue biopsies, are cut into several small pieces of 1–2 mm^3 into a sterile Petri dish with a sterile scalpel. This process will freshly expose viable organisms from the inside of the samples to the surfaces of the media onto and into which they are inoculated.

Pieces of tissue samples may require a pre-treatment including a homogenization with a sterile glass homogenizer. Semiliquid or viscous samples, such as sputum or pus, are spread in a sterile Petri dish, and, eventually, visible small whitish grains or granules are picked with sterile forceps and prepared for microscopical and cultural examinations. Identical homogenization and pre-treatment protocols for the detection of bacteria, mycobacteria, legionellae, and fungi are recommended. This greatly facilitates the routine processing of specimens collected for the diagnosis of unclear pulmonary infections. Furthermore, it ensures that equivalent aliquots of a single individual specimen are available for the different investigations.

3.6 Laboratory safety aspects

All clinical specimens from the lower respiratory tract of patients must be handled with single-use gloves and processed in a biological class II safety cabinet in order to protect personnel from inhaling infectious aerosols (e.g., tuberculosis). Blood and serum samples must be handled with single-use gloves, while wearing safety goggles, mainly for the protection of personnel from hepatitis B and HIV.

Once a filamentous fungus has produced a visible colony on an agar plate or slant agar tube, the culture should be sealed with parafilm. Further processing of this isolate, e.g., inoculation of subcultures, preparation of slides for microscopy, or preparation of inoculum suspensions for susceptibility testing of the fungus, is done in a separate class II safety cabinet. Preferably, this is not the same one that is used for the primary processing of the clinical specimens. The purpose of this procedure is to protect other cultures in the laboratory from contamination and to protect personnel from inhalation of potentially hazardous airborne fungal spores ([23] and numerous national guidelines, directions, and regulations).

3.7 Report of results

Positive microscopic findings of fungal elements at sterile body sites or the detection of highly pathogenic fungi of the biohazard class 3 [24] should be reported immediately by telephone or telefax. In such cases, the results of rapid techniques, such as microscopy or antigen or DNA detection, should be reported immediately, even if the results of slower techniques are not available yet. The complete final report must include all results [25].

3.8 Emergency examinations

Many laboratory examinations for fungal diseases can wait until the next morning. However, there are some clinical settings in which certain specimens must immediately undergo mycological examination. These include specimens from patients who are not yet under appropriate antimycotic therapy, if there is a significant clinical probability for the presence of a life-threatening deep fungal infection.

Specimens that must be appropriately processed, techniques that must be appropriately applied, and results that must be appropriately reported *by emergency laboratory staff* include the following:

(1) Cerebrospinal fluid: Microscopic detection of *Cryptococcus neoformans*, e.g., by India ink, and/or detection of antigen from *C. neoformans* using a latex agglutination test (see Sections 4.5 and 9.1 of this chapter).
(2) Blood cultures growing a fungus: If a blood culture is signalled as being positive, aliquots from the bottle are aspirated for Gram and methylene blue stains, for cultures, and for preliminary susceptibility testing. The results of staining make it possible to inform physicians by telephone, as to whether a yeast or a filamentous fungus is growing. Measures for identification and susceptibility testing of the fungus must be initiated.
(3) Respiratory specimens from patients with possible invasive aspergillosis, such as bronchoalveolar lavage fluids, bronchial or tracheal secretions, or transbronchial or other pulmonary biopsies, require immediate microscopic examination for filamentous fungi by calcofluor white staining (see Section 4.4 of this chapter).

4 Direct microscopy

For the diagnosis of non-culturable organisms, such as *Pneumocystis jiroveci*, *Lacazia loboi*, and others, direct microscopy remains the gold standard of diagnosis. For many other fungal diseases, including superficial candidosis, microscopic examination of a stained smear is the single best diagnostic test [9].

After inoculation of the culture media, a microscopical slide is prepared. A wet mount or a methylene blue-stained slide will easily disclose cells or organisms that may or may not be fungal elements. Special stains, such as India ink for the demonstration of the capsule of *Cryptococcus neoformans*, are useful only if there are suspicious round elements in a methylene blue- or Gram-stained smear.

4.1 Wet mount

The fastest and simplest way to have a microscopic view of a clinical sample is to look at a wet mount. A cover slip is placed on top of the droplet of a processed specimen, and the slide is examined under a light microscope with closed aperture, for better contrast, at a magnification of 400×.

4.2 Methylene blue stain

The one-minute, single-step, methylene blue stain will quickly disclose almost any microorganism, including intracellular bacteria and fungi.

4.3 Gram stain

The Gram stain shows gram-positive and gram-negative bacteria and the gram-positive yeasts. However, it may miss filamentous fungi and other fungal elements and must therefore be supplemented with a special fungal stain.

4.4 Calcofluor white stain

Calcofluor white, diluted 1 to 1000 in a 10% potassium hydroxide solution, is recommended for the staining of fungi [26, 27]. It visualizes the chitin cell wall of the fungi. However, it requires the use of a fluorescent microscope with an excitation wavelength below 400 nm and a barrier filter at 420 nm. Skin scrapings and scales, nail clippings, tissue homogenates, pellet suspensions of liquid specimens, and virtually all specimens can be subjected to the calcofluor white stain. If it is used with 10% KOH, it will at the same time dissolve mammalian cells and other non-fungal debris, whereas the hardy fungal cell walls remain intact. The identification of possible fungal elements depends on the recognition of characteristic micromorpologic fungal features by trained personnel.

4.5 India ink

Mixing the sediment of centrifuged CSF with a small drop of India ink reveals the capsules of *Cryptococcus neoformans* as a clear halo around the spherical yeast cells. Thus, *C. neoformans* blastospores can be easily distingiushed from lymphocytes or other round elements of similar size.

5 Histopathology

Since fungi are eucaryotes, they can, in principle, be recognized in histological thin sections with low-power magnification because of their sheer size – with few exceptions, such as histoplasmosis. When examining for deep-seated opportunistic fungal diseases, positive cultures from non-sterile body sites may indicate nothing more than commensalism, colonization, or superficial disease. Therefore, the histological documentation of tissue invasion by fungal elements remains the ultimate diagnostic tool [28]. Unfortunately, the standard histological stain, hematoxylin and eosine, does not easily disclose fungal elements. Thus, many fungi are actually missed when using an H&E stain only. Periodic acid Schiff's (PAS) reagent is widely used for staining of fungi, but PAS staining may miss non-viable fungal elements.

The best stain for fungi in histological sections is Gomori's methenamine silver stain as modified by Grocott (GMS [29]). It is impossible to rule out an invasive fungal infection without the use of this silver stain. Once they are detected, visible fungal elements often allow an amazingly accurate diagnosis, sometimes right down to the species level, e.g., in cases of histoplasmosis, coccidioidomycosis, blastomycosis, paracoccidioidomycosis, and others. Briefly, yeast infections show characteristic forms of budding, *Aspergillus* infections show septate hyphae that are dichotomously branched in 45° angles, and members of the class Zygomycetes have non-septate hyphae of variable diameters with often rectangular branching. The silver stain, however, conceals the natural pigmentation of the hyphae. Thus, additional H&E staining is necessary for differentiation of melanized fungi (phaeohyphomycetes) from hyaline fungi, including most of the yeasts and the more common moulds, such as *Aspergillus* [21, 30], *Fusarium* [31], and the Zygomycetes [32–35].

6 Culture and isolation

6.1 Use of multi-purpose, non-selective media and methods

High-quality media for fastidious bacteria, such as chocolate agar, allow the growth of almost all of the clinically relevant fungi. The fungi grow even faster on these media than on widely used mycological media like

Sabouraud's glucose agar. Furthermore, 2-day cultures at 35–37 °C in either normal atmosphere or in 5% CO_2 – the common conditions for the culture of bacteria – are sufficient for most of the clinically relevant yeasts and moulds to produce macroscopically recognizable colonies [36]. Hence, for *Candida* and *Aspergillus* a set of standard plates and broths for regular bacteria, e.g., blood and chocolate agar plates plus brain-heart infusion broth, incubated for 2 days at 37 °C in an atmosphere containing 5% CO_2, will suffice. In fact, there is no need for any additional fungal media, whether solid or liquid, for the vast majority of clinical samples that need to be examined for bacteria and fungi. It is acceptable to miss low numbers of yeasts in specimens from non-sterile sites with a heavy physiological bacterial flora, such as throat swabs or sputum samples. If there are larger numbers of yeasts, the colonies appear within the bacterial flora at the latest on the second day and thus they become detectable.

6.2 Specific requirements for fungi

Reasons for the use of special, selective fungal media and/or special incubation conditions include situations in which, empirically, the following can occur:

(1) Suppression of fungal growth by more rapidly growing bacterial pathogens in specimens from non-sterile sites, e.g., *Pseudomonas* in wound swabs.
(2) Markedly slow growth of the fungus.
(3) Markedly better growth of the fungus at 25 °C or failure to grow at 35–37 °C.

Thus, cultures for dermatophytes require media containing antibiotics and cycloheximide and prolonged incubation times of up to 21 days at a reduced incubation temperature of 25 °C [37, 38]. Fungi causing deep infections grow at 37 °C. Therefore, with the exception of dermatophytes, there is no need for primary fungal cultures at a temperature other than 35–37 °C.

However, with numerous fungal diseases, there is only a small number of viable fungal elements in the specimen available for investigation. Thus, on rare occasions, macroscopically visible colonies on agar plates or turbidity in broth may be produced only after 3 to 7 days incubation. Therefore, plates and broths inoculated with CSF, vitreous humor, bone marrow, or tissue biopsies should be kept and observed for 7 days, before a negative result is reported.

The use of Sabouraud's glucose (2%) agar containing autoclavable antibiotics, such as aminoglycosides and chloramphenicol, selectively allows the growth of fungi featuring their individual macro- and micromorphological characteristics. Sabouraud's broth containing antibiotics may enable the isolation of low numbers of fungi which have been damaged by the host defense or antimycotic drugs. These often fail to produce colonies on the surface of solid media.

7 Identification of fungal isolates

Each clinically relevant isolate should be identified to the species level, because certain fungal species within a given fungal genus may have a significantly higher incidence of resistance to particular antifungal drugs.

7.1 Yeasts

Candida albicans can be identified morphologically, as it produces germ tubes in serum or albumin at 37 °C within 2 hours and chlamydospores at 25 °C on rice agar within 24 hours. *Candida dubliniensis* shares multiple phenotypic properties with *C. albicans*. However, *C. dubliniensis* is darker green on chromagar, produces chlamydospores more abundantly, and fails to grow at 42 °C [39]. Non-*C. albicans* yeasts are identified by testing a set of 5 to 40 physiological properties, i.e., mainly fermentation or assimilation of carbohydrates at 30 °C in regular atmosphere for 24 to 48 (to 72) hours [8, 10, 40, 41].

Numerous methods for the rapid and easy presumptive identification of *C. albicans* and other clinically relevant yeast species include enzymatic tests, which are performed on colonies after primary isolation or directly on differential isolation plates, such as chromagar *Candida*. Kits are commercially available and have sensitivity and specificity values between 95% and 99% [41] and thus can be recommended for routine use.

7.2 Moulds, dermatophytes, and dimorphic fungi

The filamentous fungi, which include moulds and dermatophytes, and the dimorphic fungi are identified macro- and micromorphologically, with the help of a few physiological properties, such as urease production, or by sequence analysis of fragments of their ribosomal genes [42, 43]. For dimorphic fungi, so-called exoantigen test kits are commercially available for species identification [44]. Despite some cross-reactions, these kits perform well with extracts of inactivated fungi. Thus, the possibly hazardous handling of the endemic high risk agents [24] can be avoided. Furthermore, there is no time delay for the production of characteristic conidia, as the exoantigen tests can be performed with sterile mycelia.

8 Typing of fungal strains

Several fungal diseases can occur in outbreaks. For the diagnosis of a true outbreak rather than frequent occurrence of a fungal disease by incident, it is necessary to prove the clonality of the causative fungal strain. Typing of strains also helps to illuminate routes of transmission and eventually helps in preventing the further spread of an outbreak.

Special care must be taken to conserve fungal isolates for later typing, because moulds do not survive many common methods of bacterial preservation, such as freezing at –20 °C in 10% skim milk. Strains of filamentous fungi should be kept frozen at –70 °C in 10% glycerol before being recultured for typing.

Different fungi require different typing methods to achieve the desired discriminatory power. A whole set of phenotypic and genotypic methods, including karyotyping by pulsed field gel electrophoresis (PFGE) and random amplification of polymorphic DNA (RAPD), has been modified for the typing of different fungi, e.g., PFGE for *Candida albicans* and *Candida glabrata* [45] and RAPD for *Aspergillus fumigatus* [46]. In principle, typing methods are available for every clinically relevant epidemiological question. However, they are often cumbersome to perform (time-consuming sample preparation and running of PFGE, problems with reproducibility of RAPD). In addition, reliable typing results will require a combination of two or more methods in many cases.

9 Detection of fungal constituents and products

The detection of fungal constituents and products does not depend on the presence of viable organisms in the specimen. It is also independent of the patient's humoral immune response. Furthermore, detection facilitates the indirect quantitative measurement of the fungal load of a patient. Thus, it represents a tool for monitoring the course of an infection and the success of therapy. The assays can be performed within less than 24 hours after collecting the specimen from the patient [47].

9.1 Antigen

The detection of cryptococcal capsular glucuronoxylomannan antigen in the CSF by latex agglutination was described already 40 years ago [48]. Both specificity and sensitivity of this test are approximately 99%. For invasive asper gillosis, the galactomannan antigen EIA is highly specific (>95%) and presently is still superior to PCR assays for circulating *Aspergillus* DNA [49, 50]. It is recommended to perform this test twice weekly for the screening and monitoring of patients at risk [1]. For invasive candidosis, the sensitivity of an EIA for the detection of circulating mannan antigen in serum has been increased recently [51]. However, this test fails to discriminate between invasive candidosis, superficial candidosis, and *Candida* colonization.

A test for the detection of circulating β-glucan, which is a constituent of the cell wall of a wide range of medically relevant fungi, is commercially available. However, the sampling of blood for β-glucan testing requires extraordinary care. Therefore, the test has not been clinically accepted yet. Furthermore, it needs additional evaluation [52].

9.2 Metabolites

The detection of arabinitol and mannitol, both metabolites of *Candida* spp., has never been introduced into clinical practice. Obviously it is non-specific, as there are background levels in the healthy population [53].

9.3 DNA

The detection of fungal DNA in the bloodstream or in normally sterile body compartments is a particularly attractive tool because it is fast, specific, and sensitive due to the possible use of PCR technology. Quantitative analyses, such as the determination of the fungal load in the bloodstream by real-time PCR performed in a light cycler, appear to be possible [54]. However, as of August 2002, there still was not a single commercial PCR kit available for the diagnosis of any fungal infection.

10 Detection of antifungal antibodies

Indirect methods to diagnose a fungal infection depend on the host's immune response. Therefore, they require a functional immune system of the patient, and they will be positive only some time following the actual infection. Usually, there is a delay of at least 2 to 7 days.

Nevertheless, fungal serology, specifically, the detection of circulating antibodies of the immunoglobulin classes G, A, and M directed against fungal epitopes, may be useful in a number of clinical settings [55, 56].

For instance, the detection of anti-*Histoplasma*, -*Coccidioides*, -*Blastomyces*, and -*Paracoccidioides* antibodies is a valuable tool outside the endemic areas [53, 57]. The presence of a so-called M band in the immunodiffusion test for histoplasmosis specifically indicates active fungal disease rather than previous immunization [58].

With ubiquitous mycoses of worldwide distribution, such as candidosis and aspergillosis, the diagnostic value of antibody tests is much less conclusive. The results of most of the commercially available anti-*Candida* antibody detection assays are clinically virtually meaningless. In several recent studies, distinct profiles of the antibody status, e.g., IgM rather than IgG, or the presence of antibodies directed against specific epitopes of internal fungal antigens, have been attributed to invasive disease rather than superficial infection, colonization, or mere inapparent immunization. However, these data have not been confirmed and need further evaluation. In the future, it appears to be possible to develop assays for the detection of highly specific antifungal antibodies that, if present in high quantities, may be significantly linked to the presence of invasive fungal disease that requires therapy [59].

11 Conclusions

Accurate laboratory diagnosis is a keystone for the management of most of the deep fungal infections. Without laboratory tests, the correct diagnosis may be missed, and the patient may die without appropriate treatment.

In the majority of invasive fungal diseases, large numbers of viable fungi are present at the patient's infected body sites. Thus, the best diagnostic methods are direct microscopy and culture of appropriate specimens, because they are rapid, simple, cost-efficient, and often successful. Assays for the detection of fungal antigen, metabolites, and DNA should be attempted if conventional methods fail. Antibody tests are valuable in areas with a non-immune population.

References

1 D.W. Denning, E.G.V. Evans, C.C. Kibbler, M.D. Richardson, M.M. Roberts, T.R. Rogers, D.W. Warnock and R.E. Warren: Eur. J. Clin. Microbiol. Infect. Dis. *16*, 424 (1997).

2 A. Glasmacher, G. Marklein, G. Just-Nübling, C. Leuter and S. Ewig: Dtsch. Med. Wschr. *123*, 157 (1998).

3 M.R. McGinnis (ed.): Laboratory Handbook of Medical Mycology, Academic Press Inc, New York 1980.

4 H.P.R. Seeliger and T. Heymer (eds.): Diagnostik pathogener Pilze des Menschen und seiner Umwelt, Thieme, Stuttgart, New York 1981.

5 E.W. Koneman and G.D. Roberts (eds.): Practical Laboratory Mycology, Williams & Wilkins, Baltimore 1985.

6 J.W. Rippon (ed.): Medical Mycology, W.B. Saunders Company, Philadelphia 1988.

7 E.G.V. Evans and M.D. Richardson (eds.): Medical Mycology. A practical approach, IRL Press, Oxford 1989.

8 C. Seebacher and R. Blaschke-Hellmessen (eds.): Mykosen. Epidemiologie – Diagnostik – Therapie, Gustav Fischer Verlag, Jena 1990.

9 K.J. Kwon-Chung and J.W. Bennett (eds.): Medical Mycology, Lea & Febiger, Philadelphia 1992.

10 W. Meinhof and J. Müller, in: F. Burkhardt (ed.): Mikrobiologische Diagnostik, Georg Thieme Verlag, Stuttgart, New York 1992, 441–486.

11 M.D. Richardson and D.W. Warnock (eds.): Fungal infection. Diagnosis and management, Blackwell Scientific Publications, London 1993.

12 D.W. Denning (ed.): Opportunistic fungal infections, Science Press, London 1994.

13 J.T. Crissey, H. Lang and L.C. Parish (eds.): Manual of medical mycology, Blackwell Scientific, Cambridge MA 1995.

14 E.S. Beneke and A.L. Rogers (eds.): Medical Mycology, Star Publishing Company, Belmont CA 1996.

15 C.C. Kibbler, D.W.R. Mackenzie and F.C. Odds (eds.): Principles and practice of clinical mycology, John Wiley & Sons, Chichester 1996.
16 G. Darai, M. Handermann, E. Hinz and H.-G. Sonntag (eds.): Lexikon der Infektionskrankheiten des Menschen, Springer-Verlag, Berlin, Heidelberg, New York 1997.
17 F.W. Fischer and N.B. Cook (eds.): Fundamentals of diagnostic mycology, W.B. Saunders, Philadelphia 1998.
18 P.R. Murray, E.J. Baron, M.A. Pfaller, F.C. Tenover and R.H. Yolken (eds.): Manual of clinical microbiology, ASM Press, Washington 1999.
19 I.F. Salkin, M.R. McGinnis, C.R. Cooper, J.W. Rippon and E.S. Beneke: J. Med. Vet. Mycol. *32* (Suppl. 1), 309, 1994.
20 J.A. Horvath and S. Dummer: Am. J. Med. *100*, 171 (1996).
21 R. Kappe and D. Rimek, in: A.A. Brakhage, B. Jahn and A. Schmidt (eds.): *Aspergillus fumigatus*, Karger, Basel 1999, 88-104.
22 G. Haase, M. Borg-von Zeppelin, H. Bernhardt, W. Fegeler, D. Harmsen, R. Kappe, H.C. Korting, A. Kuijpers, R. Rüchel, M. Schaller et al., in: H. Mauch and R. Lütticken (eds.): MIQ. Qualitätsstandards in der mikrobiologisch-infektiologischen Diagnostik, Urban & Fischer München, Jena 2001, Band 14.
23 J.Y. Richmond and R.W. McKinney (eds.): Primary containment for biohazards: Selection, installation and use of biological safety cabinets, U.S. government printing office, Washington, D.C. 1995.
24 G.S. de Hoog: Mycoses *39*, 407 (1996).
25 G. Haase, M. Borg-von Zeppelin, H. Bernhardt, W. Fegeler, D. Harmsen, R. Kappe, H.C. Korting, A. Kuijpers, R. Rüchel, M. Schaller et al., in: H. Mauch and R. Lütticken (eds.): MIQ. Qualitätsstandards in der mikrobiologisch-infektiologischen Diagnostik, Urban & Fischer München, Jena 2001, Band 15.
26 G. H. Hageage Jr. and B.J. Harrington: Lab. Med. *15*, 109 (1984).
27 R. Rüchel and M. Schaffrinski: J. Clin. Microbiol. *37*, 2694 (1999).
28 S. Ascioglu, J.H. Rex, B. de Pauw, J.E. Bennett, J. Bille, F. Crokaert, D.W. Denning, J.P. Donnelly, J.E. Edwards, Z. Erjavec et al.: Clin. Infect. Dis. *34*, 7 (2002).
29 R.G. Grocott: Am. J. Clin. Pathol. *25*, 975 (1955).
30 K.B. Raper and F.I. Fennell (eds.): The genus *Aspergillus*, Williams & Wilkins, Baltimore 1965.
31 E.I. Boutati and E.J. Anaissie: Blood *90*, 999 (1997).
32 J.A. Ribes, C.L. Vanover-Sams and D.J. Baker: Clin. Microbiol. Rev. *13*, 236 (2000).
33 R.D. Baker (ed.), in: E. Uehlinger (ed.): Handbuch der speziellen pathologischen Anatomie und Histologie, Band III/5, Springer-Verlag, New York 1971.
34 F.W. Chandler, W. Kaplan and L. Ajello (eds.): Color atlas and text of the histopathology of mycotic diseases, Year Book Medical Publishers, Chicago 1980.
35 K. Salfelder, T.R.D. Liscano and E. Sauerteig (eds.): Atlas of fungal pathology, Kluwer Academic Publishers, Dordrecht, Boston 1990.
36 A.J. Morris, T.C. Byrine, J.F. Madden, L.B. Reller: J. Clin. Microbiol. *34*, 1583 (1996).
37 I. Weitzman and R.C. Summerbell: Clin. Microbiol. Rev. *8*, 240 (1995).
38 J. Kane, R. Summerbell, L. Sigler, S. Krajden and G. Land (eds.): Laboratory Handbook of Dermatophytes, Star Publishing, Belmont CA 1997.
39 K. Tintelnot, G. Haase, M. Seibold, F. Bergmann, M. Staemmler, T. Franz and D. Naumann: J. Clin. Microbiol. *38*, 1599 (2000).

40 C.P. Kurtzman and J.W. Fell (eds.): The yeasts, a taxonomic study, Elsevier, Amsterdam 1998.
41 A.M. Freydière, R. Guinet and P. Boiron: Med. Mycol. *39*, 9 (2001).
42 G.S. de Hoog, J. Guarro, J. Gené and M.J. Figueras (eds.): Atlas of clinical fungi, Centraalbureau voor Schimmelcultures/Universitat Rovira i Virgili, Utrecht/Reus 2000.
43 D. Larone (ed.): Medically important fungi, ASM Press, Washington 2002.
44 L. Kaufman and P.G. Standard: Annu. Rev. Microbiol. *41*, 209 (1987).
45 P. Hamal, R. Kappe and D. Rimek: J. Hosp. Infect. *49*, 37 (2001).
46 P.M. Rath, G. Marggraf, H. Dermoumi and R. Ansorg: Mycoses *38*, 429 (1995).
47 S.F. Yeo and B. Wong: Clin. Microbiol. Rev. *15*, 465 (2002).
48 N. Bloomfield, M.A. Gordon and D.F. Elmendorf Jr.: Proc. Soc. Exp. Biol. Med. *114*, 64 (1963).
49 D. Stynen, A. Goris, J. Sarfati and J.P. Latgé: J. Clin. Microbiol. *33*, 497 (1995).
50 S. Bretagne, J.M. Costa, E. Bart-Delabesse, N. Dhédin, C. Rieux and C. Cordonnier: Clin. Infect. Dis. *26*, 1407 (1998).
51 B. Sendid, M. Tabouret, J.L. Poirot, D. Mathieu, J. Fruit and D. Poulain: J. Clin. Microbiol. *37*, 1510 (1999).
52 T. Mori, H. Ikemoto, M. Matsumura, M. Yoshida, K. Inada, S. Endo, A. Ito, S. Watanabe, H. Yamaguchi, M. Mitsuya et al.: Eur. J. Clin. Chem. Clin. Biochem. *35*, 553 (1997).
53 R. Kappe and H.P.R. Seeliger, in: M. Borgers, R. Hay and M.G. Rinaldi (eds.): Current topics in medical mycology, Vol. V, Prous Science, Barcelona 1993, 247–280.
54 J. Loeffler, N. Henke, H. Hebart, D. Schmidt, L. Hagmeyer, U. Schumacher and H. Einsele: J. Clin. Microbiol. *38*, 586 (2000).
55 L. De Repentigny: Clin. Infect. Dis. *14* (Suppl. 1), S11 (1992).
56 R. Kappe, A. Schulze-Berge and H.-G. Sonntag: Mycoses *39*, 13 (1996).
57 D.F. Palmer, L. Kaufmann, W. Kaplan and J.J. Cavallaro (eds.): Serodiagnosis of mycotic diseases, Thomas, Springfield, IL 1977.
58 L.J. Wheat: Semin. Respir. Infect. *16*, 131 (2001).
59 J. P. Martinez, M.L. Gil, J.L. Lopez-Ribot and W. LaJean Chaffin: Clin. Microbiol. Rev. *11*, 121 (1998).

Antifungal Agents – Advances and Problems (E. Jucker, Ed.)

Antifungal therapy – state of the art at the beginning of the 21st century

By Annemarie Polak

Spitzenrainweg 45, CH-4147 Aesch, Switzerland

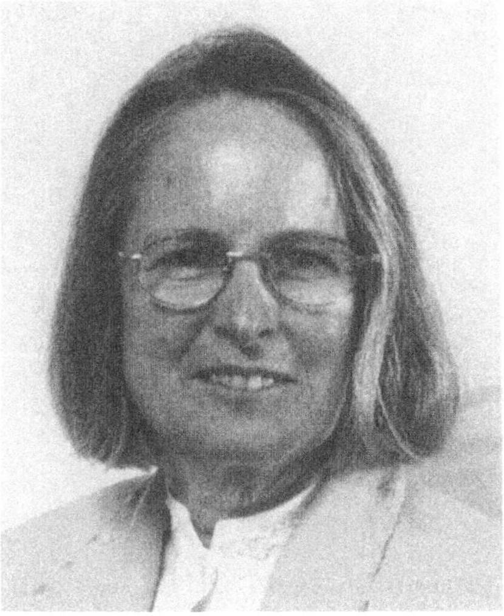

Annemarie Polak

received her Ph.D. in microbiology from the Eidgenössische Technische Hochschule (ETH), Zürich, Switzerland, in 1969. In the same year, she joined Hoffmann LaRoche as a microbiologist in the tropical medicine group. Her research interest included mode of action studies and detecting new antifungals. She became a specialist in the field of research on antifungals and was later promoted to Scientific Expert, a cadre position at Roche. In 1989, A. Polak did her "Habilitation" at the Institute of Microbiology and Hygiene in the Medical Faculty of the University Freiburg i. Br. (Germany) and received a professorship for medical mycology in 1995.

Summary

The most relevant information on the present state of the art of antifungal chemotherapy is reviewed in this chapter. For dermatomycoses a variety of topical antifungals are available, and safe and efficacious systemic treatment, especially with the fungicidal drug terbinafine, is possible. The duration of treatment can be drastically reduced. Substantial progress in the armamentarium of drugs for invasive fungal infections has been made, and a new class of antifungals, echinocandins, is now in clinical use. The following drugs in oral and/or intravenous formulations are available: the broad spectrum polyene amphotericin B with its new "clothes"; the sterol biosynthesis inhibitors fluconazole, itraconazole, and voriconazole; the glucan synthase inhibitor caspofungin; and the combination partner flucytosine. New therapy schedules have been studied; combination therapy has found a significant place in the treatment of severely compromised patients, and the field of prevention and empiric therapy is fast moving. Guidelines exist nowadays for the treatment of various fungal diseases and maintenance therapy. New approaches interfering with host defenses or pathogenicity of fungal cells are being investigated, and molecular biologists are looking for new targets studying the genomics of pathogenic fungi.

Contents

Keywords
Invasive fungal infections, dermatomycoses, amphotericin B, fluconazole, flucytosine, itraconazole, voriconazole, caspofungin, terbinafine, ciclopirox, amorolfine.

Glossary of abbreviations
Amph B, amphotericin B; L-Amph B, Ambisome®; ABLC, Abelect®; ABCD, amphotericin B in colloid dispersion; VECH, anidulafungin; Amor, amorolfine; CAS, caspofungin; C, ciclopirox-olamin; 5FC, flucytosine; Flu, fluconazole; Itra, itraconazole; Keto, ketoconazole; MICA, micafungin; Ter, terbinafine.

1 Introduction

In the early 1990s, A. Polak and P. Hartman [1] had some hope that we would be able to win the fight for an effective antifungal therapy in dermatology as well as in deep mycoses. Seemingly, the old gold standard amphotericin B (Amph B), with its broad antifungal efficacy but its package of frequent and severe side effects, would be replaced by well-tolerated, efficacious triazoles. Six years later [2] A. Polak noticed, that despite the great improvement in antifungal therapy, the fungus always seems to be one step ahead of pharmaceutical and medical research.

In this article the newest level of antifungal therapy is summarized. During the last 10 years, clear progress is notable, even if the optimal antifungal treatment has not yet been found. New drugs are established in the workday of practicians and clinicians, and new treatment schedules with a high compliance by the patients are introduced.

Fungal diseases fall into three major classes: superficial, subcutaneous, and invasive mycoses. Throughout this book the author will adhere to this division, not for microbiological reasons but because the problems associated with the three classes are completely distinct. No overwhelming problems remain in the field of dermatomycoses and gynecological infections, and indeed, high success rates are now obtainable because of the recent development of highly active fungicidal compounds with special pharmacokinetic properties. In this field we may be winning.

The situation is completely different in the field of deep mycoses. Fungal cells can induce enormous damage on a terrain of immunosuppression; medical help comes often too slow or is too weak. It will be a long time before the ideal strategy is found for an ideal prophylaxis or for the optimal therapy of deep mycoses; probably the battle will never end.

The problems encountered in antifungal therapy can be described as an interactive triangle or as a vicious circle among the fungus, the patient, and the drug.

The fungus: The ability of fungi to colonize and invade human organs is impressive, and the list of fungi causing human infections continue to grow at an enormous speed. An increased number of fungi once thought to be harmless for humans are now recognized as human pathogens. The difficulty of killing an eukaryotic cell invading host cells without damaging the host proved to be a nearly non-bridgeable task for research in human chemotherapy.

The patient: Patients with invasive fungal infections often have to fight against underlying malignant diseases or general immunological/physiological disorders. The list of predisposing risk factors is long, and the mycosis is very often set against the complex background of an underlying disease and its treatment. This phenomenon is not only true for established opportunistic fungal infections like candidosis, cryptococcosis, and aspergillosis; even the pathogenic fungus *Histoplasma capsulatum* behaves like an opportunistic fungus, especially in patients with AIDS. An increasing number of cancer, leukemia, transplant, surgery, and AIDS patients are keeping their diseases under control only to become victims of opportunistic fungal infections because of their weakened immune status. The situation is complicated because the host's defense against fungal invasions varies. Some fungal infections, like aspergillosis or deep candidosis, are granulocyte dependent; others like cryptococcosis or oral candidosis, are T- cell dependent.

The drug: The wonder drug to prevent or cure invasive fungal infections does not yet exist; all drugs available have benefits and drawbacks. Amph B, the agent with the broadest spectrum, unfortunately is associated with a toxicity that would rule out its use if there were a genuine alternative. Similarly, the resistant problem of flucytosine reduces its use to combination therapy. The new generation of triazole has clearly gained respect, but it has not yet reached the goal of replacing Amph B in the antifungal field.

2 Superficial mycoses

2.1 Dermatomycoses

The treatment of infections of the skin or hair is no longer a problem. The era of dyes is fortunately over, and griseofulvin, the first detected antifungal, is no longer the first line of defense, as allylamines and triazoles have revolutionized the therapy of dermatomycoses.

Not only is an enormous, still increasing palette of agents at hand but also numerous and varied galenical forms are available, e.g., tablets, creams, tinctures, sprays, powder, shampoos, and nail lacquers. For topical treatment, a variety of chemical classes (azoles, allylamines, tolnaftate, tolciclate, amorolfine, ciclopirox/olamin, etc.) [2–4] are in wide use and have become well established. All show high efficacy and a low incidence of adverse events.

There are fewer choices for oral treatment of dermatomycoses. Three agents are in use: terbinafine (Ter, an allylamine) and the two triazoles itraconazole (Itra) and fluconazole (Flu). Ter is the most efficacious agent for infections caused by dermatophytes [3], whereas Flu, a compound that is highly efficacious against yeasts, has not yet reached full acceptance in the field of dermatomycoses [5, 6].

Ter and Itra are well tolerated and highly effective against most forms of dermatomycoses in adults [6-8], Ter being superior to Itra in all comparative studies. Ter was also highly effective in the treatment of children with tinea capitis [9] and is well tolerated by small children [10]. It also showed high cure rates in tinea imbricata, a chronic recurrent *Trichophyton concentricum* infection that is characterized by concentric rings of papulosquameous plaques and is endemic to village populations of Indonesia [11]. Thus, even recurrent dermatophytic infections seem to be under control. Oral Ter also showed effectiveness in cutaneous alternariosis [12].

Treatment schedules have become easier and shorter. Once daily treatment is now standard; the duration of therapy, originally as long as 6 months, is now often as short as 2 weeks [13, 14]. Attempts are ongoing to improve compliance and to reduce the duration of treatment even more. The duration of therapy, however, cannot be reduced in all instances. *Microsporum* infections need a higher dose and a longer duration of treatment [15–17].

The rationale for this treatment reduction is based on the properties of the new agents: both Ter and Itra have a high affinity to keratinous tissues, where they remain for a long time. Therefore, higher drug levels are found in tissues than in plasma. Additionally, Ter exerts a stronger fungicidal activity than Itra against dermatophytes and thus is more efficacious than Itra. The strategy for the treatment of dermatomycoses could be drastically changed based on this fungicidal property of the new agents. Traditionally, fungal infections were treated for several days after complete disappearance of clinical signs and symptoms. Since the new agents reach fungicidal and long-lasting tissue levels in the skin and hair, the treatment can be stopped long before the clinical symptoms disappear, because the antifungal curative effect is continually nourished from the tissue levels of the agent long after therapy is stopped.

2.2 Onychomycosis

Onychomycosis is a non-life-threatening, non-aesthetic-appearing, chronic fungal infection of the nail, slowly destroying the whole nail plate and matrix. Dermatophytes (mainly *T. rubrum*) are by far the most common pathogens, accounting for 80–90% of all infections. Toenails are more frequently affected than fingernails. In the past, pedal onychomycosis was considered an incurable disease. Therapy was lengthy, usually unsuccessful, and perceived to be mainly for cosmetic purposes. Oral griseofulvin, discovered in 1958, traditionally was the only antifungal agent prescribed for this infection. Topical therapies became available 15 years ago; however, their clinical efficacy was not sufficient, especially when a significant proportion of the nail plate or matrix was diseased. Until recently the only curative alternative was the surgical avulsion of the nail followed by application of an antifungal cream. In the last 10 years, however, significant progress has been made not only in systemic treatment but also in topical treatment of nail infections. Today it would be a mistake for a doctor to remove an infected nail as therapy. Four entities are mainly responsible for revolutionizing the treatment of onychomycosis: the oral agents Ter, Itra, and Flu and the topical nail lacquers with amorolfine (Amor) and ciclopirox (Cprox).

The drugs Ter, Amor, and Cprox, mainly used for dermatophytic infections, will be discussed in these sections, whereas Itra and Flu, with a broader clinical spectrum, will be considered in the section on invasive mycosis.

2.2.1 Oral treatment

2.2.1.1 Terbinafine

Ter possesses *in vitro* a broad antifungal spectrum against a wide variety of pathogenic fungi, including non-dermatophytic moulds causing onychomycosis such as *Alternaria* spp., *Scopulariopsis brevicaulis, Hendersonula,* and *Acremonium* sp. The antifungal efficacy is especially strong against dermatophytes (minimal inhibitory concentration [MIC] 0.003–0.2 μg/ml) [2, 3]. Besides this strong fungistatic effect, Ter also exerts a strong fungicidal activity, the minimal fungicidal concentrations being in the same range as the MIC. This property makes Ter an outstanding antifungal agent, since most of the antifungals (excluding Amor) have either only fungistatic activity (Flu) or a degree of fungicidal activity that is significantly lower than the fungistatic one (Itra).

Ter is a sterol biosynthesis inhibitor that interferes with the ergosterol pathway at the level of squalene epoxidase. This interaction leads to depletion of ergosterol and accumulation of squalene. A clear correlation exists between growth inhibition and degrees of sterol biosynthesis inhibition. The fungicidal effect is not directly related to depletion of ergosterol, but instead seems to correlate with the high intracellular accumulation of squalene. Changes in the lipid content are known to disrupt chitin synthesis. The cell walls of dermatophytes contain higher amounts of chitin than the wall of yeasts. Thus, this sequelae of the mode of action may explain the great sensitivity of dermatophytes to Ter [18, 19]. A new biochemical effect of Ter was observed and presented at the last ISHAM congress. Ter also inhibits the production of reactive oxygen species in yeasts [20].

Generally Ter is well tolerated in adults and children [19, 21–24, 24a]. In a prospective, open post-marketing study, only 10.5% of 25,884 patients showed some adverse effects, and these were primarily GI (4.9%) or dermatological (2.3%) in nature. The GI events were mainly nausea (1.3%), abdominal pain (0.8%), or dyspepsia (0.6%). All GI events were mild, transient, and reversible. The dermatological events were mainly rash (0.9%), pruritis (0.3%), urticaria (0.25), or eczema (0.2%). Hepatobiliary side effects appeared in 0.25% and taste disturbance or loss appeared in 0.7% of the patients. Serious adverse events probably or possibly related to Ter were observed in only 0.046% of the cases [25]. Severe events are observed in various organs: cardiovascular; neoplasia; GI; respiratory; urinary; musculoskeletal; hematological; central/peripheral nervous system; hepatobilary; psychiatric; hearing; reproductive; and skin with cutaneous eruption such as erythema, multiforme, or toxic epidermal necrolysis [25–30]. Ter is also excreted in mother's milk; therefore, nursing mothers should not be treated with Ter.

Ter has, in contrast to Flu and Itra, a low interaction profile. H.I. Katz [31, 32] describes in his summary tables only the following interactions: cimetidine and terfenadine increase Ter levels, whereas rifampicin decreases Ter level. Ter increases the level of caffeine and decreases the level of cyclosporin. In healthy volunteers, Ter showed no interaction with warfarin; however, one case of an elderly patient with gastrointestinal bleeding probably related to the concomitant treatment with Ter and warfarin has been reported.

Several clinical studies have revealed that the fungicidal and pharmacokinetic properties of Ter have an important impact on the efficacy of the agent and on the rapid onset of mycological cure in dermatophytic infections. The drug accumulates to high concentrations in adipose tissues, skin, and nails and is only slowly metabolized and released from the sites. Ter reaches the nail plate rapidly and persists there for several months after cessation of active treatment. It is detectable in the distal nail within 1 week of starting therapy and reaches concentrations well above the MIC for dermatophytes. Whereas plasma levels rapidly decrease after termination of treatment, Ter was detected in the nails as long as 30 weeks after termination of treatment [33].

Treatment duration in all dermatophytic infections, including onychomycoses, could be drastically shortened as a result of Ter's high fungicidal activity and its pharmacokinetic properties [20, 34–36]. Disappearance of the symptoms is ongoing after therapy has been stopped.

A great number of publications describing high cure rates in onychomycoses show that treatment with Ter is well accepted by physicians and patients [18, 37–39a]. The long-term effect of Ter is excellent: 3 to 6 years after termination of treatment, over 70% of the patients had no or minimal dystrophic nails changes or negative mycological findings [39, 40]. Pharmacoeconomic analyses have shown that oral Ter has a cost-effectiveness ratio superior to that of Itra, Keto, or griseofulvin, since the relapse rate with Ter is lower and therapy with Itra has to be repeated more often [18, 41, 42].

In vitro, Ter exerts excellent activity against most pathogenic fungi; this high antifungal effect is unfortunately lost in animal models, since Ter is rapidly metabolized and strongly binds to proteins. Clinical case reports show, however, that – under certain circumstances – Ter may be efficacious in subcutaneous or even systemic mycoses [43]. A successful outcome was seen in a case of lung aspergillosis [44]. Ter also had a potential to cure chromomycosis or cutaneous leishmaniasis [45, 46]. The lesions of *Paecilomyces lilacinus* in a heart transplant disappeared under Ter, while Itra, Amph B, and Flu failed [47]. Ter also showed efficacy in lymphocutaneous sporotrichosis [20]. A combination of oral and topical Ter cured an *Aspergillus versicolor* infection of the external auditory canal [48]. A patient with painful, malodorous lesions of Paracoccidiomycosis was successfully treated with oral Ter [49].

2.2.1.2 Itraconazole and fluconazole

Itra has pharmacokinetic properties comparable to Ter; it also has a high affinity to adipose tissue, skin, and nails and is therefore also active in onychomycosis [7, 36]. Based on the advances in understanding of the pharmacokinetics of Itra and Ter, new, innovative dose regimens have been studied [50]. For Ter the duration of treatment could be significantly reduced; for Itra a pulse therapy was established (1 week per month over a time period of 3–4 months) [36, 37, 39a].

Itra pulse therapy (200 mg twice daily for 1 week per month for 3 consecutive months) is well tolerated and effective in toe onychomycosis with complete cure, marked improvement, and mycological cure in 64%, 88%, and 64% patients, respectively. *Candida* onychomycosis as well as onychomycosis associated with non-dermatophyte moulds also respond well to treatment with Itra [36, 51, 52]. The long-term follow-up also shows good results: 77 patients (88.5% of the treated patients) showed microscopical and culture cure after 6 months of treatment, and only 6.5% relapsed during a 3-year follow-up; no relapse occurred after the first few years [52a].

Generally, continuous Ter application is more efficacious than pulse Itra application, as was demonstrated in the LION and other clinical studies [53-56]. Significant differences are also seen in long-term observations [53, 57]. Recently, a new type of pulse therapy – two pulses of Itra (200 mg twice daily for 1 week) followed by a pulse of terbinafine (250 mg twice daily for 1 week) – was tested in onychomycosis of the fingernails and showed high success rates with a low profile of side effects [58].

This year, Flu just got approval for the treatment of onychomycosis. The phase III studies have been published in a supplement to J. Am. Acad, Dermatology [58a]; Flu administered once weekly for various periods of time (2–9 months) is safe and effective in eradicating distal subungual onychomycosis of the toe- and fingernails. For toenail onychomycosis the clinical and microbiological response was best after a 9-month treatment. Follow-up after 2 years showed cure rates between 64% and 70%; recurrence occurred only in 6.9% [58b].

2.2.2 Therapy with nail lacquers

In the past, topical therapy has met with little success, mostly due to poor penetration of the antifungal into nail tissue. This obstacle could be overcome by a new formulation, a nail lacquer, containing either Amor or Cprox. Topical treatment has the advantage that no systemic adverse reactions and no drug-drug interactions occur. Topical efficacious antifungal regimens can additionally be used for prevention of reinfections or relapses.

2.2.2.1 Amorolfine

The morpholine derivative Amor possesses a broad antifungal spectrum, including dermatophytes; yeast dimorphic fungi; dematiacaeae; and non-dermatophytic moulds causing onychomycosis such as *Alternaria* spp., *Scopulariopsis brevicaulis, Hendersonula, Acremonium* spp. etc. However, it is inactive against aspergilli. The highest degree of activity is seen against dermatophytes (geometric mean MIC 0.02 μg/ml) [2, 3, 59–61]. Amor exerts both fungistatic and fungicidal activity against most fungal species, i.e., in contrast to Ter it is also fungicidal against yeasts, the MFC being very close to the MIC [59, 61]. Amor exerts its fungicidal effect like Cprox even against non-growing cells.

Both Amor and Ter are highly suitable for treating dermatophytic infections, whereas Amor is more effective against skin infections caused by yeasts because of its essential fungicidal activity against yeasts.

Like all sterol biosynthesis inhibitors, Amor causes depletion of ergosterol and accumulation of the unplanar sterol ignosterol. The agent interferes at two levels in the essential ergosterol biosynthesis pathway, the Δ_{14}-reductase and the Δ_7–Δ_8 isomerase, with IC_{50} of 2.39 μM and 0.0018 μM, respectively. Thus, a natural synergistic effect is built into the molecule so that the risk of appearance of resistant mutants is low and the activity of Amor is high [62]. The fungistatic activity is clearly correlated with the depletion of ergosterol and not with the accumulation of ignosterol [59]. Although the basis of the fungicidal effect is not fully understood, two hypotheses have been suggested to explain its mode of action. At high doses of Amor, squalene is accumulated and this accumulation may lead, as with Ter, to a fungicidal effect. Electron microscopic studies, on the other hand, have revealed an extreme accumulation of chitin in the membrane [63]. Thus, severe chitin synthesis disturbance may be the cause of this distinct fungicidal effect.

Because of its favorable pharmacokinetic properties, Amor has fulfilled its promise as an agent for topical treatment of onychomycosis [36, 64]. Amor (from 5% lacquer) penetrates rapidly into the nail. As expected, the kinetics of the penetration follows an exponential law; the level of Amor measured in the upper levels of the nail exceeds the MIC of most fungi causing onychomycosis after 24 h of contact. Even the lower part of the nail shows measurable microbiological activity within 24 h [36, 60, 65]. Penetration into the deepest nail slice is also observed in patients with severe onychomycosis treated for 4 weeks with Amor nail lacquer. The level of Amor obtained in the deepest layer ranged in the same order as in the upper levels; thus, a steady-state concentration – well in excess of the MFC against most dermatophytes and yeasts – is reached after this time period. Amor applied topically is detectable in the nail earlier than Ter or Itra after oral application. Amor additionally has a high vapor pressure; thus, it overcomes hollows (air chambers) in the nail and penetrates rapidly through heavily diseased nails.

Amor should be used only in cases of onychomycosis characterized by less than 80% of affected nail surface and an intact matrix and lunula. In patients treated with Amor nail lacquer once weekly for 6 months, clinical cure or improvement was achieved in 77.6% of all toenails and in 83.7% of fingernails by 3 months after the end of therapy [20, 36, 37, 39a, 59, 66–69]. Generally, eradication rates for *T. rubrum* were slightly lower than those for *T. mentagrophytes*; the same phenomenon has been observed with Ter and Itra. Local adverse events have been recorded in less than 1% of patients. *Candida onychomycosis* with chronic paronychia seems to respond especially well to Amor [36, 63].

The practicable therapy schemata (oral and topical) were studied in a multinational (Canada, France, Germany, Italy, UK) pharmacoeconomic analysis: Amor was in second place behind Cprox, and the efficacy cost relation was less favorable for oral therapy with Ter and Itra [64]. In a retrospective cost-efficacy analysis for general practices in the UK, Amor stood again in second place (£312), whereas this time oral Ter (£258) treatment stood in first place, griseofulvin and Itra being more expensive [69].

2.2.2.2 Ciclopirox/olamin

The antifungal and antibacterial effects of ciclopirox/olamin (Cprox) are attributed to the hydroxypyridone group. Cprox possesses a broad antifungal spectrum including dermatophytes, yeasts, and-non dermatophytic moulds causing onychomycosis, such as *Scopulariopsis brevicaulis* and *Scytalidium hyalinum*, with MICs between 0.4 and 4 μg/ml. Aspergilli are less sensitive to the drug than dermatophytes and yeasts [66].

The degree of activity of Cprox is lower than that of Amor, Ter, and Itra, i.e., a higher concentration in the lacquer (8% vs. 2%) and a more frequent application schedule (once daily vs. once weekly) than with Amor are needed for clinical use. Cprox has, in contrast to azoles, a relatively good antibacterial activity and, like Ter, exerts an anti-inflammatory activity [70].

Cprox is one of the few antifungals that do not interfere with sterol biosynthesis. The mechanism of action of Cprox is diverse, targeting different metabolic processes in the fungal cell. The major interference seems to occur on the level of trivalent cation; Cprox shows a high affinity to Fe^{3+} ions, which are essential cofactors in enzymes such as cytochromes. As a consequence of this action, Cprox impairs the microbial metabolism by affecting mitochondrial electron transport processes in the course of energy production. Additionally, the activity of catalase and peroxidase is reduced [70]. The details of the different modes of action are not yet fully understood; however, it is clear that the complexity of Cprox's mode of action significantly reduces development of resistant mutants.

The good penetration of Cprox through nail tissues was demonstrated in various *in vitro* models, which are nicely summarized in the paper by M. Bohn and K. Th. Krämer [70]. As with Amor, a good penetration of the active ingredient was evident after 24-h contact. After 7 days of treatment, a steady state with high biological activity was achieved in all layers of toenails; the same was seen after 14 days of treatment in fingernails. It seems that Cprox is eliminated from the nail tissue more rapidly than Amor, Ter, or Itra. Fourteen days after treatment was stopped, the amount of Cprox present in the nail was below the limit of detection (40 μg/g).

Clinical studies conducted worldwide demonstrate the efficacy of Cprox nail lacquer (8%) for the treatment of finger- and toenail onychomycosis with a good safety profile [39a]. Cprox is applied daily for a duration of 6 months in Europe and 48 weeks in the U.S. [37]. In two U.S. studies performed for FDA approval, mycological cure (negative KOH and negative culture) was achieved in 29-36% of the patients, negative culture was seen in 84% of the cases, and clinical cure or improvement was observed in 12% to 20% of the patients [71]. In the U.S., the Cprox nail lacquer shows a better cost efficacy than the oral antifungal therapies Ter, Itra, Flu, or griseofulvin. The cost of regimen for Cprox was $325 compared to $881–$1413, and the relative cost-effectiveness was 1.0 vs. 1.19–3.13 [72].

2.2.3 Combination therapy in onychomycosis

It has always been a matter of contention whether one should burden the body with an oral drug when an effective topical treatment is available. Until recently, no equivalent topical treatment existed for onychomycosis; nowadays, however, we have that choice. Both treatment schedules – systemic and topical – still have their drawbacks. Thus, it has always been of interest to search for new treatment strategies. A combination of two drugs that have synergistic activity is one possible advance towards achieving higher cure rates in difficult cases with extensive diseased areas and matrix involvement. Combination of a topical and an oral treatment schedule may additionally reduce the number of severe side effects [39a, 64, 71, 73].

Amor has shown an additive or even synergistic *in vitro* effect with several antifungals, including Keto, Itra, Ter, and griseofulvin; both the fungistatic and the fungicidal activities were augmented. The synergy between Amor and other sterol biosynthesis inhibitors was predictable, but the positive effect with griseofulvin is surprising from the biochemical viewpoint. The synergy observed *in vitro* also translates into chemotherapeutic activity, the degree of synergy being even more pronounced *in vivo* than *in vitro* [64, 74]. In murine trichophytosis, combination of Amor with griseofulvin, Ter, Itra, and Flu was always more efficient than monotherapy.

In extensive onychomycosis, the beneficial effect of local treatment with Amor combined with a short oral treatment of griseofulvin [75], Ter [76], or Itra [2] was proven in various clinical trials. In an open comparative study,

339 patients with severe onychomycosis (affecting lunula and matrix) received either a combined treatment with Amor nail lacquer (twice weekly for 12 months) and griseofulvin (500 mg b.i.d. for 2 months) or griseofulvin alone (500 mg b.i.d for the first 2 months and q.d. for the remaining 10 months). Three months after the end of the treatment, the clinical cure and improvement rate was more than 90% in both groups. Mycological cure was quicker and better in the combination group than in the griseofulvin group (78% vs. 61%) The most common adverse events were headache, nausea, and vomiting, all attributed to griseofulvin. The results of this first combination study showed that the duration of griseofulvin therapy can be drastically reduced with the same clinical response but a quicker mycological cure [75].

Later, the combination of Amor with Ter was studied in two clinical trials [76, 77]. The combination of Ter (250 mg q.d.) for 12 weeks plus Amor nail lacquer (once weekly for 15 months) showed a clear beneficial effect over the control group, which received Ter monotherapy (250 mg q.d. for 12 weeks). After 15 months 64% of the patients treated with combination therapy were cured, whereas only 42% of the patients treated with monotherapy were cured [76]. A cost-effectiveness study additionally showed that the combination of Amor plus Ter (12 weeks) is the most cost-effective way to treat severe onychomycosis with matrix involvement [76, 78]. In Switzerland, various treatment schemata were compared in a multi-center open study with 305 patients. The combination of Amor plus Ter was applied for 6 or 12 weeks; additionally, Amor was combined with Itra pulse or continuous Itra. The most effective treatment schedule regarding clinical cure and mycological findings was again the combination of Amor with Ter for 12 weeks: 97.2% of the diseased nails were cured or at least significantly improved. The patients also showed the best compliance under this regimen. The outcome under the combination of Amor with Itra was generally lower: cure and improvement were seen in only 84.9% to 88.9% of the nails.

Furthermore, the clinical efficacy of a combination of Amor plus Itra was compared to Itra monotherapy in a clinical trial in Spain, comparing the following treatment schedules: Amor nail lacquer (once weekly for 6 months) combined with Itra (200 mg q.d. for 6 weeks or 3 months) or Itra monotherapy (200 mg q.d. for 6 weeks or 3 months). Again, the same trend was seen, i.e., the combination therapy being better than the corresponding monotherapy. The combination additionally had a marked cost per patient cured advantage [78a].

Combination of Cprox with Itra showed increased efficacy in patients with onychomycosis not responding to monotherapy. The combination was successful in mycological terms in all cases, but the appearance of healthy nails was directly dependent on the absence of blood flow disorders [78b].

In conclusion, combination therapy may be particularly helpful for very severe nail infections. Above all, the duration of the oral therapy may be significantly reduced, and, consequently, the risk to the patients of lengthy oral therapy may be minimized. To date, the combination of Ter and Amor has proved to be the most efficacious and cost-effective treatment.

A totally new concept of combination therapy in onychomycosis was recently presented by a Belgian working group: they combined an antifungal with a device boosting germination of fungal propagules in order to render these cells more responsive to treatment. Patients applied Amor nail lacquer onto the diseased nail once weekly, and every second day for the rest of the week, they applied a piece of Sabouraud agar enriched with cycloheximide and chloramphenicol to the nail plate, securing it in place for 24 h. After 1 week the patients used regular, once-weekly Amor for 3 weeks, and then the whole procedure was repeated for a second time. Only 2 of the 13 patients were not cured after this therapy, and no relapse was seen in the 6 follow-up months [79].

2.3 Pityriasis versicolor and seborrhoeic eczema

Pityriasis versicolor and seborrhoeic dermatitis are the most widespread superficial infections. They are both benign but cause unpleasant aesthetic disorders and show a strong tendency to relapse. The epidemiology of seborrhoeic dermatitis is not yet fully understood, but the lipophilic, keratinophilic yeast *Malassezia furfur* seems to play an important role in the course of seborrhoeic dermatitis, as it clearly does in pityriasis.

Because of their high relapse rate, pityriasis and seborrhoeic eczema have not been curable with one single treatment. In the last 10 years however, significant progress has been made in winning the battle against these unaesthetic diseases. Azoles [80] and especially Keto [81] (locally applied in the form of gel, cream, or shampoo) have shown high cure rates and have significantly reduced the relapse rates. One single application of 20 g Keto gel moussant on affected skin for 5 min (while taking a shower) has proven to be curative in several studies. Keto was also safe and curative for seborrhoeic eczema in children [82]. Oral Itra and Flu [80, 83, 84] are also highly efficacious in this clinical setting and significantly reduced the relapse rate. Oral Ter, the most potent antifungal drug for superficial infections caused by dermatophytes, has no efficacy in pityriasis versicolor but seems to have some effect in seborrhoeic eczema after a 4-week treatment duration with daily 250 mg Ter [85]. However, local treatment with Ter as gel or solution is highly effective (70–80% cure rate) in pityriasis versicolor [18, 86, 87]; moderate activity was also seen in seborrhoeic dermatitis after treatment with Ter 1% solution [18]. After a treatment duration of 6 weeks, Cprox shampoo (1%) also showed good efficacy in mild to moderate seborrhoeic eczema [88]. Cprox administered in a cream also demonstrated a good therapeutic value in mild to moderate facial seborrhoeic eczema [89]. Thus, the armamentarium of therapy possibilities for these indications has significantly enlarged in the last decade.

2.4 Vaginal candidosis

Vaginal candidosis is a common gynecological complaint. Indeed, estimates show that 75% of women experience at least one episode of vaginal candidosis during their lifetime. *Candida albicans* is the typical causative agent; however, *C. glabrata* is increasingly isolated. This organism is associated with a lower clinical response to standard therapy and with a higher relapse rate. Various risk factors may predispose women to vaginal candidosis: pregnancy, oral conceptives, diabetes, antibiotic therapy (especially with cotrimoxacole), and HIV infection [90, 91].

The choice for a successful therapy is extensive; a broad spectrum of pharmaceuticals similar to those used for the treatment of dermatomycoses is available with the two chemical classes azoles and polyenes. Various galenical forms can be used at the patient's convenience: vaginal tablets, ovula, pressaries, creams, lotions, and normal tablets. Both topical and systemic treatments have proven high efficacy in acute vaginal candidosis. Developments in recent years have not been so much in the improvements of efficacy (clotrimazole, the first azole available back in 1970, achieved a cure rate of more than 80%) but in decreasing the duration of therapy: a 1-day treatment period is the standard today. A single tablet of 250 mg Flu or a daily dose of 2 × 200 mg Itra has shown the same degree of efficacy as topical treatment with a single dose of a newer azole [2, 92, 93].

Scientific discussions today deal mainly with the potential benefits and liabilities of topical *versus* oral therapy. As a rule, it is preferable to treat local disorders with topical therapy. Most women, however, prefer systemic treatment in spite of the increased risk of interactions or adverse events. Topical therapy is clearly safer, since the drugs are only poorly absorbed and scarcely reach the circulation, and is advisable during pregnancy and breast-feeding. Women, especially HIV-positive patients, receiving therapy with other drugs that could interact with oral azoles should also be treated with topical agents [93].

In summary, the therapy for acute vaginal candidosis is unproblematic and highly efficient. However, some women suffer from chronic recurrent vaginal candidosis over periods of months and years and endure associated physical and physiological stress. The pathogenesis of the disease is still not fully understood. Intensive studies have not yet clearly revealed distinct risk factors. Despite the consideration of all known predisposing factors that may induce acute vaginal candidosis, no reason for frequent recolonization could be identified in the majority of these women. However, in recent years the observation was made that early stages of HIV infection may constitute a possible risk factor [89].

The optimal treatment of recurrent vaginal candidosis has not yet been defined. Several approaches have been tried, including treatment with transfer factor and immunotherapy with *Candida* vaccines [2]. In recent years so-called maintenance therapy or prophylaxis has been promoted as a successful approach. Generally, the acute symptoms are treated topically or orally up to their disappearance, then a maintenance therapy is initiated for a certain period of time. The drug of choice is given weekly or monthly, locally or orally. The efficacy of this regimen is measured in terms of reduction in recurrence. During maintenance therapy, the rate of relapses is generally significantly reduced; however, many patients experience a relapse after the treatment ends. A proper cure has not yet been achieved [20, 92, 93]. For example, during the 12-month phase of prophylaxis, recurrence was seen in 68% of the placebo-treated patients but in only 42% of the Flu-treated patients. Two months after discontinuation of therapy, more patients (94% vs. 84%) remained disease-free in the Flu group [92].

Thus, there is some hope for future success based on the promising results with suppressive therapy; however, the disease is not yet fully curable, and the pathology and risk factors not fully understood.

3 Subcutaneous mycoses

Three fungal infections – Madura feet (mycetoma), chromomycosis, and sporotrichosis – fall into the category of subcutaneous mycoses. The distribution of the three infections is mainly in tropical and subtropical areas. Skin trauma is the portal of entry for the fungal spores of all three infections, and most cases of Madura feet and chromomycosis occur in male agricultural workers working barefoot.

3.1 Madura feet

The term "mycetoma" is used to denote any tumor due to fungal infection. This group of infections is caused by a variety of unrelated fungi found on plants or in soil. Subcutaneous infections of this type are not common but are difficult to treat and tend to be chronic. Mycetoma can be caused by filamentous bacteria (actinomycetes) or by a fungus. The infection is classified according to the appearance of "grains" that are composed of microcolonies of the causative fungus or actinomycete filaments found within the lesions [94]. The diagnosis is done by imaging methods or histology; the causative agent is seldom isolated. In those parts of the world in which the infections are endemic, the morbidity of the condition can pose a problem for the patient as well as for the community.

The therapy for both types of mycetoma differs according the causative agent: if the infection is due to a bacterial strain of actinomycetes, antibacterial therapy must be used. A two-step treatment schedule – starting with an intensive phase of therapy with penicillin, gentamicin, and co-trimoxazole for some weeks, followed by a maintenance therapy with amoxicillin and co-trimoxazole for several months – seems to be an effective therapy for this therapy-resistant disease [95].

Therapy for fungal infection is more difficult. Surgery or even amputation has been the standard for a long time and is still in use. In recent years, Keto and especially Itra have been successfully used [96, 97]. More successful than an antifungal monotherapy is the combination of surgery or of curettage plus antifungal therapy. The optimal therapy for Eumycetoma is not yet defined, but there is evidence that azoles are of significant benefit [98].

3.2 Chromomycosis

Chromomycosis is a chronic fungal infection of the subcutaneous tissues caused by a group of dematiaceous fungi. Direct examination of biopsy or potassium hydroxide preparation show the deeply pigmented, thick-walled sclerotic cells typical of dematiaceous fungi. The course of the disease is chronic; the time of inoculation is often years before the symptoms are apparent.

A general direction for the optimal therapy of chromomycosis does not exist, although traditional schedules and new approaches are described in the literature. The rare disease chromomycosis, caused by a variety of fungal species, demands the creativity of physicians, since many strains do not respond to conventional antifungal therapy with Itra monotherapy.

The treatment of choice for early localized lesions is surgical removal by excision or destruction by means of cryotherapy, cautery, or diathermy. In more chronic cases, systemic Amph B therapy was not curative; however, combination therapy with 5FC plus Amph B or Keto was in some cases beneficial [2, 99]. Itra alone was successful in many cases of chromomycosis, especially that caused by *Cladosporium carionii*. Itra combined with 5FC or local 5FU cream or Itra plus thiobendazole seems to be needed for a complete cure in infections caused by *Fonsecaea pedrosoi* [2, 100–103]. Flu was also curative in some cases [104]. Additional to the more conventional therapy reports with Itra, interesting positive case reports are found in the literature that demonstrate the creativity of the various physicians: a patient responded to local therapy of 5FU cream [105]. A rare case of chromomycosis due to an unidentified species of *Phialophora* has been reported that was eventually cured by topical Amor and local hyperthermia after recurrence following initially successful Itra and local Amph B cream and then treatment with Itra and Cprox [106]. Compassionate long-term oral Ter was highly curative in a pilot study of 42 patients [107]. Colleagues from Venezuela described the various therapy schedules for 422 patients: topical monotherapy with 5FU cream showed 44% cure rates; combined with excision, the success was 61%. Itra was curative in 94% of the cases, whereas Ter had the lowest success rate, with 50%. For the first time the curative effect of topical Ajoene was described for this indication [20].

It is very difficult to find a single optimal therapy for a disease that can be caused by a large variety of fungi showing various degrees of resistance; therefore, the battle against this disease is not yet won. Some progress has been made, especially because of the efficacy of Itra, but there is still a long way to go.

3.3 Sporotrichosis

This fungal infection involves the lymphatics and subcutaneous tissues and is caused by the dimorphic fungus *Sporotrix schenckii*. The sporotrichosis lesions spread *via* lymphatics from the original wound and form nodules and pustules that quickly ulcerate. In some cases, sporotrichosis disseminates to organs and bones; sporotrichosis is often seen in alcohol addicts.

Potassium iodide has been the therapy of choice for many years and is still used in many countries despite its frequent side effects (nausea and flow of tears). A study published in 1996 [108] showed that cutaneous sporotrichosis was cured by a single dose of potassium iodide in 80% of the cases. In recent years, Itra has been set up as standard therapy for cutaneous and lymphatic sporotrichosis [109–111]. The trade name of Itra, Sporanox, is based on its efficacy in this indication. C.A. Kauffman and colleagues have recently presented guidelines for the management of patients with various forms of sporotrichosis [112].

Amph B was and still is used in the more disseminated cases [2, 109]; success is, however, also seen under Itra therapy [113]. Treatment of pulmonary sporotrichosis with Amph B or Itra has been disappointing, with low response rates of 30–50%. Some patients may need lifelong suppression with Itra. Especially aggressive therapy is needed in HIV patients with sporotrichosis: both Amph B and Itra showed the same – not overwhelming – efficacy in this difficult setting [114]. A case of disseminated osteoarticular sporotrichosis in an AIDS patient was successfully treated with Amph B [115]. Flu seems to be only moderately active in sporotrichosis and will never replace Itra in this indication [116].

4 Systemic mycoses

4.1 The causative agents

Fungi are eukaryotic cells, structurally and biochemically similar to human cells. Biochemical studies have identified a number of potential targets for antifungal chemotherapy, including cell wall synthesis (the only fungus-specific target), membrane sterol biosynthesis, nucleic acid synthesis, metabolic inhibition, and macronuclear biosynthesis. However, most antifungal drugs interfere with the enzymatic steps of sterol biosynthesis that are common for fungi and human cells.

Sterol biosynthesis seems to be the Achilles' heel of the fungus cell, since ergosterol, the essential component of the fungal membrane, exerts two functions: it is a bulk membrane component and it regulates growth and proliferation. Finally, the glucan synthesis inhibitor caspofungin (CAS), an antifungal drug interfering with the sole specific target, the synthesis of cell wall, is on the market.

Agents of the deep mycoses can be divided into two groups according to their ability to infect a healthy, immunocompetent host. Those that are able to do so are known as primary pathogens; these include *Coccidioides immitis, Histoplasma capsulatum, Histoplasma duboisii, Blastomyces dermatitidis, Paracoccidioides brasiliensis*, and *Sporotrix schenckii*. Opportunistic pathogens such as *Candida, Aspergillus, Cryptococcus, Trichosporon*, and Zygomycetes cause invasive infections only if specific predisposing risk factors (immune deficiency, long and broad antibacterial therapy, severe underlying diseases, etc.) are present.

Although in the past most fungi have been clearly placed into one of the two categories, the borders have recently been effaced. The primary pathogen *Histoplasma capsulatum*, which causes outbreaks in endemic areas, behaves like an opportunistic fungus in patients with AIDS. The old, seemingly cured infection suddenly flares up when AIDS has weakened the patient's immune system. This phenomenon also happens in non-endemic areas and is therefore entirely dependent on the immune status of the host and not on the environment.

Classifying some rare fungi as primary pathogens or opportunists has always been difficult. No clear correlation between pathogenicity and immunological state has been demonstrated for dematiaceous fungi, which cause chronic subcutaneous infections as well as acute brain infections.

Primary dimorphic pathogens cause serious fungal infections in normally immunocompetent hosts. Epidemics are often observed in endemic areas. These species are to a large extent resistant to the defense mechanisms of the host. Their spores, inhaled by the host, overcome the alveolar macrophages that play the main role in the primary defense mechanism against parasites. Converted to the invasive tissue form, the fungi also seem to be resistant to human neutrophils. The phenomenon of recurrent histoplasmosis in AIDS patients may be explained by the fact that a functional, active population of T-cells is needed to control the overtly cured disease. In the case of disturbance of the T-cell function, the latent fungal infection causes a secondary severe invasion. Many questions regarding the nature of the immunological defense mechanism towards primary pathogenic fungi still remain unsolved.

The opportunistic pathogen is a danger only if the immune defense has been weakened. Observations of which infections are associated with which form of immune inadequacy have contributed significantly to our understanding of the natural defense mechanism against mycoses. The former scarce knowledge regarding the host defense mechanism towards *Cryptococcus neoformans* has significantly increased in recent years since this fungal species has become prominent among opportunistic pathogens causing invasive disease in HIV patients. It has become clear that the main defense against *Cryptococcus* must be based on T-cells and not on neutrophils. Which fungal species can cause a systemic infection in immunocompromised patients is not something that can be stated with confidence, but many are potential candidates. Beside the typical opportunistic fungi (*Candida, Aspergillus, Cryptococcus*, Zygomycetes), the primary pathogenic fungi, usually causing little sickness in healthy individuals, can be devastating in the immunocompromised patient. Other fungi that have always been regarded as non-pathogenic and harmless for humans are now causing life-threatening mycoses. It is necessary to look closer at a few of the "newer" pathogens, as doing so it gives some indication of the problem the physician faces when trying to determine the most probable diagnosis.

4.1.1 Emerging pathogens

As mentioned earlier, it is slowly becoming impossible to find a fungal species that has not been reported in the literature to cause severe infections in humans, but certain fungi have made themselves more visible than others. The emergence of uncommon opportunistic fungi in immunocompromised patients and its relevance as a new nosocomial threat was recently summarized [117]

Saccharomyces cerevisiae could be considered the least dangerous of the fungi; nevertheless, several cases of invasive, life-threatening infections have been caused by this harmless baker's yeast [1, 2]. *Rodotorula* has generally been regarded as having low pathogenicity; however, several cases of bloodstream infections related to use of indwelling central catheters have recently been reported [2]. A successful therapy should include removal of the catheter plus antifungal therapy. 5FC (alone or in combination with Amph B) is the first-line antifungal drug, since *Rodotorula* is highly susceptible to 5FC but only moderately to Amph B. Recently, a *Rodotorula* meningitis was diagnosed in an HIV patient [118]. Deep mycoses like this meningitis case require maintenance therapy with an azole (e.g., Itra) after the initial treatment in order to avoid relapses.

In recent years it has become apparent that *Fusarium*, a well-known plant pathogen, is able to cause severe infections in humans, mainly in leukemia patients. These infections are difficult to control in neutropenic patients since most *Fusarium* species are relatively resistant to all antifungals used in human chemotherapy [119–121]. Up to now several antifungal treatment schedules (mono- and combination therapy) have been used; however, no regimen was unambiguously superior to the others. Combination therapy with a new azole plus immunostimulators, increasing the host defense activity, may improve the fatal prognosis of this invasive disease in the future.

Another unusual pathogen is *Trichosporon beigelii*, which has been shown to cause sepsis in premature infants [2]. A cluster of sepsis cases has been observed in a neonatal intensive care unit [122]. Other known risk factors for this disease are neutropenia, valve replacement, ambulatory peritoneal dialysis, and AIDS [2]. *Trichosporon beigelii* is *in vitro* relatively Amph B resistant; however, successful treatments with Amph B alone or in combination with rifampicin, 5FC, or triazoles have been reported [2]. Flu proved to be the best therapy in murine trichosporosis [123], and it was successful in a *Trichosporon* infection refractory to a combination therapy with Amph B plus 5FC [124].

Penicillium marneffei, a fungus endemic in Southeast Asia and Japan, causes disseminated fungal infections, especially in HIV-positive patients [125–127]. About 550 cases of *P. marneffei* infections were diagnosed in

Japan up to 1995. Most patients responded to appropriate antifungal therapy (such as Amph B, Flu, Itra, or Vori) *P. marneffei* is highly susceptible *in vitro* to Itra, Keto, and 5FC but appears to be less susceptible to Amph B and Flu. In HIV-positive children, Keto was successfully used as prophylactic therapy to prevent relapses [126]. Disseminated *P. marneffei* infections in AIDS patients have also been diagnosed in Europe in subjects returning from a visit to certain areas of Southeast Asia [128, 129]. In AIDS patients, mild and moderately severe infections should be treated with Itra or Keto, and severely ill patients should be treated with Amph B. However, the failure rate in AIDS patients is substantial. Suppressive therapy should be considered in advanced AIDS patients, since relapses are common after the treatment has been stopped.

Hansenula anomala is another emerging fungal species causing fungemia in children and neutropenic adults. This infection is often associated with a central catheter and total parenteral nutrition [130–132]. Removal of the catheter is essential for successful therapy; some patients recovered without antifungal treatment, but only because the catheter was removed [120]. Amph B or Flu therapy seems to be successful in this clinical setting (always inclusive removal of the catheter). However, a breakthrough fungemia due to *H. anomala* has been observed in a leukemia patient under Flu prevention [133]. The patient responded favorably to Amph B treatment.

Malassezia sp. is another fungal species able to cause bloodstream infections in premature infants or in neutropenic adults who receive parenteral nutrition and/or intravenous lipids [134]. For example, a nosocomial outbreak of *M. pachydermatis* in a neonatal intensive care unit was studied epidemiologically: the transmission occurred most likely from person to person *via* the hands of the medical staff [135]. Treatment consists of discontinuing the parenteral lipid emulsion and removal of central venous catheter. Non-immunocompromised patients seldom require antifungal therapy once the catheter is removed and the lipid emulsion is discontinued. If antifungal therapy is necessary, systemic azoles are preferred to Amph B, since they are considered to be more efficacious.

Pseudoallescheria boydii infections are known to be resistant to Amph B treatment; however, miconazole has been the therapy of choice for this disease for many decades despite the fact that miconazole has severe safety liabilities. Recently, successful treatment has been reported with Keto, Itra, or newer triazoles [2, 136]. In the future new triazoles with higher efficacy and better safety margins will replace miconazole for *Pseudoallescheria* infections; Vori alone cured a chronic case of meningitis due to *P. boydii* [137], and Vori combined with surgical drainage was successful in an Amph B- and Itra-refractory brain abscess [138].

Aspergillus ustus [139] and *Aspergillus terreus* [20] also belong to the emerging opportunistic fungi causing cutaneous or even deep mycoses in immunosuppressed patients. Infections due to *Aspergillus terreus* are extremely difficult to treat since this species is Amph B resistant [20]. The same is true for the *Acremonium* sp. [117, 140].

During recent years, all the above-mentioned fungal species have been observed to cause fatal infections in immunocompromised patients with a disquietingly increasing frequency. Certain other fungi are rarely seen but nevertheless cause deep concern in the medical world: *Scedosporium prolificans (inflatum)* causes deadly disseminated infections in patients with various immunosuppressions (AIDS, leukemia, lymphoma, etc.). *S. prolificans* strains are *in vitro* resistant to Amph B, 5FC, and older azoles, but are susceptible to newer triazoles like Vori and Sch 56592. Disseminated infections seem to respond to Vori or Sch 56592 [20, 141]. In 1992, a case of fatal dissemination due to *Maceliophthora thermophilia* was diagnosed post mortem. *Trichoderma pseudokonigii* in a bone marrow transplant proved to be resistant to Amph B, Flu, and Lip Amph B plus 5FC. A liver transplant developed a fatal infection due to *Trichoderma viride*. A fungal infection due to *Scytalidium* on a granulocytopenic child responded well to Amph B [2]. *Pytium insidiosum* caused fatal arthritis in six patients with thalassemia. Early recognition and radical amputation are at present the only chance of surviving [142]. A-six-year-old child without an apparent risk factor died after an infusion contaminated with *Blastomyces capitus* [143]. A patient with short bowel syndrome as a consequence of multiple intestinal resections for Crohn's disease had a port system implanted. One year later she presented fever, weakness, and nighttime sweating, and *Metschnikowia pulcherrima* was isolated [144]. The weak plant pathogen *Neocosmospora vasinfecta* induced ostheoarthritis after a multiple trauma [145]. In India, *Ascotricha chartratrum* was diagnosed as agent of sinusitis [146]. A case of fungemia due to *Paecilomyces lilacinus* was reported in a non-neutropenic adult, 120 days after a bone marrow transplant [147]. Four cases of exogenous endophthalmitis caused by Amph B-resistant *P. lilacinus* responded to Keto and Miconazole [148]; a cutaneous infection in a renal transplant was temporarily cured by Vori [149].

In conclusion, the physician is confronted not only with an increasing number of agents but also with an uncertainty regarding the susceptibility of the fungal strain. Physicians have to be aware that the fungal cell has an incredible potency to invade practically any organ in the presence of an overwhelming number of risk factors.

4.2 The patient

The major factor in the increase in systemic mycoses is undoubtedly immunodeficiency. There is an expanding community of people with weakened or even non-existent immune systems due to underlying diseases, medical treatment, surgical intervention, or transplantation (especially bone marrow transplantation). Although travel to endemic areas is becoming more common, and disease caused by primary pathogens is more often diagnosed, it is the increase in opportunistic infections that has completely changed the significance and necessity of antifungal therapy.

The fungi have not changed their habitat, but the factors that turn a saprophyte into a virulent pathogen have become more varied and more common. For instance, immune suppression in organ transplant patients and antitumor therapy in cancer patients have become rather frequent; however, it was the AIDS pandemic that changed the whole picture of opportunistic infections. The division between primary and opportunistic pathogens is blurred, as colonization or asymptomatic infections can flare up into life-threatening diseases in a host whose immune system is weakened from day to day.

HIV-positive patients are at the highest risk of falling ill with infections caused by traditionally recognized opportunistic fungi, an emerging new pathogen, or a recognized primary pathogen. In AIDS patients, all fungal infections, superficial or deep mycoses, display a more severe clinical course with frequent therapy resistance in comparison to normal or less strictly immunocompromised patients.

Seborrhoeic dermatitis, which in normal patients can be kept under control by an array of compounds active against *Malassezia furfur*, is a clinical problem in HIV-infected patients. Dermatophytic infections require a longer treatment duration, and relapses are common. The recurrent form, not the acute form, of vaginal candidosis, is observed in HIV-positive females.

Before the emergence of AIDS, oropharyngeal candidosis was seen only in patients of extreme age (babies or very old people). In the years before a highly active antiviral therapy (HAART) was used, oropharyngeal candidosis was the most common infectious disease in HIV patients, affecting 90% of the patients with a 60% recurrence rate within 3 months [150]. Oral candidosis appears at an early stage of HIV infection, whereas oesophageal infections are seen in those with more advanced disease. Eradication of the clinical manifestation of candidosis is the major goal in treating mucosal candidosis of HIV-positive patients. As follow-up action, suppression of recurrence was the ultimate goal. *Cryptococcus meningitis* was the most frequent manifestation of deep mycoses. During the past few years, the frequency of cryptococcal meningitis significantly decreased thanks to a highly efficacious antiviral therapy and a widespread use of Flu prophylaxis [151, 151a]. The disease takes a more severe course and a long suppressive therapy is necessary because the prostate and the meninges act as nidi of infection despite successful therapy. Optimal initial treatment should aim to immediately stop the fungal infection in order to prevent further immunosuppression of the host by cryptococcal polysaccharide, which is known to be immunosuppressive. Additionally, it has been shown that cryptococcal polysaccharides significantly enhance HIV infectivity, further depleting residual CD4 cells [152]. Two of the four major endemic mycoses of the U.S., histoplasmosis and coccidioidomycosis, have increasingly appeared as HIV-associated opportunistic infections. Penicillosis (caused by *P. marneffei*) is known to be one of the most frequent opportunistic infections in AIDS patients in Southeast Asia.

In a setting of neutropenia, severe diabetes mellitus, or use of broad spectrum antibacterials, the main opportunistic infections are caused by *Candida* and *Aspergillus*. Treatment is often ineffective unless the underlying disease can be controlled. As soon as this control is working, antifungal therapy is successful and no maintenance therapy is necessary.

In recent years, more knowledge has accumulated about the way the human body defends itself against fungal infections and about the particular risk of specific groups of patients. Oropharyngeal candidosis is seen in T-cell disturbance, whereas *Candida* infection of organs is mainly observed in neutropenic patients. *C. tropicalis* and *C. krusei* have an affinity for leukemia patients and are increasingly isolated from AIDS patients in the late stage of the disease. *Mucor* has an affinity to diabetes mellitus and *Fusarium* to neutropenic patients. Despite increased understanding regarding host-fungus interactions, there is still a long way to go until we understand the host defense mechanism towards fungi in detail. Until our knowledge regarding the immunology of fungal disease becomes more detailed, the most important advance will remain the increased awareness of the medical world of the power and danger of fungal infections in the ever-growing population of the immunocompromised.

In conclusion, AIDS patients are at a very high risk of contracting severe fungal infections, of experiencing a relapse, or even of dying from opportunistic fungal infections. Thus, it is of importance to initiate suppressive therapy for all deep fungal infections after the initial therapy has proven successful, even if the niche of the fungus is not known, since relapses in patients without broad antiviral therapy are extremely frequent as soon as antifungal therapy is stopped. The detailed experience of systemic antifungal therapy in neutropenic and AIDS patients will be discussed in the section for each drug.

4.3 The drugs on the market

Ten years ago only three established drugs for the treatment of systemic mycoses existed; today this number has increased to seven: Amph B (with the new formulations taken as one single entity) 5FC, Keto, Flu, Itra, Voriconazole (Vori), and Caspofungin (Cap).

4.3.1 Amphotericin B, the conventional antifungal

Although hundreds of macrolide polyenic antibiotics are synthesized by actinomycetes, only one, Amph B, is used in systemic antifungal therapy. It is produced by *Streptomyces nodosus*. Amph B has an extremely broad *in vitro* spectrum (fungicidal and fungistatic) that includes the established opportunistic fungi (*Candida* spp., *Cryptococcus neoformans*, *Aspergillus* spp., *Mucoraceae*) and the primary pathogens (*H. capsulatum*, *Coccidioides immitis*, *Paracoccidioides brasiliensis*). Dermatophytes, the dematiaceous fungi and species of *Madurella*, are considered to be resistant [2, 153].

4.3.1.1 Resistance

It was always easy to isolate resistant mutants in the laboratory [154]. The Amph B mutants are generally distinguished from parent strains by alterations of the lipid composition or the cell wall [155, 156]. Previously, it was generally accepted that secondary resistance of *Candida albicans* to Amph B is rare despite its extensive use in chemotherapy for more than 40 years. This may be explained by the fact that the changes in the sterol composition of the membrane leading to *in vitro* resistance reduce virulence and slow cell growth rate. No resistance or increased MICs to Amph B have been observed in 43 isolates of a surveillance study in bone marrow transplant recipients treated prophylactically with Amph B [157]. Over the last 10 years, however, secondary Amph B resistance has been documented in *C. albicans* and *Cryptococcus neoformans* [158, 159]. This phenomenon seems to be related to prolonged use of azole prophylaxis in cancer and AIDS patients [156, 160]. Additionally, new species, primary resistant to Amph B, have been isolated from highly immunocompromised patients, i.e., *Aspergillus terreus* shows high Amph B resistance [161].

4.3.1.2. Mode of action

The current model for the mechanism of action is based on the formation of 1:1 Amph B/sterol aggregates, which associates into a transmembrane barrel with a large –OH-lined aqueous pore down the middle [2, 162–164]. The result of interaction between Amph B and the sterols is a disturbance of the ergosterol function leading to increased permeability, disruption of the proton gradient, and leakage of potassium ions. At low levels of Amph B, non-aqueous channels are built, leading to K^+ leakage. At higher Amph B concentrations, these non-aqueous channels react with ergosterol to form transmembrane aqueous pores. Non-aqueous channels are permeable to urea and monovalent cations, aqueous pores are permeable to monovalent cations and anions and divalent cations. The complete mechanism of action of Amph B is still not fully understood. New hypotheses are being framed, and many researchers studying the interaction with natural membranes or artificial bilayers are trying to prove them. Conflicting membrane-permeability data suggest a multiplicity of Amph B channel structures and modes of action [163]. Oxidative damage to the cells seems to be involved, and the drug appears to induce a cascade of oxidative reactions linked to its own oxidation. The fungistatic activity is correlated with permeability changes, i.e., the potassium efflux; the lethal activity is more dependent on the oxidative challenge, e.g., irreversible inhibition of ATPase, induced by the aqueous channels. The complexcity of the mode of action of Amph B will probably keep generations of biochemical researchers busy.

4.3.1.3 Safety and toxicity

Amph B has a higher specificity for ergosterol than for cholesterol, the mammalian sterol; this is considered the key to the relatively low toxicity of Amph B to the human host in comparison with other polyenes like nystatin and candicidin. Nevertheless, the major drawback for broader use of Amph B is the frequent occurrence of adverse events. Amph B does induce reversible and chronic side effects that are unpleasant and, in many cases, menacing [2, 153, 159, 163]. Acute toxicity to Amph B – usually fever, chills, rigor, or nausea – can be ameliorated by concomitant administration of meperidine, acetaminophen, or hydrocortisone. There is additionally the possibility of tailoring time and duration of the infusion to the individual patient, since the acute reactions vary significantly. The incidence of side effects is dependent on the infusion rate, being higher under rapid infusion. Reversible anemia develops in 75% of patients. The potential value of co-administration has not yet been fully evaluated [153]. Chronic toxicity of Amph B is mostly due to renal damage. Hypokalemia, hypomagnesemia, and increased creatinin are common and troublesome [153, 159]. Nephrotoxicity does not appear to be strictly dose-related and can occur with standard therapy as well. The knowledge regarding this chronic adverse event has significantly increased, and prevention of the chronic tubular injury seems feasible: making certain that the patient is eunatremic appears to mitigate nephrotoxicity. The reversal of sodium depletion by salt loading gained full acceptance in clinical practice. This can be achieved either by a special salt diet or by combination therapy with 5FC infusion, which contains 0.9% saline. Using this combination therapy avoids not only the nephrotoxic effects of Amph B but also coincidentically improves efficacy against several opportunistic fungal infections based on the proven synergism between Amph B and 5FC (see details in Section 4.3.7). An interesting phenomenon has been observed: patients with higher serum LDL cholesterol concentrations were more susceptible to Amph B-induced renal toxicity than patients with lower LDL cholesterol levels [165]. In AIDS patients, a combination of Amph B and foscarnet (an antiviral drug) should be avoided, since this combination rapidly induces renal insufficiency [166]. Nephrotoxic drugs like aminoglycosides, cyclosporine and pentamidine should not be combined with Amph B. Amph B-induced hypokalemia may increase the toxic effect of digitalis and increase the activity of neuromuscular inhibitors [167]. The incidence of adverse events is meanwhile known to be rather high: Amph B therapy caused side effects in 46% of 102 patients with fungal infections. Acute side effects (chills, nausea, etc.) occurred more often in patients aged less than 50 years, whereas laboratory abnormalities (hypokalemia, renal insufficiency) occurred more often at higher doses [168]. The incidence of renal adverse reactions in AIDS patients is not higher than in normal patients: 67% of the patients showed no renal impairments, 20% showed moderate dysfunctions, and 1.3% showed severe renal dysfunctions [169]. The incidence of nephrotoxicity in 239 immunosuppressed patients with aspergillosis was investigated. Elevated creatinin associated with Amph B therapy was not only a marker for renal dysfunction but also was associated with a substantial risk for the use of hemodialysis and a higher mortality rate [170]. The attitude towards the use of Amph B has drastically changed through increased knowledge. Most clinicians have lost their fear of prescribing Amph B, and they now use the drug, despite its toxicity, with confidence for highly immunosuppressed patients with fungal disease. Courageous medics have successfully treated AIDS patients with *Candida* endophthalmitis with i.v. Amph B at home. Renal function deterioration was observed, but all side effects were reversible. These authors conclude that patients requiring i.v. Amph B therapy can be treated at home under hospital supervision, with considerable savings for the clinic [171].

Research has detected another way to avoid major side effects of Amph B without losing the efficacy. The renal toxicity rates are drastically reduced if Amph B is embedded in liposomes or associated with lipids (see Section 4.3.2).

4.3.1.4 Therapy

Despite its toxicity, Amph B is still used as superior therapy for a wide range of systemic mycoses: its fungicidal effect makes it irreplaceable for disseminated infections in highly immunodeficient patients, at least as initial therapy. It must, however, be mentioned that even after 40 years of clinical use, no general agreement exists regarding the optimal dose, the duration of therapy, or method of administration. The therapeutic or pharmacokinetic rationale for optimal Amph B dosing is lacking [172]. In the last 10 years – despite the introduction of triazoles – Amph B has kept and probably will keep its leadership role in the area of severe fungal infections in highly immunocompromised patients, including HIV-infected patients. Amph B monotherapy remains the drug of choice for the initial therapy in disseminated histoplasmosis [150] and coccidioidomycosis of AIDS patients [150, 173, 174]. The optimal initial treatment for cryptococcal meningitis aiming to rapidly halt the infection in order to prevent further immunosuppression remains combination therapy with 5FC [150, 174, 175] (for detailed description, see Section 3.4.6). Amph B prevails in the therapy of mucormycosis (zygomycosis), since all Zygomycetes are resistant to azoles. Despite the fact that Flu has gained its own place for the treatment of candidosis, Amph B is still used for candidemia, hematogeneously disseminated *Candida* infection, and *Candida* meningitis. 5FC should be administered concurrently with Amph B in patients whose condition is not improving under monotherapy [176]. Catheter-related funguria is eradicated only by a combination of Amph B bladder irrigation plus catheter change; *Candida* thrombophlebitis requires Amph B plus surgery for a complete cure [177, 178]. In 1996, the crude mortality and rate of response to Amph B therapy of invasive aspergillosis were reviewed in 1223 immunocompromised patients [179]. The response rate of pulmonary aspergillosis was not overwhelming, and was dependent on the underlying disease and the duration of the treatment. Only patients treated for more than 134 days had any real chance of being cured. Pulmonary aspergillosis responded in 33% of the bone marrow transplant patients, 54% of the leukemia cases, and 83% of the heart or renal transplant patients. *Aspergillus* sinusitis cases responded with 49% and cerebral aspergillosis with 33%. Thus, Amph B is in no way a "wonder drug" for aspergillosis therapy, but it is still not clear whether i.v. Itra, a new triazole, or one of the new Amph B formulations will ever be superior to Amph B. In conclusion, Amph B has not yet lost its place in human chemotherapy.

4.3.2 Amph B in new clothes

The first publication of clinical experiments with liposomal Amph B was that of Lopez-Bernstein in 1984. Meanwhile, three lipid-associated forms – namely, liposomal Amph B (Ambisome®, Lipo-Amph), Amph B lipid complex

(ABLC, Abelect®), and Amph B colloidal dispension (ABCD, Amphocil, Amphotec®) – are on the market and have found their niche indications during the last 10 years. The properties of the three lipid-based Amph B preparations and their usefulness for antifungal chemotherapy have been reviewed comparatively in several articles [180–182], the last one in 2001 [183].

Beside the three FDA-proven Amph B lipid formulations, a variety of other new formulations exist, all being individually mixed in hospitals or small laboratories. The interested reader finds Amph B poly micelles [184], admixtures with Intralipid or Lipofungin [185], and new triglycerid emulsions [186] or new delivery systems for Amph B with nanosphere [187] or cochleates [188]. In the last 10 years, a diversity of reports appeared dealing with these individually prepared formulations of Amph B and describing their efficacy *in vitro* or in animal models, the pharmacokinetic properties, the therapeutic indices, and the cure rates observed under these treatments. Not all Amph B lipid admixtures are usable for chemotherapy: when a solution of Amph B in water was mixed with a lipid emulsion and run through an infusion pump, there was a considerable decrease in the effluent Amph B concentration due to a substantial accumulation of the drug in fat emulsion droplets that had accumulated in the bottle and the tubing [189]. Generally, all Amph B-lipid preparations are less toxic than the conventional Amph B, and, therefore, higher doses are applicable in animal models, leading to higher efficacy. Amph B-lipid formulations also may have an increased effect on the immune response in murine aspergillosis [190], e.g., Amph B/cholesterol hemisuccinate increased in *Aspergillus* infected animals the interferon γ levels, leading to an inhibition of TH2 cytokine response, a decreased fungal load, and better survival. In human chemotherapy both the free Amph B and its new formulations show the same efficacy with a better tolerability in most [191, 192] but not all [193] cases. The intensive research for new Amph B-lipid formulations is probably so intensive because the approved Amph B-lipid formulations are too expensive for most countries and hospitals.

The properties of the three marketed lipid formulations differ in terms of the amount of Amph B and lipid used as well as their physical form and the pharmacokinetic properties, especially their serum clearance and acute infusion-related toxicity [183]; however, they are similar in that they permit Amph B to bypass the kidney and to concentrate in other organs (reviewed in [182, 183, 194–196]). The *in vitro* activity, mode of action, toxicity, and efficacy will be reviewed in this section. Most published data are available for

Ambisome®, which was the first on the market for salvage therapy in patients experiencing toxicity with free Amph B; however, in the last 6 years the other two formulations have become equally established in the field of antifungal therapy.

4.3.2.1 Mode of action

The *in vitro* activities of L-Amph B, ABLC, and ABCD are comparable to that of traditional Amph B. All Amph B-lipid formulations are less damaging to phagocytic host cells without losing their antifungal power [180, 181].

Much work has been done investigating the physical biochemistry of Amph B liposomal complexes and the mechanism by which toxicity is reduced. The details of these investigations are beyond the scope of this review, but more information can be found in [181, 182, 197]. The essentials are that Amph B in any formulation consists of complexed and free substance in equilibrium, and it is only the latter that is active. The job of the liposomes is to bring the drug into close contact with sterol-containing membranes in tissue, where the greater affinity of ergosterol ensures better transfer of active substance to the fungal cell. Less free Amph B is available to cause toxic side effects.

In vitro and *in vivo* studies have clearly demonstrated that L-Amph B accumulates at sites of infections. Empty and drug-containing liposomes equally attach to the surface of fungal cells, but only Amph B-containing liposomes interact with the fungal cells. This interaction results in the disruption of liposomes releasing Amph B and causing the death of the cell within 2 to 4 hours. In the case of ABLC, fungal lipases act to release Amph B in the tissues, i.e., the formulation is engulfed by phagocytic cells of the liver with release of free Amph B into the circulation [181, 198]. As with the free Amph B, not every detail of the mode of action of liposomal or lipid Amph B is understood, but some aspects of the interactions became clear from the intensive study of L-Amph B. Amph B is anchored in the liposome so that no dissociation of free Amph B from the liposome takes place in aqueous medium.

4.3.2.2 Plasma pharmacokinetic

L-Amph B remains intact in circulation for a long period of time [198], whereas lipid-based formulations are more rapidly cleared from the circulations. Especially ABLC is rapidly taken up by the reticuloendothelial system and is concentrated in liver, spleen, and other organs of the body [180]. Total systemic exposure expressed as area under the curve for plasma levels is significantly larger for L-Amph B than for ABCD or ABLC [181]. All lipid formulations accumulate in tissue with significantly higher levels than in the plasma [181].

4.3.2.3 Safety and toxicity

All three marketed new formulations of Amph B have a better safety profile than the conventional Amph B (Fungizone®) [159, 181–183, 199–201].

Ambisome, L-Amph B: The safety of L-Amph B has been studied in patients with AIDS, hematological malignancy (bone marrow transplants), and those receiving liver or heart/lung transplants [2, 180–183, 199]. The tolerability profile of Lipo-Amph B in adults and children is superior to that of conventional Amph B: both the infusion-related toxicity and the nephrotoxic side effects are significantly reduced. Rapid administration of a high daily dose of L-Amph B is feasible without the well-known acute adverse effects of traditional Amph B, e.g., fever was observed in only 14% of patients treated with L-Amph B vs. 43% of patients treated with Amph B; chills and rigors were reduced from 56% to 20% [181]. Furthermore, the use of premedications necessary to reduce the infusion-related toxicity of Amph B can be significantly lowered [181]. The influence on renal function is also significantly reduced: in an European study, no change in serum creatinin levels was seen in 99 of 121 (81%) patients. However, 11 (15%) episodes were associated with increased creatinin concentrations, evenly distributed among various cumulative doses of L-Amph B. It should be stressed, however, that in 17 (34%) of the patients, the initially high creatinin level was reduced to normal during L-Amph B therapy. A multi-center study in the U.S. demonstrated that nephrotoxicity, defined as a 100% or more increase in baseline serum creatinin, was significantly more prevalent with a 24% incidence under Amph B regimen compared with 10% for 1 mg/kg L-Amph B and 12% for 3 mg/kg L-Amph B. The same degree of reduced toxicity regarding nephrotoxicity (19% vs. 34%), fever (17% vs. 44%), and chills/rigors (18% vs. 54%) was seen in a randomized study with 687 neutropenic patients; however, the hepatoxicity was similar in both groups, namely, 18 vs. 20% [202]. The safety of L-Amph B also has been evaluated in 187 transplant patients who were concomitantly treated with cyclosporin [203].The major problem using Amph B in these patients is the synergistic nephrotoxic effect between Amph B and cyclosporin. Dramatic increases in serum creatinin have been seen in transplant patients treated with Amph B plus cyclosporin. Furthermore, Amph B as well as L-Amph B cause a substantial increase of the cyclosporin level in blood. When conventional Amph B was replaced with Lipo-Amph B in transplant patients, an improvement in renal function was observed. Lipo-Amph B was also successfully used in a case of Amph B-induced nephrogenic diabetes insipidus [204]. Chest discomfort mimicking myocardial infarction or pulmonary embolism while receiving Lipo- Amph B has been observed in some patients [205].

Amph B in colloidal dispersion (ABCD): The adverse event profile is the same as for conventional Amph B, but the incidence differs [206]. ABCD was safely applied in doses up to 7.5 mg/kg/day over 6 weeks to bone marrow transplant patients without any renal toxicity. No nephrotoxicity was observed; 32% of the patients tolerated the drug extremely well. Acute adverse events (chills/rigors or fever) with a scoring of 2 occurred in 52% of the patients, with a scoring of 3 in 5% [207]. The adverse event profile of ABCD is mainly based on the experience of 572 patients with systemic fungal infections treated with mean doses of 3–6 mg/kg/day for 1–409 days [200]. No chronic renal toxicity was observed, but in >5% of the patients, adverse events such as chills (50%), fever (33%), increased creatinin level (12%), tachycardia (10%), hypotension (10%), nausea (8%), etc. were observed. Generally, ABCD shows less nephrotoxicity than conventional Amph B; however, the infusion-related side effects are relatively frequent, i.e., in the same order as for Amph B; therefore ,ABCD is not suitable for prophylaxis and has still to find its niche [183].

Abelect®; ABLC: Generally, ABLC as the other lipid formulations is safer than traditional Amph B [159,180, 208, 209]. Minimal or no renal and hepatic toxicity was observed in the various phase clinical studies conducted in adults and children with fungal infections [209]. The drug also can be safely administered to bone marrow transplant patients [208]. Infusion-related side effects, mainly fever, were seen in 29% of the treated cases. The requirement for dialysis – necessary due to renal toxicity of Amph B therapy – is known to be associated with a reduced survival of patients with aspergillosis. ABLC significantly reduces the need for dialysis and therefore leads to an increased survival of patients with aspergillosis [209]. Interestingly, the cause of infusion-related toxicity of ABLC seems not to be the same as that of traditional Amph B: a patient showed severe and life-threatening reactions associated with the first infusion of ABLC, despite previous uneventful treatment with traditional Amph B. After switching back to normal Amph B, no undesirable effects were seen and the patient was discharged one week later [210].

In summary, all three marketed formulations have the advantage of a better safety profile over conventional Amph B; this is a major step forward in the battle against fungal diseases.

4.3.2.4 Efficacy

All three lipid formulations are FDA approved for second-line therapy of fungal diseases, i.e., for patients who did not respond to conventional antifungal therapy, who showed severe side effects to Amph B, or who suffered from renal impairment. L-Amph B also has approval for empirical therapy and can reasonably be considered for prophylaxis because toxicity is reduced in all measured parameters [180–183, 206].

The efficacy of L-Amph B is meanwhile clinically broadly established. During phase II/III studies, European and American investigators have had extensive experience with the use of Lipo-Amph B in immunocompromised patients with probable and proven fungal infections, in both adults and children [180, 183, 210]. The most common fungal pathogens isolated were *Candida* and *Aspergillus* species. Patients with underlying hematological malignancies or AIDS and bone marrow and solid organ transplant recipients were the most commonly treated. Several patients with documented invasive fungal infections who had previously failed treatment with Amph B recovered from the disease under L-Amph B therapy. L-Amph B is also safe and highly efficacious in children [180, 211, 212]. Ten years ago Schneeman [213] summarized the early clinical experience with L-Amph B as follows: L-Amph B was curative in 37 of 52 (71%) candidosis cases, in 12 of 35 (34%) aspergillosis cases, and in 7 of 8 (88%) cryptococcosis cases. The EORTC antifungal group studied two different doses of L-Amph B infusions (1 or 4 mg/kg/day) in the treatment of invasive aspergillosis in 87 neutropenic patients. The outcome of the trial showed no advantages for the higher, more expensive dose; the mortality due to fungal infection in both groups was ca. 20%. However, in a subgroup evaluation – patients with proven mycosis – L-Amph B showed clearly better efficacy than the traditional Amph B: 58% clinical response in the L-Amph B group vs. 37% in the Amph B group and 8% vs. 37% death [183, 214]. In an other study [183, 215] L-Amph B generally compared favorably with conventional Amph B in the treatment of documented or suspected neutropenia-associated invasive fungal infections: more patients (64% vs. 16%) achieved a cure with L-Amph B, and L-Amph B was associated with a lower incidence of nephrotoxicity. L-Amph B seems to lead to a faster sterilization of the spinal fluid in patients with cryptococcal meningitis (7–14 days vs. >21 days). A fast sterilization of blood culture has also been seen in patients with histoplasmosis. In a comparative study between L-Amph B and Itra therapy for histoplasmosis, the cure rates at week 2 were identical under both regimens, but the blood culture became sterile faster under L-Amph B therapy. In the future the following treatment schedule may be used: a short treatment with L-Amph B followed by oral Itra.

Several successful treatments with L-Amph B for rare infections are known. Rhinocerebral zygomycosis, pulmonary zygomycosis [182], and disseminated mucormycosis in a child with leukemia responded well to the therapy; in the latter case, antifungal therapy was combined with surgery [216]. A case of neonatal trichosporosis [217] and a case of Madura feet were cured [2]. In Leeds [218] L-Amph B was used in children with fungal infections at home. Additionally, L-Amph B received approval from the FDA for treatment of visceral leishmaniasis [182, 219].

In the last few years, L-Amph B has found its place in antifungal therapy and has achieved remarkable response rates with minimal side effects [220]. The only prohibition for a broader use of L-Amph is its substantially higher cost. Pharmacoeconomic studies are contradictory: in a Swedish and Dutch study, the use of L-Amph B was clearly associated with extra costs [182], whereas another study showed no great cost difference between a 3 mg/kg L-Amph B therapy and a 1 mg/kg Amph B therapy, because of the reduced requirement for expensive salvage treatment under L-Amph B [183].

Clinical trials with ABCD for established infections are still relatively rare [206]. In a phase I study [221], ABCD proved to be efficacious in patients with invasive fungal infections after bone marrow transplantation. The complete or partial response across dose levels and infections types was 52%. For fungemia, the curative rate was 55% and for pneumonia, 37%. ABCD treatment afforded better responses, lower mortality, and less renal insufficiency than did conventional Amph B among 343 patients with invasive aspergillosis of the lung. The response rate (complete + partial) was 48.8% in patients treated with ABCD *versus* 23.4% inpatients receiving Amph B [222]. Based on this positive data, ABCD received FDA approval for second-line treatment of invasive aspergillosis. ABCD was also efficacious in infections caused by *Can-*

dida; disseminated candidosis responded less (14%) to the drug than did *Candida* sepsis (66%) Furthermore, ABCD was effective in 73% of the patients infected with *C. albicans* or *C. parapsilosis* but in only 46% of those infected with other *Candida* species [223]. ABCD could also be an alternative treatment for Zygomycosis [224, 225], whereas the degree of activity in paracoccidioidomycosiss is questionable [226]. ABCD was efficacious in animal models of leishmaniasis [206]. Since ABCD is clearly less well tolerated than L-Amph B or ABLC [159, 183], its place in the clinical world is not yet clearly defined.

The beneficial effect of ABLC for invasive fungal infections has been studied in hundreds of patients with various underlying diseases (cancer, bone marrow transplantation, AIDS, hematological malignancy) according a well-defined "emergency use" protocol [167, 180, 183, 227]. Unpublished results of these studies in 228 patients suggest clinical cure rates of 78% for candidosis and 60% for aspergillosis [167]; some of the open-labeled studies are published. For example, in cancer patients ABLC was effective in 75% of the cases [228]. ABLC was also highly effective in the treatment of cryptococcal meningitis [229]. ABLC was successfully used for a case of rhinocerebral mucormycosis [230] and fusariosis [231]; it showed a beneficial effect in disseminated coccidioidomycosis [232] and recurrent blastomycosis [233]. It cured an infection caused by *Apophysomyces elegans* [159], and an intraabdominal abscess due to *Candida norvegiensis* associated with a Gore-Tex mesh infection responded well to treatment with ABLC [234]. However, failures are also reported: a case of *Candida* endophthalmitis worsened under ABLC [235].

Unfortunately, only a few prospective comparative trials are available and published. The first comparative clinical efficacy results with ABLC were not highly impressive; ABLC was not more efficacious than modest doses of conventional Amph B [236]. Newer data, however, show equal or sometimes even better cure rates under ABLC treatment than with Amph B for aspergillosis and candidosis. Equal efficacy was seen in a study of 153 patients with invasive candidosis; 68% of the patients responded to ABLC and Amph B treatment, ABLC being significantly safer than Amph B [180]. Results of a comparative trial for cryptococcal meningitis in AIDS patients also showed equal activity [180].

Trials comparing the three liposomal formulations are extremely rare. An open-labeled trial evaluated the efficacy of L-Amph B on patients who were refractory to or intolerant of ABCD or ABLC. Most of the 27 patients enrolled had ABLC as primary therapy. Success was seen in 21 patients, improvement in 22, and failure in 14; according to the fungal infections, the outcome was satisfactory in 68% of the aspergillosis cases, in 80% of the candidosis and cryptococcosis infections, and in 100% (2 cases) of mucormycosis [181]. In another study with bone marrow transplant patients, L-Amph B was directly compared with ABLC: both formulations were equally efficacious (71% L-Amph B vs. 78% ABLC). However, ABLC showed significantly more infusion-related side effects [237]. A serious infusion-dependent adverse event, rigor, has been seen after unrecognized substitution of ABLC by ABCD in a patient who tolerated ABLC over several days. Once ABCD was switched back to ABLC, the infusions were again well tolerated [238]. Recently, a multi-center database was queried to identify patients who failed under treatment with L-Amph B prior to treatment with ABLC. Twenty-five patients have been identified, 10 under empiric treatment and 15 with various laboratory-confirmed fungal infections. ABLC was beneficial in all cases of aspergillosis, cryptococcosis, or candidosis; however, the drug was unsuccessful for histoplasmosis, zygomycosis, and a case of a mixed infection with *Candida* and *Aspergillus* [239].

In conclusion, the use of all three new formulations of Amph B results in an overall improvement of the therapeutic index. This step forward is of the greatest importance for all patients with fungal infections of known or new pathogens. The possibility of reducing the toxic side effects of Amph B has given new life to the old standard, which still has the broadest antifungal spectrum. Whether one or more of the three formulations will ever totally replace conventional Amph B is dependent not only on the proven clinical efficacy but also on pharmacoeconomic considerations. All three formulations are significantly more expensive than conventional Amph B: a European pharmacoeconomic evaluation of Itra, Amph B, and L-Amph B showed that the acquisition cost of L-Amph B was too high in proportion to its benefits [240].

4.3.3 Flucytosine

Flucytosine (5-fluorocytosine, 5FC), a mock pyrimidine, is the only antifungal drug that acts as true antimetabolite. Its antifungal spectrum is limited to species of *Candida, Cryptococcus,* which are highly sensitive (MIC 0.1–2 μg/ml), and *Aspergillus* and *Dematiaceae,* which are only moderately sensitive (MIC 1–25 μg/ml). 5FC shows fungistatic and fungicidal activity against yeasts and *Dematiaceae* but is only fungistatic against aspergilli [2].

4.3.3.1 Mode of action

Exposure of sensitive fungi to 5FC almost immediately induces inhibition of the synthesis of DNA and RNA. In yeasts and dematiaceous fungi, cell growth continues with carbohydrate and protein overproduction; this unbalanced growth is defined as thymineless death. In aspergilli the inhibition of nucleic acid synthesis causes immediate inhibition of growth, and the lack of overproduction of protein and carbohydrates is probably the reason that 5FC is not fungicidal to this species [241].

The metabolic pathway of 5FC has been carefully studied by using various mutants resistant to the drug. 5FC is taken up actively by cytosine permease, which is normally responsible for the uptake of adenine, guanine, hypoxanthine, and cytosine [241, 242]. Inside the cell 5FC is immediately deaminated to 5 fluorouracil (5FU), which is the active principle responsible for killing the fungal cell. This step is essential for the antifungal activity of 5FC, since fungi lacking the cytosine deaminase are resistant to the drug. The low toxicity of 5FC in humans is due to the absence of cytosine deaminase in mammalian cells [243]. Normal enteric bacteria, however, are capable of deaminating 5FC [244]; the resulting 5FU is fortunately poorly absorbed from the colon.

5FU acts along two different pathways. It is converted by uridine monophosphate pyrophosphorylase into 5FUMP, which is finally incorporated into the RNA (a step that is antagonized by uridine). Simultaneously, it is converted to 5-fluorodeoxyuridine monophosphate, a potent inhibitor of thymidylate synthetase; this step leads to the inhibition of DNA synthesis. 5FU itself cannot be used as antifungal therapy, since its uptake by most of the fungal cells is poor, and its toxicity for mammalian cells forbids systemic use of the high dose necessary to kill the fungal cell. The details of the modes of action of 5FC were reviewed in 1990 [220, 241].

What is remarkable about the action of 5FC is that the fungal cell itself produces the fungicidal principle from the inert compound by internal metabolization causing its own death, a situation unique in medical mycology. However, the length of the metabolic pathway and the several different enzymes involved are also the reason for the frequent appearance of 5FC-resistant mutants.

4.3.3.2 Resistance

Primary and acquired resistance to 5FC may result from absence, dysfunction, or deletion of one or more enzymes not essential to fungal survival. In every normally sensitive population of fungi, there is a minority that is resistant to 5FC. The absolute number of primary resistant cells is species dependent; the lowest resistance frequency is seen in *Candida albicans* (2.7×10^{-7}), and the highest, in aspergilli (3.5×10^{-5}). A highly significant correlation also has been found between the incidence of primary resistance to 5FC and the serotype of *C. albicans*, the incidence being significantly greater in *C. albicans* of serotype B [1, 245, 246]. During lengthy monotherapy with 5FC, the proportion of resistant cells can so increase that the population as a whole becomes resistant [245]. Because there is a clear correlation between therapy failure and the appearance of secondary (acquired) resistance, 5FC monotherapy is no longer used in long-term chemotherapy but is always used in combination with another antifungal (see Section 4.3.7).

Most mutants isolated (clinically or in the laboratory) lack uridine monophosphate pyrophosphorylase. However, resistance also may be due to changed cytosine permease or deaminase or to an overproduction of pyrimidine. A clear segregation between highly resistant and partially resistant mutants has been observed [247] in experiments showing that *C. albicans* is a diploid organism. It was clearly demonstrated that the mutation in partially resistant strains is located on only one allele, whereas totally resistant strains have the mutation on both alleles.

It is not clearly proven whether the appearance of 5FC resistance does or does not influence the virulence of the strains. The degree of virulence may be dependent on the enzyme altered. Dysfunction of the cytosine deaminase and uridine transport seem to induce loss of virulence [248]; however, the uridine monophosphate pyrophosphorylase dysfunction seems to have a minor effect on virulence [249]. The loss of virulence is at any rate less pronounced than that seen with Amph B- or azole-resistant isolates.

4.3.3.3 Safety and tolerance

The actual clinical relevance of 5FC is controversial. Some clinicians emphasize it and speak of it as if it were a major problem. Others have a different opinion, stating clearly that adverse affects are uncommon and are rarely severe or irreversible.

It was assumed that the toxicity of 5FC is related in some way to the internal production of 5FU; yet no direct correlation was ever found to the 5FU levels measured in serum. The frequency of adverse events is, however, directly correlated with 5FC concentrations above 100 μg/ml for a sustained time period [2, 3, 250]. This correlation has been observed in all patients suffering from side effects during controlled studies with combination therapy [251, 252]. Most important, since 5FC is entirely excreted by the kidneys, even a minor impairment in renal function (e.g., by combination with the Nephrotoxic drug Amph B) leads to elevated 5FC levels. Thus, it is important to monitor 5FC levels and adapt the dose to actual kidney function. This reduces the toxic effects of 5FC to acceptable levels [253].

Anorexia, nausea, vomiting, diarrhea, and/or abdominal pain occur in 6% of treated patients. Hepatic disturbance (liver enzyme elevation) may occur with or without hepatomegaly in about 5% of patients. Of greater concern is the potential for bone marrow depression (seen in 5% of cases, all with elevated 5FC levels), which is not always reversible, especially if not recognized early enough. This aspect of 5FC toxicity is often overplayed, and more careful monitoring would decrease fears. A. Vernes [253a] and colleagues have investigated the efficacy and accuracy of an early derived relationship between thrombocyte nadir and mean creatinin clearance and have found a possibility to predict 5FC-related thrombocytopenia.

5FC was temporarily abandoned after a warning that it may cause myelotoxicity in AIDS patients. However, a retrospective analysis of the clinical outcome of cryptococcal meningitis suggested that 5FC is tolerated in AIDS patients at least as well as in cancer patients [253]. As with Amph B, exact evaluation of toxicity is complicated by the fact that patients are invariably suffering from an underlying disease that disturbs metabolic function and that all patients are treated concomitantly with other potentially toxic drugs [2, 3].

4.3.3.4 Efficacy

Despite its narrow spectrum and resistance problems, 5FC remains a useful agent for the treatment of opportunistic fungal infections in combination with Amph B or another antifungal. It has found its place as an ideal combination partner in the battle against opportunistic fungal infections in highly immunosuppressed patients (see Section 4.3.7).

4.3.4 Old imidazole derivatives: miconazole and ketoconazole

Intravenous miconazole was the first imidazole derivative used for the treatment of invasive fungal infections. It was soon followed by oral Keto. Both drugs have shown activity and opened up a new era of research, as well as human chemotherapy. They are, however, losing their pioneer role and have been or are going to be replaced soon by more specific, less toxic, and more efficacious triazoles for all fungal infections in immunosuppressed patients.

4.3.4.1 Mode of action

The imidazoles and triazoles appear to operate *via* a common mechanism of action. They disturb the function of the cell membrane by interfering with cytochrome P450-dependent lanosterol C_{14} demethylase, leading to depletion of ergosterol and accumulation of lanosterol in the membrane. At the molecular level, one of the nitrogen atoms of the azole ring binds to the heme moiety of cytochrome P450. Only compounds with higher specific binding to the fungal cytochrome than to the human one can be used as antifungal drugs. Compared with the imidazoles, the triazoles have a much higher affinity for the fungal cytochrome than for the human cytochrome P450 enzyme steps [3].

The fungistatic activity of all azoles is related to inhibition of lanosterol C_{14} demethylase, leading to depletion of ergosterol. Ergosterol has two fundamental functions in the fungal cell membrane: it is the major bulk material, giving the membrane its essential structure, and it has an important regulatory function [162]. The depletion of ergosterol alters fluidity, thereby reducing the activity of membrane-bound enzymes (e.g., chitin synthetase, lipid metabolism, and oxidative steps) and initiating increased permeability. Depletion of ergosterol also reduces cell membrane sites for the interaction of polyene antifungal agents, leading to antagonism with Amph B (see Section 3.7).

In addition to the main interaction with the P450 cytochrome, azoles may inhibit cytochrome C oxydase and peroxidative enzymes; they also may interact with phospholipids and inhibit the transformation of yeast to mycelial growth. The fact that miconazole and Itra are fungicidal is thought to be the result of a direct interaction with the membrane, leading to the loss of cytoplasmic constituents [162, 254]. The mode of action of azoles has been intensively studied; a detailed review of all the accumulated knowledge is beyond the scope of this paper (for more information, see [162, 254, 255]).

4.3.4.2 Miconazole

Over a long period of time, miconazole has retained its niche indication of treating the invasive infections caused by *Pseudoallescheria boydii.*

4.3.4.3 Ketoconazole

Neither primary nor secondary resistance was a great problem with Keto. However, the necessity of using a high dose of Keto for various indications has led to crucial toxic problems. Nausea and vomiting are the most frequent adverse reactions; they increase in severity with increased doses. Endocrinopathies – manifested in males as gynecomastia and in females as irregular menses – were seen. Hepatotoxicity is rare, usually reversible, but some lethal cases have been observed [3, 256, 257]. These adverse reactions have been limited ever since the broad use of oral Keto in dermatology, especially onychomycosis.

A number of meaningful interactions between Keto and other drugs are known, and new ones are continually observed. Most interactions occur by means of one of two basic mechanisms:

- inhibition of absorption of the azole leading to lower bioavailability; or
- interference with the activity of hepatic microsomal enzymes, which alters the metabolism and the plasma levels of the azole, the interacting drug, or both.

Keto significantly prolongs the elimination half-life of cyclosporin A by inhibition of cytochrome P450 enzymes. It also increases the levels of warfarin, digoxin, terfenadine, astemizole, phenytoine, indinavir, ritonavir, and tolbutamide, leading to unwanted toxic effects of the concomitant drug. Absorption of Keto is influenced by H2-receptor-antagonists and sucralfate. The serum levels of Keto are significantly decreased with concomitant administration of rifampicin and isoniazid. Tirilazad mesylate levels are significantly increased in the presence of Keto [3, 31, 258].

Keto was and still is highly useful in chronic mucocutaneous candidosis. However, Keto should be used only for deep fungal infections in non-immunosuppressed patients. Keto has shown its beneficial value in endemic fungal infections such as paracoccidioidomycosiss, blastomycosis, and histoplasmosis, provided the patients were not immunosuppressed. Amph B remains the standard treatment for all these infections in patients with decreased host defenses. All meningeal infections are excluded due to the poor penetration of Keto into the cerebrospinal fluid. Keto is inactive against aspergillosis and should therefore not be used for prophylaxis in hospitals with a great risk of *Aspergillus* infection. Keto is also not recommended for empirical antifungal therapy for suspected candidosis, since Amph B proved to be more efficacious in a randomized trial [256, 259].

4.3.5 Fluconazole

Flu has some properties that are unique among azoles. It is highly soluble in water or saline; it shows a high bioavailability and is distributed in all body fluids; and especially high concentrations are reached in the stratum corneum and in the urine. No CNS or ocular barrier exists, and it is scarcely metabolized and is primarily excreted by the kidneys as unchanged mother drug.

Flu is active *in vitro* against dermatophytes, true pathogenic fungi, and opportunistic fungi: *Cryptococcus neoformans* and *Candida* spp. belong to the most sensitive species, while aspergilli are resistant. The species cluster *C. albicans, C. tropicalis,* and *C. parapsilosis* has distinctly higher susceptibility than *C. krusei* or *C. glabrata; Aspergillus* spp. are resistant to the drug. The significance of sensitivity testing was disputed in the past, since no proper correlation could be observed between *in vitro* and *in vivo* data. Generally, all fungal species tested showed a higher sensitivity in animal models or in the clinic than *in vitro.* Most fungi showed high MICs when tested in conventional standard media. However, recent advances in standardization of susceptibility testing of *Candida* spp. [260] have improved the reproducibility of these tests, which now show low MICs and lead to a better correlation with animal data or with the actual clinical response [256, 257, 261, 261a] (for details, see the chapter by Seibold and Tintelnot).

4.3.5.1 Resistance

Until the late 1980s, the development of clinically important resistance to azoles was rare. However, during the last few years treatment failures due to appearance of resistant isolates have increasingly been reported, especially in AIDS patients who were receiving intermittent or continuous Flu therapy for oropharyngeal candidosis [257, 262, 263]. Various risk factors predisposing resistance to azoles, particularly to Flu, have been observed and studied in clinical trials: they are HIV infection, advanced stage of immunosuppression (low number of CD4 T-cells), recurrent oral candidosis, prior azole use, previous tuberculosis, and treatment with antituberculous drugs [262–266, 266a].

Therapeutic failure of antifungal therapy is based either on microbiological resistance due to the fungus or on clinical resistance due to host factors. Clinical resistance may be seen in extremely immunosuppressed patients who fail to respond to therapy despite high susceptibility of the fungus and adequate concentrations of the drug or in patients with unfavorable drug interactions. Microbiological resistance is based on two mechanisms: the originally sensitive fungus has become resistant, or a new agent has appeared with a lower susceptibility to the drug. In this section only the appearance of microbiological resistance is discussed.

Microbiological resistance of *Candida* to Flu has been appearing surprisingly fast in AIDS patients with recurrent oropharyngeal candidosis. In France an increase in MICs combined with the first clinical failures have been observed only 4 years after the first clinical trials with Flu. Before 1987 all *C. albicans* strains isolated from AIDS patients were highly sensitive; however, in the period of 1990–1991 roughly 40% of the isolated strains showed an MIC >12.5 µg/ml [262]. Gradual increases in MIC values, together with therapeutic unresponsiveness, also have been observed in other parts of the world after intermittent or continuous use of Flu for oral candidosis in AIDS patients [263, 267–269]. Oropharyngeal candidosis also may be caused by a mixed population of sensitive and resistant yeasts, and under Flu therapy the resistant species may become dominant [263, 268, 270]. An AIDS patient suffering simultaneously from oral candidosis and from *Candida* meningitis was found to harbor two different but resistant strains of *C. albicans*; one strain caused the oral and the other caused the disseminated disease [271]. Transmission of strains between HIV-positive partners can occur [268, 272], but it remains unclear whether azole-resistant strains of *C. albicans* can persist if transmitted to HIV-negative persons.

Not only *C. albicans* strains but also other yeasts may become resistant to Flu. For example, three cases of resistant *Cryptococcus* strains have been diagnosed under prolonged maintenance therapy with Flu [268]. The problem is so important that researchers have studied the dynamic and heterogeneous mutations to Flu resistance in *Cr. neoformans* [273].

It seems that acquisition of resistance to Flu caused a major problem in AIDS patients with relapsing oral candidosis and less so in other immunosuppressed patients who received Flu therapy for a short term. Only a few reports describe the appearance of resistance to Flu in HIV-negative patients [267, 273, 274], but they are of great concern. Breakthrough candidemia during antifungal prophylaxis or therapy with Flu or Amph B was caused mainly by non-*Candida albicans* species; prior Flu therapy was associated with the appearance of *C. krusei* and *C. parapsilosis*, while prior Amph B therapy was associated with *C. glabrata* [264]. Especially *C. krusei* and also *C. parapsilosis* show an intrinsic resistance to Flu. Of great concern is the fact that primary Flu-resistant *C. albicans* strains could be isolated from non-HIV-infected patients who were never before exposed to Flu [274].

The pattern of strains causing invasive infections is changing since the introduction of Flu. A. Kunova and colleagues [275] claimed that use of Flu is not associated with a higher incidence of *C. krusei* or other non-*C. albicans* species. M.F. Price and collaborators [276], however, studied the distribution of species isolated from blood over a 5-year period and found a clear change in the pattern: the susceptibility to Flu remained the same, but the number of *C. albicans* decreased, whereas *C. glabrata*, *C. tropicalis*, and *C. parapsilosis* increased. The emergence of new, non-*C. albicans* strains in patients with candidemia also was observed by other authors [264, 264a]. In some hospitals, however, the fraction of *C. albicans* has recovered during the last 3 years and has reached – after a decline over at least 5 years – the pre-fluconazole level [264b].

The mechanism of resistance to Flu is intensively studied by biochemists and geneticists. Three major mechanisms of resistance have been identified in various pathogenic fungi (*Candida* spp., *Cryptococcus*, *Histoplasma*): decreased binding affinity to the P450 cytochrome [277–280], increased production of the target cytochrome [281]; and, most important, decreased accumulation of Flu in the fungal cell due to reduced uptake or increased efflux [262, 265, 281–284]. Other mechanisms of action have been identified. Up-regulation of Erg genes can be the cause for resistance to Flu [285]; resistant mutants of *C. glabrata* had a respiratory deficiency caused by mitochondrial DNA deletions [286].

The molecular mechanism of the efflux mechanism is intensively studied by geneticists especially in *C. albicans*; they found several molecular mechanisms including increased m-RNA levels for two types of efflux pump genes: the ATP binding cassette transporter CDRs and the major facilitator MDR1 [287–291].

The presence and absence of cross-resistance between azoles may be explained on the basis of the different mechanism causing resistance. Fungal isolates have been observed with a 10-fold increase of MIC for both Flu and Itra; other isolated strains were found to be resistant to Flu but remained more or less sensitive to Itra. This phenomenon may be related to the hydrosolubility or liposolubility of the two drugs or to the underlying mechanism of resistance (affinity to the enzyme, transport) [267, 292–294]. Oral candidosis in AIDS patients, with a strain resistant to Flu, was often curable under Itra therapy. Recurrent candidosis due to Flu-resistant *C. albicans* was cured by initiation of the new aggressive triple therapy for HIV infection combined with switching to Itra therapy [295].

Sensitivity to Flu seems to be correlated with adherence capacity. Flu-resistant *C. albicans* showed slightly less adherence to buccal epithelial cells than did sensitive ones. Similar findings have been observed with 5FC-mutants [249]. It may be that Flu-resistant fungal cells are less virulent. This would explain why the rapid appearance of resistance to Flu is seen only in severely immunosuppressed AIDS patients and not so often in more immunocompetent cancer patients and why transmission of resistant strains to HIV-negative persons has not yet been described. In contrast to these above-mentioned observations stands the following finding: a laboratory mutant of *Candida albicans* with a high resistance to Flu (MIC >80 μg/ml) was superior to the original strain in all the virulence traits (germination, adherence, secretion of proteinases, mouse model) tested [296]. In this case the development of resistance was associated with significant changes in morphology and physiology. Whether these changes also occur in patients and not only under artificial conditions is not yet proven. The clinical experience supports the hypothesis that resistant mutants are normally less virulent than the wild type.

4.3.5.2 Safety and tolerance

Flu is generally better tolerated than Keto. Nausea, vomiting, rash, and asymptomatic elevations of plasma aminotransferases occur in less than 5% of the patients [3, 24a, 256, 257]. The drug is also safe for children [297] and newborns [298]. High doses of Flu are also well tolerated; one patient was treated over 86 months with a total of 1997 g of Flu without any safety problems [299]. The adverse effects on levels in the liver and the endocrine system are significantly lower and less severe than with Keto; hepatoxicity [300] is rare, and inhibition of the steroid genesis has not yet been detected. However, Flu has been reported to worsen liver function in the case of antecedent hepatitis [301] and in a patient with severe impairment of the kidney induced acute hepatic necrosis [259].The risk of hepatotoxicity is also reported to increase in HIV-positive patients or alcoholism [302].

A short course of Flu during the first trimester of pregnancy (mainly for vaginal candidosis) seems not to increase the risk of congenital disorders in infants [303, 304]. In another prospective study [305], no increase in miscarriages, congenital abnormalities, or low birth weights was seen; however, an increased number of abortions (12.6% vs. 2%) were documented. Prolonged treatment with Flu for coccidioidomycosis induced congenital abnormalities in triplets; only one survived [306]. Similar abnormalities were seen in another newborn. The abnormalities in all four infants share some characteristics with the Antley-Bixler syndrome. Flu apparently has a teratogenic potential leading to specific malformations when applied after the first trimester and over a longer period of time [307].

4.3.5.3 Drug interactions

Possible drug interactions in the presence of azoles are intensively studied. Flu shows a significantly lower potential for interactions than Keto and Itra; however, a number of interactions with Flu are known [31, 32, 256, 257]. H.I. Katz [32] wrote an excellent review on drug interactions and alerts the physician to be aware of the potential for interaction of all azoles and to read carefully the individual package insert or to perform a careful monitoring. Flu has a dose-dependent ability to inhibit human P450 enzymes, especially CYP3A4 and CYP2C9; therefore, concomitant use of substrate drugs (e.g., nifepidine, digoxin, felopidine, simvastatin) should be avoided. Additionally, all substrates with low bioavailability (such as HMG-CoA reductase inhibitors) and those with extensive first-pass metabolism (astemizole ansd cisapride) and/or a narrow therapeutic window (warfarin, digoxin, phenytoin and sulphonylureas) also should be avoided. Co-administration of rifampicin or cimetidine reduces plasma levels of Flu [32, 308]. Hydrochlorthiazide, however, increases the plasma level of Flu by 40% [31.] Flu causes a rise of plasma levels of various drugs, increasing their activity or toxicity (phenytoin [309], theophyllin, alfentanil [310], nifedipine [311], amitriplin, midazolam, digoxin, diazepam, triazolam and terfenadine, zolpidem, cyclosporin, tolbutamide, and some sulfonylureas) [31, 32]. Under Flu therapy, the protrombin time of warfarin is increased by 12%; Flu significantly reduces the metabolism of losartan and therefore negatively influences the bioavailability of E3174 [312]. A combination of cisapride and astemiozole with azoles is contraindicated. Flu may also reduce the activity of some contraceptives by interfering with the hormonal status of the patients. Concomitant use of other nephrotoxic drugs should be avoided, since Flu is eliminated by the kidney and needs a functional renal system. At any rate, the dose has to be adopted to the renal function to avoid Flu toxicity [259]. Fortunately, there is no interaction with H2 receptor antagonists and the antiviral drugs indinavir [313] and delavirdine [314].

4.3.5.4 Therapeutic indications in opportunistic mycoses

Candidosis: Oropharyngeal candidosis was the most frequent complication of HIV infections, affecting 80–90% of the patients at some point during the disease. With the aggressive triple combination of antiviral therapy and the wide use of prophylactic Flu, the incidence of this disorder is slowly decreasing. Symptomatic esophageal candidosis becomes common as CD4 count drops below 100/ml [262, 263]. During recent years, the relatively good safety of azoles has led to their widespread use as a first-line treatment for this indication. Flu at doses of 50–100 mg/day has become the first choice, since it has proven to be superior to Keto [173, 256, 315]. Oral Flu administered for 7–21 days cured 71% and improved 16% of 103 HIV-infected patients with oral candidosis [316]. Even short-term Flu treatment for 5 days showed favorable clinical success in 85% of candidosis episodes [267]. Flu also proved its beneficial effect in esophageal candidosis; the long-term efficacy has been proven in 1105 AIDS patients, Flu being curative in more than 80% of the cases 2 weeks after the treatment started. At months 6 and 12, endoscopic and clinical cure were observed in 97% of patients [317]. High clinical response with Flu was also reported in cancer patients with esophagitis. The efficacy of Flu appears to be equivalent to that of Amph B but with the advantage of fewer side effects and better compliance [318–320].

It may be argued whether prevention (suppressive) therapy for symptomatic recurrence of thrush is advisable. In 1994 [321], a study showed that the probability of recurrent oral candidosis was significantly reduced in patients continuing long-term therapy with Keto or Flu. Some authors even claim that empirical Flu treatment would be a more cost-effective strategy than one starting treatment only after confirmation of the disease [322]. Both continuous and intermittent therapies with Flu showed excellent responses, reducing relapses and colonizations significantly; the continuous schedule is slightly better than the intermittent (relapses: 0 vs. 4.1 episodes per year; sterile cultures 38% vs. 11%). Resistance occurred under both regimens [323]. Other clinicians [324] controlled the intermittent therapy by a non-endoscopic procedure and found that a 2-week dose regimen is insufficient for maintaining systemic sclerosis patients free of *Candida*. These authors had no problems with appearance of resistance.

The introduction of aggressive antiviral treatment with a combination of protease inhibitors changed the epidemiology of oral candidosis. The incidence of recurrent oral candidosis in AIDS patients treated with HAART is significantly reduced; therefore, suppressive therapy for thrush can be discontinued. The rare appearance of recurrent thrush under HAART responds well to reinstatement of a short therapy with Flu [325]. However, it should be mentioned that HAART antiviral therapy has little impact on thrush recurrence unless it is accompanied by both viral load suppression and a sustained rise in CD4 cell counts [326].

The appearance of clinical resistance combined with decreased *in vitro* susceptibility in AIDS patients with oral candidosis forced the clinician to use new treatment strategies. In most cases Flu resistant oral candidosis responded either to high doses of Flu or was cured under therapy with Itra [327–329]. Additionally, a new oral formulation of Amph B exists that could be used for highly Flu-resistant infections of the oral cavity [262]. The suspension, a new formulation of Flu, has the advantage of producing higher levels in saliva, achieving better local efficacy for oral candidosis than the tablets. The oral suspension of Flu showed equal activity and tolerance to oral Amph B, and a prospective study showed that the clinical response to the suspension was substantially more rapid than under the conventional tablets and the degree of activity [330–332]. Flu is also available as suppositories and in this form is well tolerated and efficacious for the treatment of oral candidosis [333].

Thanks to better tolerance and good efficacy, Flu has replaced Amph B in its position as first choice for the treatment of candidemia due to *C. albicans* in patients without neutropenia [334–336]. Similar efficacy of Flu compared with Amph B was also reported for hematogenous candidosis in cancer patients, surgical patients, or in patients under treatment for hematological malignancy [337–340]. Systemic candidosis in neutropenic or otherwise severely immunocompromised patients should still be treated with the fungicidal drug Amph B alone or combined with 5FC [341]. Flu has become for some clinicians the fist choice for the treatment of neonatal candidosis (fungemia, lung and CNS candidosis), since Flu showed a high clinical response without severe adverse effects in contrast to Amph B, which is poorly tolerated in neonates [342–347]. Some other clinicians are still using Amph B as first-line therapy since its activity is excellent and since comparative trials proving that Flu is as efficacious as Amph B in severe neonatal candidosis are lacking [347a]. The syndrome of hepatosplenic candidosis is rather slow in responding to therapy. The best regime seems to be initial therapy with Amph B with or without 5FC followed by Flu [348].

Ocular fungal infections respond favorably to treatment with flu, since this drug is evenly distributed in all body fluids, including ocular fluid. Flu has been successfully used for *Candida* endophthalmitis in heroin addicts [349]. Flu as sole long-term therapy achieved a 94% cure rate in 15 affected eyes, including five infections complicated with vitreitis [350].

Flu also shows high efficacy with no major side effects for neurosurgery-related fungal infections [351]. Flu cured an auricular case of *C. parapsilosis* chondritis [352], a case of spondylodicitis caused by *C. albicans* after unsuccessful treatment with Amph B [353], and a case of candidal osteomyelitis refractory to L-Amph B therapy [354]. The use of Flu in the management of fungal infections of artificial implants also seems to be of beneficial value [355].

Flu is also of great value in treating complicated and uncomplicated fungal urinary tract infections. The observed high efficacy is based on the pharmacokinetic properties of Flu, which is mainly excreted as unchanged drug by the kidneys; thus, high concentrations are achieved in the urine [356]. Flu has proven to be a safe and more efficacious alternative to Amph B bladder irrigation [357–360]. A short course of Flu has resulted in a prolonged clearance of yeasts, whereas intermittent bladder irrigation with Amph B has resulted in prompt but short-lived clearance [361]. We note, however, that the appearance of Flu-resistant species has been observed, and these cases must of course be treated with Amph B [362].

Flu also may show beneficial effects in infections caused by newly emerging pathogens, e.g., a case of *T. beigelii* prosthetic valve endocarditis has been successfully treated with Flu [363].

Cryptococcosis: Overall Flu has proven to be as effective as Amph B monotherapy for primary therapy of cryptococcal meningitis in patients with AIDS. The sterilization of the cerebrospinal fluid was, however, more rapid under Amph B treatment than with Flu. Since Amph B combined with 5FC has shown better cure rates than Amph B alone, this combination should remain the standard for the initial therapy of cryptococcal meningitis in HIV-positive patients [356, 364, 365]. The correlation between the daily dose of Flu and the clinical outcome was investigated in AIDS-related cryptococcosis: the higher daily dose of > 400 mg Flu for initial therapy as well as for maintenance therapy leads to a better clinical and microbiological outcome, lower mortality, and lower relapse rates [366]. A combination of Flu + Amph B may be used for this indication, especially if the patients develop severe side effects under the standard combination of 5FC + Amph B [367, 368]. Flu has found its place as initial therapy for mild cryptococcosis, e.g., 11 of 14 AIDS patients with non-meningeal cryptococcosis were cured under monotherapy with Flu [367]. Flu was also as efficacious as Amph B monotherapy for cryptococcosis in HIV-negative patients [369, 370]. Prospective studies investigating the optimal therapy for cryptococcosis in non-AIDS patients are still lacking. The combination of 5FC + Amph B seems still to be the most effective therapy for meningeal cryptococcosis (see also Section 7.4).

Chronic suppressive therapy was essential for all AIDS patients to avoid relapses of meningeal cryptococcosis. The prostate and meningen act as nidi of infection, inducing frequent relapses despite successful primary therapy. Flu has become the agent of first choice for this suppressive therapy in AIDS-related cryptococcal meningitis [150, 173, 257, 356]. Since the new antiviral therapy HAART is widely used in the western world, the relapse rate of cryptococcosis is drastically decreasing. Martinez and colleagues [370a] concluded from a prospective study that secondary prophylaxis may be safely discontinued in HIV-infected patients showing successful immunological response to HAART.

Chronic prophylactic treatment with Flu for recurrent oral candidosis has been reported to influence the incidence of meningeal cryptococcosis in AIDS patients. Under weekly Flu maintenance therapy, only 4% of treated patients developed disseminated cryptococcosis compared to 14% of untreated patients [371]. However, long-term, low-dose therapy with Flu does not invariably prevent a clinical manifestation of severe cryptococcosis. In France [372] two fulminate cryptococcal infections have been diagnosed in AIDS patients on Flu, and in Spain [373] a relapse occurred under suppressive therapy with Flu. It should be mentioned that the incidence of cryptococcal infection in AIDS patients has significantly decreased since the introduction of the aggressive antiviral therapy HAART [374]. In the future a chronic suppressive therapy may be no longer necessary.

Aspergillosis and other mould infections: Flu is not recommended for invasive mould infections, since its therapeutic value is limited, even at extremely high doses (1600 mg/day) [375].

4.3.5.5 Therapeutic indications in endemic mycoses

The addition of Flu and Itra to the antifungal armamentarium has clearly been of benefit in the treatment of endemic deep mycoses, both drugs being less toxic and easier to handle than Amph B. Flu seems to be less active than Itra in the area of endemic mycoses and should, therefore, be considered as second-line therapy [376–380].

Favorable responses have been observed in immunocompetent patients with histoplasmosis, coccidioidomycosis, sporotrichosis and/or paracoccidioidomycosiss [2, 356, 376–378]. Flu seems to be only moderately efficacious against blastomycosis; relatively high doses (400–800 mg) are needed to see positive clinical effect [380–383]. Flu was less active than Amph B or Itra for histoplasmosis in AIDS patients [384].

Both Flu and Itra are efficacious in pulmonary or extrapulmonary coccidioidomycosis; however, there is a trend toward slightly better efficacy with Itra. Itra was clearly superior to Flu in skeletal diseases [377, 385–387]. Flu has become the first-line therapy for meningeal coccidioidomycosis [377]. Unfortunately, an extremely high relapse rate has been observed after azole therapy was stopped, and lifelong suppression therapy is needed for this indication [376]. An optimal therapy schedule for meningeal coccidioidomycosis is not in view.

Amph B therapy remains the standard for all endemic infections in severely immunocompromised patients. Flu is recommended as second choice after Itra for histoplasmosis and blastomycosis in patients who cannot tolerate Itra. AIDS patient maintenance therapy is always necessary after an initial successful therapy with Amph B. Which of the drugs on the market is the best for this purpose is still intensively discussed: some clinicians are of the opinion that Flu is the optimal suppressive drug, others prefer Itra, and some even use Amph B.

4.3.6 Itraconazole

In contrast to Flu, Itra is highly lipophilic and nearly insoluble in water. These properties have been the reason for some drawbacks: no optimal galenical formulation existed over a long time period, and the bioavailability varied not only from patient to patient but also within the same patient, being strongly dependent on the intake of food. Itra has a broader antifungal spectrum than Flu, including dematiaceous fungi and moulds, especially *Aspergillus* spp. Itra, a representative of the second azole-generation, has a unique characteristic: it is fungicidal against aspergilli. This fungicidal effect is not associated with the typical mode of action, the inhibition of sterol biosynthesis, but is due to direct interaction of the molecule with the fungal membrane [388, 389].

Today three different galenical formulations exist: a capsule, an oral solution, and an intravenous solution [51]. The pharmacokinetic properties and their efficacy have been intensively studied in order to have guidelines for clinicians to use the optimal formulations for the respective disease or location. The bioavailability of the capsule is perfectly adequate in volunteers and patients with dermatophytic disease. Itra is, however, poorly absorbed in severely ill patients; to facilitate absorption, the drug has to be taken shortly after a meal. Taking Itra capsules on an empty stomach reduces the bioavailability, and consequently the efficacy, by half. Significant, unpredictable variation in plasma levels in patients often caused problems, and monitoring to assure adequate plasma levels was essential, especially in neutropenic patients [390]. Dose splitting over one day increased the clinical efficacy in neutropenic patients [391]. The combination of Itra with the enabling vehicle, cyclodextrin, in the oral solution formulation has improved the pharmacological profile of Itra: in contrast to the capsules, absorption is better when the solution is taken without food, and the total bioavailability is significantly improved, reaching nearly 100%. Furthermore, efficacious levels of the drug are achieved in the saliva [51, 220, 392–395]. A great step forward and a real progress for severely ill patients is, additionally, the introduction of intravenous Itra. Adequate steady-state plasma levels are rapidly achieved after administration of i.v. Itra in volunteers and patients with various underlying diseases and, consequently, severe immunosuppression ([51, 220], reviewed in [395, 396]).

Itra is tightly bound to plasma proteins; therefore, concentrations in most body fluids are low. However, the distribution of Itra into tissue is excellent: in tissues such as kidney, liver, bone, stomach, skin, etc., effective concentrations, higher than plasma levels, are achieved. Itra is especially accumulated in pus, fat, and keratin; it is excreted in sebum and sweat [3, 256]. Surprisingly, Itra's binding to proteins does not reduce its antifungal activity [397]. Itra is extensively metabolized by the liver and mainly excreted in the bile. Hydroxy-itraconazole, the major metabolite, is antifungally active and accounts for the antifungal effects in the blood. Less than 1% of the mother compound and 34% of the inactive metabolites are excreted in the urine [3, 51, 256].

4.3.6.1 Resistance

Most molecular mechanisms leading to resistance are similar to the one discussed with Flu; the same species show reduced susceptibility, and cross-resistance is not a rare event [398]: 39.9% of *C. glabrata* and 66.6% of *C. krusei* were relatively resistant to Itra in an international epidemiological fungemia study [399]. Another survey in Spain also found a relatively high degree of resistance in clinical isolates: 8.5% of *C. albicans*, 34.3% of *C. tropicalis*, 4.4% of *C. glabrata*, and 1.5% of *C. parapsilosis* were resistant to Itra [2]. Generally, the development of resistance to Itra has not yet caused the same levels of concern as with Flu. The lower incidence of resistance may be due to the less widespread use of Itra for prevention or therapy of *Candida* infections in HIV-positive patients.

4.3.6.2 Safety and tolerance

Like Flu, Itra is relatively well tolerated with a significantly better safety profile than Amph B in adults and children. Nausea is the most common side effect (2.4–10.6%); less frequent are vomiting, abdominal pain, diarrhea, headache, and skin rashes [3, 24a, 400]. Even after long-term therapy, no effect on steroidal hormones has been observed [401]. There have been some reports on hypertension and hyperkalemia; one case of severe cholestasis due to Itra has been reported [3, 402]. Asymptomatic abnormalities of hepatic function occur in less than 3% of patients. Reversible, apparently idiosyncratic, hepatitis is rare. A retrospective study showed that no hepatic disorders were seen in patients treated with Itra alone; however, several patients treated with the combination of Amph B + Itra showed abnormal liver function [403]. Congestive heart failure can be associated with Itra; therefore, the labeling of Itra has been changed recently and the drug is now contraindicated for the treatment of onychomycosis in patients with evidence of ventricular dysfunction [403a]. Itra did not cause a difference in the rate of major malformations in a prospective cohort of 198 women. There were differences between the Itra and control group regarding the rates of live birth, spontaneous abortion, therapeutic abortion, and fetal death. Relative risk for any pregnancy loss in the treated group compared to the control group was 1.75 [403b]. The use of Itra is, however, limited to 30 days in many countries, and periodic liver function tests may be necessary if Itra is given over a longer period of time [3, 256]. The oral and intravenous solution of Itra are also well tolerated, and the addition of cyclodextrin does not significantly add to the known side effects [395, 404]. Cyclodextrin shows, however, some osmotic activity in the gastrointestinal tract after a dose of Itra of > 400 mg. Few additional adverse events are associated with the i.v. formulation; most are related to the type of administration, namely, injection-site reactions and vein disorders [394–396]. Long-term safety studies for the carrier cyclodextrin after i.v. application are, unfortunately, not yet available.

4.3.6.3 Drug interactions

Clinically significant interactions of Itra with other drugs are less frequent and less severe than with Keto, but they are more significant than with Flu (see tables and review in [31, 32]). Like Flu, both Itra and its major metabolite can inhibit the human P450 enzyme CYP3A4 in a clinically significant manner with routine dosing; therefore, concomitant use of substrate drugs (e.g. nifedopine, digoxin, felopidine, simvastatin) should be avoided. Additionally, all substrates with low bioavailability (such as HMG-CoA reductase inhibitors) and those with extensive first-pass metabolism (astemizole and cisapride) and/or a narrow therapeutic window (warfarin, digoxin, phenytoin, and sulphonylureas) should also be avoided. H2 antagonists, ormeprazole, cimetidine, and all other drugs increasing intragastric pH, including those formulations with buffering agents such as didanosine, significantly decrease the absorption of Itra. Combinations of these drugs should be avoided in order not to hamper the already poor absorption of Itra in the capsule formulations. Itra is also extensively metabolized by hepatic CYP3A4; decreased bioavailability of Itra may occur if given with CYP3A4 inducers such as carbamazepin, dexamethasone, phenobarbital, phenytoin, prednisone, rifampin, etc. These drugs reduce the plasma concentration of Itra to undetectable levels [405]. Other drugs such as didanosine or isoniazid also negatively influence the plasma concentration of Itra. Itra, on the other hand causes a rise in plasma levels of various drugs, increasing their activity or toxicity (alprazolam, astemizole, cisapride, cyclosporine, diazepam, digoxin, felodipine, levostatin, midazolam, nifedipine, pimozide, simvastin, triazolam, and warfarin) [32, 406, 407]. The same interaction (increase in plasma level) is seen under co-administration of the following drugs: atirvastatin, buspiron, bupivacaine, busulan lignocaine, methylprednisolon, pimozidem, sildenafil, tacrolismusterfenadin, theophylline, tolbutamide, and vincristine [32, 408–410]. The plasma level of all these drugs, when co-administered with Itra, have to be monitored, and the daily dose has to be adjusted [3]. Protease inhibitors and azoles are also metabolized with the same hepatic enzyme, sometimes leading to an increase of Itra, sometimes to an increase of the protease inhibitor [411, 412]. For instance, a case of significant increase of the elimination half-life of Itra in the presence of saquinavir has been reported [413]. Fortunately no interactions exist between Itra and drugs used in diabetic patients [414].

Some of the interactions may lead to death if the pharmacodynamic effect of the concomitant drug is too high; therefore combinations of Itra with terfenadine, astemizole cisapride, simvastin, levostatin, or vincristine are contraindicated.

4.3.6.4 Therapeutic indications in opportunistic mycoses

Recent studies showed that the efficacy of the new formulations of Itra are improved compared with the capsules, probably because of the enhanced bioavailability; additionally, high concentrations of Itra have been found in the saliva under treatment with the oral solution. Thus, the recent introduction of the oral solution and especially of the parenteral formulation has substantially increased the options of Itra for the battle against fungal diseases.

Candidosis: For oropharyngeal candidosis, oral solutions of Itra are significantly more efficacious than its capsules, which were only marginally better than Keto and inferior to Flu in this indication [2, 415, 416]. Itra solution (200 mg/day) proved to be at least as effective as Flu (100 mg/day), and most of the patients with Flu-refractory *Candida* infections responded to the treatment with Itra [416–418]. Candida esophagitis also responds well to treatment with Itra (capsules or solution) [419] and leads to response rates similar to those of Flu. In 1996 a comparative study with 2213 AIDS patients was published that showed after a 2-week treatment a better efficacy of Itra capsules compared to Flu: the cure rate was 81.2% under Itra and 65.5% under Flu; the long-term observation showed for both drugs the same high efficacy, namely, 96% [317].

The situation is not as clear for disseminated candidosis as it is for thrush. In two studies, Itra capsules have been reported to be as effective as Amph B for disseminated candidosis in neutropenic patients. The widespread use of Itra capsules for disseminated candidosis in neutropenic patients is, however, not recommended because of its erratic bioavailability in neutropenic patients [390]. In Japan, Itra proved its efficacy in systemic fungal infections – mainly caused by *Candida* sp. – in patients with hematological disorders [420]. To date, no large clinical trials studying the activity of the oral or parenteral formulations of Itra in the field of disseminated candidosis exist.

Cryptococcosis: Itra was found to be active in murine cryptococcosis, and the drug (capsule) alone or combined with 5FC was efficacious in AIDS patients with meningeal cryptococcosis [421–424]. Only one study exists comparing intravenous Itra with Amph B in the treatment of cryptococcosis. Amph B was superior regarding complete cure rates and in clearing the CSF more rapidly and therefore led probably to a better prognosis [396]. Itra's definite role – after introduction of the other formulations – for the therapy or prevention of human cryptococcosis is not yet clear, as clinical comparative trials with Flu or Amph B are lacking [396]. The drug is recommended neither as the first-line treatment nor as suppressive treatment for cryptococcosis in AIDS patients. Flu proved to be the optimal drug for suppressive therapy [425].

Aspergillosis [426–428]: Invasive aspergillosis remains a devastating opportunistic infection despite Amph B therapy. An overall response rate to Amph

B of 55% has been observed in all host groups at all sites of disease [429]. The outcome of antifungal therapy in aspergillosis strongly depends on the immunological status of the host: no cure can be achieved if the immunosuppression is not overcome.

Itra represents a real step forward in the battle against various forms of aspergillosis, including pulmonary aspergillosis, disseminated aspergillosis, aspergilloma, and allergic bronchopulmonary aspergillosis. It was the first orally available, well-tolerated antifungal with efficacy against aspergillosis. Since the introduction of its intravenous formulations, the activity in this devasting disease is better and more reliable.

The first non-comparative trials suggested that the efficacy of Itra (capsules) is similar to that of Amph B, with the advantage of lower toxicity and the possibility of treating outpatients for a prolonged period if time (for details, see Suppl. 1 of *Chemotherapy* 38, 1992, and [427]).

In a thorough, well-controlled multi-center study [428], Itra (capsules) proved to be an alternative therapy for aspergillosis, with response rates similar to Amph B. The overall response rate at the end of the treatment was 39%, and the failure rate attributable to Itra was 26%. For aspergillosis, the clinical response to therapy varies widely according to the site of infection and the underlying disease . Itra failure was seen in 14% of pulmonary or tracheobronchial cases, in 50% of the sinus cases, and in 63% of the CNS cases. The highest failure rate was seen in AIDS patients (44%), compared with 14% in those with prolonged granulocytopenia and 29% in allogeneic bone marrow transplants. Post-treatment follow-up showed a relatively high relapse rate in patients who were still immunocompromised. The NIAID study [429] also concluded that Itra was an effective therapy, showing results similar to Amph B: 27% of the treated patients were cured, 36% improved, 16% remained unchanged, and 21% worsened. The EORTC multi-center prospective study [430] came to a similar conclusion: there was no discernable difference in outcome among initial therapy with Amph B, lipid-associated Amph B, or Itra. In the meantime, other studies have proven the efficacy of Itra for various forms of invasive aspergillosis [396, 430a]. Treatment with intravenous Itra as initial therapy for 14 days, followed by capsules for 12 weeks resulted in a complete cure rate of 48%. Another comparative study showed with intravenous Itra the same rate of desfervescence as with Amph B, and a slightly higher complete cure rate was observed under Itra (48% vs. 38%) [396]. Successful treatment of pulmonary aspergillosis also has been reported in patients with bone marrow transplantations [395, 431]. There are several individual case reports reporting cure under therapy with Itra, e.g., for chronic (10 year long) aspergillosi, for invasive paranasal aspergillosis [432], for primary cutaneous aspergillosis in AIDS patients [433], for necrotizing pulmonary aspergillosis [434], and as postoperative therapy for *Aspergillus* pericarditis [435]. Itra was clearly a breakthrough for the therapy of aspergilloma. Before the appearance of Itra, surgery offered the only possibility of eradicating aspergilloma. Nowadays, Itra therapy replaces surgery in all cases where there is no danger of hemoptysis [2]. The standard therapy for allergic bronchopulmonary aspergillosis was corticosteroid therapy without addition of antifungals. Addition of Itra to steroid therapy seems to improve the clinical outcome and lowers the requirement of steroids [436–438]. In patients with cystic fibrosis, Itra may be curative as monotherapy [439]. Itra has clearly found its place as second-choice therapy for all kinds of invasive and local aspergillosis.

Rare opportunistic fungal infections and phaeohyphomycoses: Several case reports exist describing successful therapy for fungal infections caused by unusual pathogens, e.g., a *Trichosporon* pneumonia refractory to Amph B therapy responded well to Itra [440], and a pulmonary infection in a bone marrow transplant patient caused simultaneously by *Aspergillus terreus* and *Pseudoallescheria boydii* was successfully treated by Itra [441]. A rhinocerebral case of zygomycosis [442], a basidio-bolomycosis [443], an *Entomophtora* mycosis [444], a sinusitis caused by *Schizophyllum commune* [445], and a fungal osteomyelitis due to *Curvularia* sp. [446] responded favorably to treatment with Itra.

Phaeohyphomycosis is a new classification for a diverse group of previously known entities grouped together on the basis of finding dematiaceous fungi in tissue. Tissue involvement may be superficial, cutaneous, subcutaneous, corneal, or systemic. The infections occur in both immunocompetent and immunocompromised patients. Itra has been dramatically successful in individual patients [447]. Cutaneous infections are caused by *Alternaria* sp. Normal and immunosuppressed patients were successfully cured with Itra [448, 449]. Itra cleared subcutaneous phaeohyphomycosis due to *Exophiala jeanselmei* in a diabetic patient, in a farmer, and in three cardiac transplant recipients. None of these patients had evidence of dissemination [450–452]. A sino-nasal *Alternaria* infection refractory to Amph B treatment markedly improved in response to Itra therapy. Itra was, however, unsuccessful in a case of cerebral phaeohyphomycosis caused by *Dactylaria* [453]. An ulcer due to *Phialophora verrucosa* disappeared under Itra therapy [454], and an osteomyelitis due to *Phomopsis* was successfully treated by Itra [455]. A case of a relapsed phaeohyphomycosis due to *Cladosporium cladosporiodis* was refractory to a treatment with the combination of 5FC + Amph B but healed under high doses of Itra [456].

The number of patients with phaeohyphomycosis is so small that no comparative trials are likely ever to occur. Thus, changes in therapy will be based on individual reports. The optimal duration of therapy with Itra is not yet determined. Relapses seem to occur if Itra is stopped too early. Despite all these unknowns, it is clear that Itra has a definite place in these rare but sometimes dangerous indications.

4.3.6.5 Therapeutic indications in endemic mycoses

Itra is of greatest benefit in endemic mycoses; histoplasmosis, paracoccidioidomycosis, coccidioidomycosis, and sporotrichosis all respond favorably to Itra therapy [257, 378–380, 457].

Histoplasmosis: before the advent of azoles, Amph B was the drug of choice in patients with chronic pulmonary or disseminated histoplasmosis. Keto and especially Itra have become safe and effective alternatives to Amph B. The response rate among patients with chronic pulmonary histoplasmosis treated for at least 2 months was 86%. Patients with disseminated histoplasmosis responded even better [396, 457]. Itra is also safe and efficacious in children with histoplasmosis [458]. An unusual case of intestinal histoplasmosis also responded to therapy with oral Itra [459]. The African histoplasmosis also responds to Itra [460].

Disseminated histoplasmosis is an increasingly recognized opportunistic fungal infection in AIDS patients [257, 457]. Even in these severely immunocompromised patients, mild to moderate histoplasmosis responds well to Itra, with a 85% cure rate; however, severe cases are preferentially treated with Amph B [461]. It is currently standard to initiate suppressive therapy in AIDS patients after a successful initial therapy: more than 90% of the AIDS patients remained relapse-free when Itra was given as maintenance therapy [462]. In summary, Itra is regarded as drug of first choice for both treatment and suppression of mild to moderate histoplasmosis [396, 378]. The impact of the intravenous form for severe histoplasmosis remains to be determined; it showed efficacy in a first small trial [378].

Blastomycosis: Itra has become the fist-line therapy for pulmonal and extrapulmonal blastomycosis in non-AIDS patients, whereas Amph B has kept its place for the treatment of CNS blastomycosis [379, 396, 463].

Paracoccidioidomycosis: Itra is also recommended for mild and moderate forms of this disease; severe cases again should be treated with Amph B [464].

Coccidioidomycosis: The appearance of azoles has markedly changed the approach to the treatment of coccidioidomycosis. A prolonged course of therapy is still needed, but this is much easier to handle with a safe oral drug than with the parenteral Amph B. Itra appears to be effective in meningeal and non-meningeal coccidioidomycosis; however, the response rates are lower than those for histoplasmosis and blastomycosis [457, 465]. A trend for superiority of Itra was seen in a comparative study (Flu vs. Itra) for progressive, non-meningeal coccidioidomycosis: at 8 months of therapy 52% of Itra- and 26% of Flu-patients were classified as responders; at 12 months of therapy 86% of all patients responded, the difference between Itra and Flu being 15% [466].

Flu may become the first-line therapy for CNS coccidioidomycosis, whereas for others forms of the disease, Itra may be more successful.

Sporotrichosis: Itra is clearly the agent of first choice for most forms of sporotrichosis. It achieved higher efficacy than Keto or Flu against this disease, reaching response rates of 90–100%. For lymphocutaneous sporotrichosis, treatment duration is usually 3–6 months with doses of 100–200 mg/day. Osteoarticular sporotrichosis is more problematic; higher doses and a prolonged treatment period are necessary, sometimes even over a year, to achieve clinical response [467]. Pulmonary sporotrichosis is refractory to all therapies. Neither Amph B nor Itra achieve high cure rates; lifelong therapy may be needed for this form of the disease. Lengthy treatment is easier to handle with an oral drug than with the parenteral Amph B [457, 468].

4.3.7 Voriconazole

Vori, the first representative of the third generation of azoles, received approval for the treatment of potentially fatal fungal infections in early 2002. It is available in oral and intravenous formulation. The approval is primarily for treatment in immunocompromised patients with progressive infections including invasive aspergillosis, Flu-resistant serious invasive candidosis (e.g., *C. krusei*), and serious infections caused by *Scedosporium* and *Fusarium*.

4.3.7.1 Preclinical data

The mode of action is typical for all azoles: it inhibits the cytochrome P450-dependent 14 α-sterol demethylase. However, Vori also inhibits the 24-methylene dihydrolanosterol demethylation in certain yeasts and filamentous fungi, explaining in part its activity against moulds, especially *Aspergillus* [469–471].

The better and broader antifungal activity of Vori in comparison to Flu has been demonstrated in diverse *in vitro* studies. The *in vitro* spectrum includes yeasts; Flu-resistant yeasts; moulds, especially aspergilli; true pathogenic fungi; and newly emerging pathogens such as *Scedasporium* sp., *Pseudoallescheria boydii*, and *Fusarium* sp. [469–472]: Vori is 124 times more active against *C. krusei*. Generally, Vori exerts a fungistatic activity against all susceptible fungi; however, it is, like Itra, fungicidal against aspergilli. Additionally, it shows fungicidal effects against dematiaceous fungi. Vori also strongly interferes at subinhibitory concentrations with the adherence or penetration of fungal cells to epithelial cells. The broad *in vitro* effect was confirmed in various animal models using normal and neutropenic animals. Vori was superior to Amph B treatment in various models of aspergillosis [470, 473].

The same mechanism for resistance may play a role as that of other azoles described in previous sections for Flu and Itra. Cross-resistance is expected but not yet determined. In some studies, however, Vori showed good activity against Flu-resistant *C. albicans* strains as well as against Flu-resistant oral candidosis [470].

4.3.7.2 Pharmacokinetics and metabolism

Vori is widely distributed through the body; has a good bioavailability (> 90%) after oral administration, reaching maximum plasma levels within 2 hours; and its elimination half-life is approximately 6 hours. Vori is metabolized by extensive hepatic metabolism *via* the cytochrome 450 P-enzymes, especially CYP2C19 and to a lesser extent by CYP3A4 and CYP2C9. Less than 5% of the mother compound is eliminated in the urine. No dosage adjustment is necessary in patients with renal insufficiency; however, in patients with mild to moderate hepatic disorder, the dose has to be adjusted, and Vori should be avoided in patients with severe hepatic impairments. The intraindividual variation of the pharmacokinetic is small; however, interindividual variations exist that are based on genetic differences [469–471].

4.3.7.3 Safety and tolerance

During therapeutic studies, visual disturbances as well as cardiac, liver, and hepatic functions were closely monitored. Generally, Vori is well tolerated: as with the existing azoles, elevations in liver function tests have been observed in 15% of the patients. In the phase III study, no trend toward increased cardiac adverse events was seen under Vori treatment. Skin reactions (rash including severe episodes such as Stevens-Johnson syndrome) may occur under treatment with Vori. The most disturbing adverse effects are the ocular findings, including decreased vision, photophobia, altered color perception, and ocular discomfort. They all seem to be transient. At present the authorities agree that visual abnormalities occurred at a frequency of 14% to 33% in the clinical database [469–471].

4.3.7.4 Drug interactions

Drug interactions similar to Keto, Flu, and Itra may occur. *In vitro*, Vori was, however, a significantly less potent inhibitor of CYP3A4 metabolism than the other azoles. The clinical experience is still limited, but the following recommendations are already certain. Rifampin, rifabutin, and phenytoin decrease the plasma level of Vori: rifampin is totally contraindicated in presence of Vori, whereas the dose of Vori should be increased in presence of rifabutin and phenytoin. On the other hand, Vori increases the prothrombin time of warfarin and increases the plasma levels and therefore the possibly toxic effects of omeprazole, cyclosporine, tacrolimus, sirolimus phenytoin, and rifabutin. In most cases the dose of the concomitant administered drug should be reduced by one-third to one-half; sirolimus is totally contraindicated [471].

4.3.7.5 Therapeutic indications

Vori showed efficacy in muccocutaneous candidosis and oropharyngeal candidosis of AIDS patients. Vori was as efficacious as Flu against esophageal candidosis in immunocompromised patients [470, 471, 474]. Vori was also successful in severe systemic candidosis. A small number of patients with invasive candidosis refractory to standard therapy were treated with Vori; 22 of 43 patients (51.2%) could be cured [471].

Vori seems to have the potential of becoming a true alternative therapy for invasive aspergillosis. First, small studies evaluated the role of Vori in the treatment of aspergillosis. At the ICAAC in 1995, B. Dupont and his group [475] and D. Denning and his group [476] presented the first positive results with an overall favorable outcome in 69% and 75%, respectively, of the patients. Later, the usefulness of Vori for the treatment of invasive aspergillosis was studied in two large clinical trials. In the first European study, Vori was compared with historical data. In this study, Vori showed favorable results to historical Amph B controls. Fifty-eight patients received Vori as primary and 54 as salvage therapy; for primary therapy patients, the satisfactory response rate was 60.3%, and for the salvage therapy patients it was 37%. The response rate was again dependent on the location of the disease and the underlying disease: 60% of the patients with pulmonary or tracheobronchial aspergillosis but only 16% of the cerebral cases responded well to the therapy; 58% of the patients with hematological disorders and 26% of allogeneic stem cell transplant recipients responded favorably to the therapy [470, 477]. The international comparative, open-labeled Phase III studies showed for Vori a significant survival advantage compared to the Amph B regimen. The probability of survival at day 84 was 0.708 for Vori vs. 0.579 for Amph B. In addition to these large clinical trials, several case reports exist showing the efficacy of Vori in various forms of aspergillosis. The comparative clinical studies prove that Vori may be an excellent alternative to Amph B for the fight against invasive aspergillosis [471].

Vori is apparently a real step forward in the battle against fungal infections due to emerging pathogens like *Fusarium* and *Scedosporium* [470, 471]. Successful outcome was observed in 59.3% of the patients with *Scedosporium* infections; some of the cured patients even had a documented CNS location of the disease. Successful outcome was also observed in 6 of 15 patients with *Fusarium* infections. Most patients received Vori as salvage therapy.

In conclusion, three potent triazoles are now on the market, clearly improving the armamentarium of clinicians against invasive fungal infection of all kinds; based on the clinical studies available today, Vori will become the first choice for treatment of invasive aspergillosis.

4.3.8 Caspofungin

In 2001, caspofungin (CAS) received FDA approval for the treatment of invasive aspergillosis in patients who are refractory to or intolerant of other therapies. No oral formulation exists; CAS is available only as a parenteral formulation.

4.3.8.1 Preclinical data

CAS, a semisynthetic derivative of pneumocandin B – a fermentation product of the fungus *Glarea lozoyensis* – is a specific non-competitive inhibitor of the 1,3-β-glucan synthetase in several pathogen fungi. This drug is the first antifungal on the market that interferes with the fungal specific target of the cell wall [478–480].

CAS shows a broad antifungal spectrum *in vitro*, including opportunistic and true pathogen fungi: it is highly active and exerts fungicidal activity against pathogenic yeasts with the exceptions of *C. guillermondii*, *Cr. neoformans*, and *Trichosporon beigelii*, which show resistance to the drug. *Zygomcetes* and *Fusarium* spp. are resistant to the drug. CAS induces in aspergilli dramatic morphological changes in hyphal elements; filaments become distorted and blunted. CAS exerts its drastic morphological changes against all five pathogen *Aspergillus* spp.; inhibition of cell wall synthesis causes death and lysis of fumigatus growing hyphal tips and branching segments, as assessed by specific fluorescent stains. This inhibitory phenomenon is, however, difficult to express in MIC values [196, 478, 479]. CAS is strongly bound to plasma albumin (80%), but this binding does not decrease its antifungal effect; on the contrary, addition of serum to CAS increased markedly the inhibitory activity of CAS against *Aspergillus fumigatus* [481]. CAS significantly inhibits the adherence of *Candida* to epithelial cells.

The good *in vitro* activity against *Candida* and *Aspergillus* was confirmed in various animal models of aspergillosis and candidosis in immunocompetent and immunocompromised animals. CAS also prolonged survival and reduced the fungal burden in a mouse model of coccidioidomycosis and was beneficial in various models of *P. carinii* – pneumonia [196, 478, 479].

Inherited resistance to echinocandin in otherwise susceptible fungal yeasts is rare (1×10^{-8}), and CAS has a low potential for induced resistance.

The overwhelming majority of mutations conferring resistance have been mapped to the FKS1 gene, the putative catalytic component of glucan synthase. The mechanism of action is so distinct from that of other antifungals that no or only a very low potential for cross-resistance is expected [478, 479].

4.3.8.2 Pharmacokinetic and metabolism

After intravenous administration, CAS exhibits dose-proportional pharmacokinetics with a short distributional α-phase immediately post infusion, followed by a β-half-life of 9–10 h; an additional longer γ-half-life of 40–50 h also occurs. After multiple doses CAS is dose-dependently accumulated in plasma up to 50%. The 70 mg/day loading dose achieves peak levels of 10 μg/ml, and the following daily dose of 50 mg achieves through levels of 1 μg/ml. The pharmacokinetics of CAS is not dependent on age, gender, or underlying condition; the dose does not have to be adapted to renal insufficiency and mild hepatic disorders. However, a dose reduction is recommended in patients with moderate hepatic disorders. CAS is distributed widely through the body with the exception of the brain and is extensively bound to serum albumin. Distribution rather than excretion or biotransformation is the predominant mechanism controlling CAS plasma clearance. CAS is slowly metabolized by peptide hydrolysis and N-acetylation. Less than 5% of the dose is excreted unchanged in the urine [478, 479].

4.3.8.3 Safety and tolerance

CAS is generally well tolerated: less than 5% of the patients in the clinical studies discontinued the therapy prematurely. There is no evidence of dose-related toxicities. The following side effects occurred in 5% of the clinical trial patients: fever (3.6–26%), phlebitis (1.5–15.7%), nausea (2.5–6%), headache (6–11.3%), and diarrhea (2.4%). Laboratory abnormalities mainly include elevated transaminases, elevated serum alkaline phosphatases, decreased hemaglobin and decreased hemocrit, and sometimes decreased serum albumin and serum potassium. CAS crosses the placental barrier and showed embryo toxicity in rats and rabbits; therefore CAS should not be used during pregnancy [478–480].

4.3.8.4 Drug interactions

In contrast to azoles, CAS is not subject to drug interactions mediated by cytochrome P450 enzymes. The drug interaction program focused on two classes of drugs: antifungals likely to be co-administered or sequentially administered and immunosuppressants used in transplant patients. Itra, tacrolimus, myophenolate, and probably Amph B have no effect on the pharmacokinetic properties of CAS. Cyclosporin A moderately increases the plasma levels of CAS, but CAS has no effect on the levels of cyclosporin A. However, CAS slightly decreases the AUC of tacrolimus. Regression analysis of patient pharmacokinetic data suggests that co-administration of inducers of drug clearance and/or mixed inducer/inhibitors, namely, nelfinavir, phenytoin, rifampin, etc., may result in clinically meaningful reductions in CAS concentrations. The manufacturer currently recommends an increase in the daily dose of CAS if patients with concurrent medication are not clinically responding to CAS therapy [478–480].

Co-administration of cyclosporin A with CAS is, however, not recommended, based on mild increases in ALT/AST in phase I studies. Further safety studies are required to clarify this interaction [479].

4.3.8.5 Therapeutic indications

CAS has been developed for the treatment of serious infections caused by *Candida* and *Aspergillus*. In phase II studies, CAS – in the dose range of 35–70 mg – was efficacious in oropharyngeal and esophageal candidosis. In a comparative study, CAS showed superiority to Amph B; clinical response of esophagitis (measured by symptoms and endoscopy) was noted in 85.1% of the patients vs. 66.7% in the Amph B group. Oropharyngeal candidosis responded even better to the therapy, reaching >90% cure. Phase III efficacy studies for invasive candidosis are under way; interim reports also indicate superiority of CAS in comparison to conventional Amph B.

The efficacy of CAS was studied in patients with invasive aspergillosis refractory to or intolerant of standard therapies. Clinical improvement of 41–50% was seen in this group of patients, who all had an extremely poor prognosis. The response rates among patients with pulmonary disease were 47% (21/45) and with extrapulmonary disease 28% (5/18). Documented relapse is uncommon up to 4 weeks after the completion of CAS therapy. CAS proved to be effective in the treatment of invasive aspergillosis when compared to historical control group receiving standard therapy. Based on these favorable results, CAS received FDA approval for the therapy of refractory invasive aspergillosis [478–480].

4.3.9 Combination therapy

The interest in combination therapy for invasive severe fungal infections is steadily increasing. At the time when Medoff and co-workers [482] detected the synergistic effect of 5FC plus Amph B, the interest was restricted to a few groups of clinicians and some microbiologists. Today combination therapy has found its place in the antifungal field, especially in the battle against severe invasive fungal infections in severely immunosuppressed patients. It should not be forgotten that a truly synergistic effect on the level of the fungus cell is not the only prerequisite for a beneficial effect in chemotherapy. The general complement of the antimicrobial and the pharmacokinetic properties of the combination partners is also of significant importance. The reason that a certain combination therapy shows higher efficacy is rather complex and often not fully understood.

Studies *in vitro* and particularly in animal models have shown that a real increase in efficacy can be achieved with certain combinations for various indications but that others should be avoided, as they are antagonistic.

4.3.9.1 Preclinical studies

The results of combination studies *in vitro* and *in vivo* strongly depend on the fungal strain, the methodology, the animal species, and the antifungal drug used. The published *in vitro* data show great variability and are rather controversial; however, the following general conclusions can be drawn: 5FC plus Amph B is additive or synergistic against most of the opportunistic fungal strains, especially against 5FC-resistant strains [483, 484]. Amph B and the azoles – and probably also other sterol biosynthesis inhibitors – usually act as antagonists when added simultaneously or when an azole is added first, but synergy has been observed in cases where the azole was added to the cells that were pre-treated with subinhibitory concentrations of Amph B [483–487]. In aspergilli, Ter + Amph B surprisingly showed an additive or even synergistic effect depending on the isolate [483, 488]. Azoles and 5FC are usually indifferent, occasionally additive or synergistic, and never antagonistic [483, 489, 489a].

On the basis of biochemical knowledge, combinations of sterol inhibitors with different mode of actions should be synergistic: Ter displayed a potent synergism with the triazoles Itra and Vori in yeasts and aspergilli [483, 488, 490, 490a]. Flu, which has no *in vitro* activity against

Aspergillus sp. surprisingly potentiated the effect of Ter [488]. Ter plus Itra is additive or synergistic against *Aspergillus* sp., and *Fusarium* [488a]. The combination of CAS and Amph B has been found to be additive or indifferent and never antagonistic against *C. albicans, Cr. neoformans*, and *A. fumigatus* [491]. CAS shows *in vitro* beneficial effects with various antifungals: depending on the strains, CAS + Amph B is synergistic, additive, or indifferent against *Cr. neoformans* and *A. fumigatus*; however, CAS + Flu is neither synergistic nor antagonistic against *Candida* sp. or *Cr. neoformans* [491a]. Vori plus various echinocandins showed synergism against *A. fumigatus* [490a]; this combination may be useful in human chemotherapy. Vori interacts synergistically with Ter against *S. prolificans* [490a]; this combination may be useful for the human chemotherapy of *Scedosporium* infections that are difficult to treat.

Several unexpected synergisms were observed: cyclosporin A significantly increases the *in vitro* activity of Flu [492]. This interaction may have a clinical impact; however, the interaction of Flu on the level of metabolism also has to be taken into account. Ibuprofen significantly increased the *in vitro* activity of Flu in Flu-resistant *Candida* species [493]. CAS plus tacrolimus or L685818 has synergistic effects against wild-type *Cr. neoformans* strains [491]. Thus, the potential for a beneficial effect in combining various drugs seems to be overwhelming. The only drawback lies in possible antagonistic interaction, which has to be tested beforehand.

Combination therapy has been and still is studied in animal models of a variety of infections in normal and neutropenic animals. The results of the animal models vary to a greater extent than those of the *in vitro* study. The outcome strongly depends on the dose, the application route, the type of infection, and the endpoints. In the past most animal work has been done with the combination of 5FC plus Amph B, but recently combinations of 5FC plus azoles or CAS plus Amph B are being intensively studied.

5FC+ Amph B improved activity in murine candidosis, cryptococcosis, wangiellosis, and, to a lesser extent, in aspergillosis. Synergism was more pronounced in infections caused by strains partially resistant to 5FC. With this combination microbiological cure can be achieved in *Candida*-infected mice, which is never achieved with realistic doses of single antimycotics in this model. Additionally, in neutropenic rabbits only this combination was able to eradicate renal candidosis, which Flu, Itra, or another single drug regimen was not able to achieve [483].

The combination of 5FC with azoles has a beneficial effect in most cases, and antagonism is observed only in few cases [483]. The degree of interaction is weak with Keto but strong with Itra and Flu. 5FC + Flu showed superiority over monotherapy in murine models of disseminated infections due to *C. glabrata* or *C. albicans* [483, 494]. The combination of 5FC + Itra had an additive effect in murine aspergillosis, and the combination of 5FC + Flu showed synergism in most studies of murine cryptococcosis; indifference was seen in only a few experiments. The synergism between 5FC plus triazoles was most impressive in murine wangiellosis [483].

Low doses of Amph B + CAS appear more efficacious than either drug alone in murine candidosis and aspergillosis, showing at least an additive effect. The combination of CAS + Flu also showed higher efficacy [479].

The situation with combinations of Amph B and an antifungal belonging to the class of azoles is controversial and strongly dependent on the fungal species. No interaction was seen between Amph+Keto or Amph B + Itra in histoplasmosis and blastomycosis measuring survival. In experiments with measurement of the fungal burden, antagonism was seen [495]. In another histoplasmosis study, antagonism was observed under the combination of Amph B + Flu, but not with Amph B + Itra [496]. Synergy was always apparent with Amph B combined with Keto, Flu, or Itra in murine cryptococcosis, but antagonism or indifference was seen in murine aspergillosis and candidosis [483, 485, 494, 497]. In *Aspergillus*-infected mice, pre-treatment with Keto for 24-48 h completely abolished the curative effect of Amph B therapy. The same antagonism was seen with Itra. In histoplasmosis, prophylactic treatment with Keto had no effect on the outcome of Amph B therapy. Absence of antagonism was demonstrated in a model of rabbit *Candida* endocarditis: Amph B as well as the combination of Amph B + Flu decreased the fungal burden and prolonged survival in comparison to untreated animals [483]. However, another study investigated the impact of the order of initiating of Flu and Amph B in sequential or combination therapy on killing of *C. albicans in vitro* as well as in a rabbit model of endocarditis and polynephritis. Flu pre-treatment reduced the clearing activity of Amph B *in vivo* [485]. The length of Flu pre-exposure and whether Amph B is subsequently used alone or in combination with Flu determine the duration of induced resistance to Amph B. In trichosporosis, the combination of Flu+Amph B proved to be more active than either drug alone. In contrast to *in vitro* results, antagonism was not observed. The combination of Amph B + Itra was antagonistic in the same model [483].

Triple combinations of 5FC + Amph B + Flu or Itra were tested in various animal models. The triple combination was the most efficacious treatment for murine cryptococcosis, whereas a slight antagonism was seen in murine aspergillosis and candidosis [483].

The strange combination of Flu + cyclosporin A shows synergism *in vitro* as well as in experimental endocarditis due to *C. albicans*; only this combination was able to sterilize the aortic valve vegetations [498].

The preclinical results of antifungal combinations have not remained in a vacuum but have shown themselves to be predictive for clinical use.

4.3.9.2 Clinical experience

For years the combination of 5FC + Amph B has been the optimal treatment for cryptococcal meningitis. The rationale was to accelerate killing of the organism and prevent emergence of 5FC resistance. The superiority of this combination over monotherapy with Amph B was proven in non-AIDS patients by two randomized prospective clinical trials [499, 500]. Faster sterilization of the cerebrospinal fluid was seen as well as a more rapid clinical response on an overall higher cure rate. Despite the search for alternative treatment schedules, especially after the introduction of Flu on the market, and despite occasionally safety problems, which can be overcome by serially monitoring the 5FC level, the combination of 5FC + Amph B remained for a long period of time the optimal treatment for meningeal cryptococcosis in non-AIDS patients [483].

The hope of having found a nearly ideal therapy for the lethal illness sank as cryptococcosis started to become a frequent secondary infection in AIDS patients. The illness proceeds more aggressively and is far more difficult to eradicate, as reservoirs of infection seem to remain especially in the prostate even after the therapy has apparently succeeded. A high relapse rate is the rule if maintenance with Flu or Itra is not installed. The optimal therapy was difficult to find in this situation, and a great variety of different treatment schedules have been studied.

In the United States alternative regimens to the standard combination of 5FC + Amph B have been sought, especially since Americans feared the myelosuppressive adverse effects of 5FC in AIDS patients. However, neither Amph B nor Flu monotherapy showed high cure rates in the acute phase of cryptococcal meningitis in AIDS patients. Flu proved to be as efficacious as Amph B monotherapy, with a 34–40% successful outcome [483]. Yet, in a retrospective study by White and co-workers [501] an aggressive combination therapy regimen with 5FC (100 mg/kg/day) plus Amph B (1.0 mg/kg/day) cured 78% of patients with AIDS and 43% of patients with neoplastic diseases. Based on these results, the combination of 5FC+Amph B was revived and is still used for high risk, at least for the acute phase of the disease. A new randomized, double-blind trial was initiated, varying both the initial and the suppressive therapy. After a 2-week initiation phase with the combination of 5FC + Amph B, a consolidation phase follows with Flu or Itra monotherapy for another 8 weeks. At 2 weeks, the cerebrospinal cultures were negative in 60% of the patients receiving the combination therapy and in 51% of the patients with Amph B monotherapy ($p = 0.06$) [502].The clinical outcome did not differ significantly between the two groups, and overall mortality was independent of the treatment schedule, 5.5% in the first 2 weeks and 3.9% in the next 8 weeks. This mortality rate is surprisingly low in comparison to other studies, reporting mortality rates of 14–25% under treatment with lower doses of Amph B. Addition of 5FC did not increase the adverse reactions. The authors concluded from the thorough study that for the initial treatment of cryptococcal meningitis in AIDS patients, the use of higher doses of 5FC + Amph B (0.7 mg/kg/day) is associated with an increased rate of cerebrospinal fluid sterilization and decreased mortality at 2 weeks as compared with regimens used in the past.

A Californian study group was interested in evaluating the combination of 5FC + Flu for the therapy of cryptococcal meningitis in AIDS patients. The rate of clinical success was significantly greater than that previously reported for Amph B or Flu monotherapy. A total of 75% of the patients had negative cultures in the cerebrospinal fluid 10 weeks after the initiation of the therapy. However, toxic side effects that were sufficiently severe to lead to withdrawal of 5FC were observed in 28% of the patients. Thus, additional trials have to be performed to define the future place of this combination in the battle against meningeal cryptococcosis in AIDS patients [483, 503]. The same Californian working group [504] later determined the relationship of cryptococcal susceptibility to Flu, along with other clinical variables, to the risk of treatment failure for patients with acute AIDS-associated cryptococcal meningitis. The authors observed that negative blood culture, a low MIC of Flu (measured by the microtiter method), and treatment with 5FC were factors independently associated with clinical success. Further clinical studies in Japan and Thailand emphasize the high efficacy of 5FC plus triazoles for cryptococcal meningitis [483]. The combination of 5FC + Itra was successfully used in Italy, and 5FC + Flu seems to be the optimal therapy for pulmonary cryptococcosis in AIDS patients.

Another problem regarding Flu treatment deserves mention: the appearance of Flu-resistant *Cryptococcus* strains is drastically increasing. In 1987 10% of the strains were resistant to Flu, whereas in 1992 50% of the strains were resistant to Flu. The emergence of resistant strains may be enhanced by the use of Flu as primary prophylaxis. It does not look as if the combination of 5FC+Flu will replace the standard combination of 5FC + Amph B in the near future.

In China a two-step regimen with an initial therapy of Amph B + Flu followed by a maintenance therapy with Flu seems to be widely used [505].

In Germany, the triple combination 5FC + Amph B + Flu proved to be highly efficacious for acute cryptococcal meningitis in AIDS, and this combination is now routinely used in most German hospitals as well as in tropical areas [483].

The large number of variations employed in just a narrow area, cryptococcosis in AIDS, clearly demonstrates that combination therapy opens up many possibilities. But it also demonstrates that this fungal disease is rather difficult to eradicate. Proper clinical trials using combination therapy exist only for cryptococcal meningitis; nevertheless, combination therapy, especially with 5FC + Amph B is recommended as the treatment of choice for other opportunistic infections, e.g., candidosis, in severely immunosuppressed patients.

Recently a case of cryptococcal osteomyelitis and paraspinous abscess was successfully treated with the combination of 5FC + Flu [483a].

Candidosis: Combination therapy also has proven its value in deep-seated *Candida* infection. The response of *Candida* infections to chemotherapy strongly depends on the localization of the infection and the underlying disease. In some cases monotherapy is sufficient to eradicate the mycosis; in others combination therapy with 5FC + Amph B is needed for the battle.

Candida fungemia may resolve spontaneously after removal of the catheter or after monotherapy, but it also may cause endophthalmitis. *Candida* endophthalmitis has been found in 28–37% of non-neutropenic patients with *Candida* fungemia. Endophthalmitis has to be treated aggressively with prolonged therapy (5FC + Amph B/5FC + Flu) to minimize visual impairment and to effect a complete cure of the infection, which in most cases has disseminated to the organs [483].

Antifungal chemotherapy for *Candida* infection in patients with neoplastic diseases is not successful as long as the underlying disease is not controlled, i.e., bone marrow recovery is necessary to achieve cure. A study in 28 neutropenic patients showed an extremely poor clinical outcome under Amph B monotherapy as well as under combination therapy with 5FC + Amph B, because the mycoses were too far advanced at the time therapy was started, and the recovery of neutrophils was achieved in only half of the patients [506]. The combination of 5FC + Amph B showed the highest degree of success in infections due to *Candida tropicalis*, a species that is regularly more resistant to Amph B than *C. albicans* [483]. Other authors also reported high success rates under the combination therapy; combination therapy generally leads to a faster elimination of the fungus.

Neonates with various forms of candidosis in most cases respond to monotherapy with Flu or Amph B (conventional or liposomal); however, several authors have observed that under combination therapy, more neonates survive the infection without sequelae than under monotherapy [483, 507].

The syndrome of hepatosplenic candidosis or chronic progressive candidosis is increasingly recognized in patients recovering from neutropenia. This form of *Candida* infection, which responds very slowly to therapy, is another candidate for an initial combination therapy with 5FC + Amph B followed by Flu monotherapy if cure is not rapidly achieved [483, 493].

Candida meningitis or encephalitis, as well as *Candida* endocarditis or *Candida* osteomyelitis, initially has to be treated with combination therapy (5FC + Amph B/5FC + Flu) [483]. If the *Candida* meningitis is diagnosed in an AIDS patient, a maintenance therapy with Flu should follow the initial combination therapy in order to avoid relapses [508]. *Candida* endocarditis in adults mostly occurring after open heart surgery or after valve replacement does not respond to antifungal chemotherapy alone. The heavy fungal burden is not removable by monotherapy alone. The best clinical success is achieved by surgery and simultaneous combination therapy with 5FC + Amph B over a long period of time. A successful treatment of fungal prosthetic valve endocarditis with 5FC + Flu was reported [483].

The optimal treatment schedule for *Candida* peritonitis is not yet agreed upon. Monotherapy without removal of the catheter never leads to clinical success. However, combination therapy (5FC + Amph B, 5FC + Keto, 5FC + Flu) leads to high cure rates (> 93%) without removal of the catheter [509]. Generally, the success of treatment is dependent on the general condition of the patient. Antifungal therapy should be combined with surgery if a dissemination is diagnosed [483, 510].

The *Candida* syndrome peculiar to heroin addicts responds well to monotherapy with Keto or newer triazoles, if the infection is restricted to the skin. However, combination therapy is needed as soon as other localizations are additionally involved. In the case of concomitant endophthalmitis, combination therapy eradicates the fungal infection sufficiently quickly to save the patient's sight, whereas under monotherapy the fungal disease is cured, but the eyesight lost [483].

Aspergillosis: Invasive aspergillosis responds poorly to antifungal therapy; therefore, more emphasis is put on prevention or empirical therapy than in other indications. For therapy, the combination seems to be superior to monotherapy, especially when the diagnosis is made early and high doses of Amph B are used. Burch and co-workers [511] reported 90% survival in granulocytopenic patients, but they used an unusually high dose of Amph B (1.5 mg/kg/day). Walsh and Pizzo [483] likewise recommend the combination of 5FC+Amph B for this fulminate infection, especially at the beginning of therapy. Several publications demonstrated the beneficial value of combination therapy of 5FC + Amph B or L-Amph B for invasive aspergillosis [483, 512]. After the introduction of intravenous Itra, the combination of 5FC + Itra should be tested in this difficult disease, since this combination has been highly efficacious in animal models. The combination of Amph B + triazoles should be avoided since antagonism can not be excluded, e.g., 2 liver transplant patients with invasive aspergillosis died under combination therapy with L-Amph B + Itra. The authors suggest an antagonistic effect between these two drugs [513]. The optimal therapy for aspergillosis does not yet exist; even the newest drugs Vori and CAS do not show overwhelming cure rates. Therefore, the fantasy should not be restricted and new combinations should be tested in the clinic, such as CAS + Amph B or even a triple combination with 5FC + Amph B + CAS.

Phaeohyphomycosis and other unusual mycoses: Phaeohyphomycosis is defined as an invasive infection due to *Dematiaceae*, a family of fungi characterized by the production of brown pigment. This infection occurs in immunocompetent and immunocompromised patients. All dematiaceous fungi are highly sensitive to 5FC, Itra, and Vori; a combination of 5FC + Itra or 5FC + Vori may become the most beneficial treatment for this rare infection. 5FC + Itra proved to be the therapy of choice in chromomycosis cases caused by *Fonsecaea pedrosoi* [483]. A case of disseminated phaeohyphomycosis due to *Exophiala spinifera* responded well to combination therapy with 5FC + Itra [514, 515]. Controlled clinical trials are not feasible because the patients are so scattered; therefore, anecdotes are likely to become the basis for any future change in the therapy for phaeohyphomycosis.

4.3.10 Immunomodulators

There is, of course, more than one way to fight opportunistic infections. The classical approach is chemotherapy with an effective, preferentially fungicidal antifungal. However, one could also use compounds that influence virulence of the fungi or the host defenses. Knowledge concerning virulence is increasing but is not overwhelming. The wide use of antiviral therapy with proteinase inhibitors (HAART) gives us substantial information about the potential of a combination with an inhibitor of virulence plus a traditional antifungal (see next section). The ability to influence the host immune system meanwhile has become a reality. Knowledge of the host defense mechanism is steadily accumulating, and research in immunology has characterized much of the body's diverse armament of interleukins (IL), interferons (IFN), colony-stimulating factors, tumor necrosis factor, etc. Various cytokines have been isolated and thoroughly investigated *in vitro* and *in vivo* to define their role in the defense against fungal infections [483, 516, 517]. Several of them have been produced using biochemical methods.

The scope of this section is too small to give a full overview on all defense mechanisms; it can only mention some of the possibilities and mainly concentrates on the cytokines available in the clinic.

Some cytokines were found to show a deteriorating capacity, increasing the acute course of fungal infection. For example, IL-4 decreases the survival in candidosis, and IL-10 reduces the killing effect of monocytes against *C. albicans*. Most immunomodulators, however, have the capacity to increase host defense and therefore cause an increase in survival time or a decrease of the fungal burden [483]. Human salivary histatins and human defensins show significant activity against *C. albicans* [518]. IL-1α and -1β prolonged survival in lethal *Candida* infections. Murine histoplasmosis is associated with depression of cellular immune response due to deficiency in the production of IL-2. This cytokine is able to enhance natural killer cell activity through induction of IFNγ. Treatment with IL-2 has, however, no influence on the course of histoplasmosis. IL-12 treatment stimulates the production of IFNγ and IL-18 in mice infected with *Cryptococcus neoformans*; this increased host defense leads to a certain resistance towards the fungal infection. The combination of IL-12 and -18 also prolongs the survival and reduces the fungal burden in *Cryptococcus*-infected mice [519]. IL-12 and IL-18 synergistically induced the fungicidal activity of murine peritoneal exudate cells against *Cryptococcus neoformans* through production of IFNγ by natural killer cells. IL-15 significantly increases the fungicidal activity of monocytes against *C. albicans* by augmentation of superoxide production [520]. IFNγ stimulates the antifungal activity of macrophages and/or polymorphonuclear neutrophils (PMN). The growth of several fungi including *C. albicans, H. capsulatum,* and *B. dermatitidis,* was significantly more inhibited in the presence of IFNγ-stimulated macrophages and/or PMNs than unstimulated ones. IFNγ was found to be an important component of normal host defense against systemic cryptococcosis [483, 521]. The most promising immunomodulators for fungal infections appear to be the granulocyte-, granulocyte-macrophage-, and macrophage colony-stimulating factors (G-CSF, GM-CSF, M-CSF), which also show activity against new emerging pathogens like *Trichosporon* [522].

It was clearly of interest to investigate whether a synergistic effect exists when cytokines are added to conventional antifungal therapy. The available *in vitro* and animal data clearly show that addition of various immunomodulators augment the beneficial effect of conventional antifungals.

In vitro experiments [483]: The combination of 5FC and an IgG1 monoclonal antibody to *Cr. neoformans* capsular glucuronoxylomannan was more effective in reducing the colony-forming units of *Cryptococcus neoformans* than either agent alone. IFNγ has been found to act *in vitro* synergistically with Amph B, increasing the intracellular killing of *Cryptococcus neoformans* in murine macrophages [523]. Flu combined with various cytokines (IL-4, IL-10, IL-1β, IFNγ, GM-CSF) generally increases the activity of human monocytes against *C. albicans* [524]. Additionally, Flu increased the intracellular antifungal activity of inflammatory cytokine-primed macrophages even though their superoxide and nitric oxide production were decreased [525].

G-CSF, GM-CSF, and M-CSF increase the activity of phagocytic cells and show synergism with several antifungal drugs. GM-CSF activated PMNL, and monocyte-derived macrophages showed enhanced synergy with Flu against *Candida albicans* cells, clearly increasing the killing capacity of the immunologically active cells. Combination of PMN, G-CSF, and fluconazole showed the same synergism. Vori combined with neutrophils inhibits hyphal growth of *Aspergillus fumigatus*. Addition of G-CSF or GM-CSF clearly enhanced this inhibition [526]. The combination of Vori + GM-CSF, however, did not increase the high-level inhibition by monocytes seen with either agent alone. M-CSF, known to enhance the anticryptococcal activity of macrophages and PMNs, showed a clear synergistic effect with Flu, drastically increasing the killing capacity.

Animal experiments: Immunomodulating agents have proven their efficacy in various animal models of bacterial and fungal infections and show synergism with various antifungal drugs [483]. The combination of 5FC and capsule-binding antibody showed a significant synergism in murine cryptococcosis. However, the infection could not be cleared. The addition of IFNγ significantly enhanced the efficacy of Amph B, reducing the fungal burden in more mice as compared to Amph B alone [483, 527]. However, no synergistic effect was seen when Flu was used instead of Amph B. The addition of IFNγ to a suboptimal regimen of Amph B also showed a beneficial effect in murine histoplasmosis; the reduction of the fungal burden in the spleen was significant. Prophylactic treatment with G-CSF afforded significant protection against systemic infection caused by *Candida albicans* and *Aspergillus fumigatus* in neutropenic, cyclophosphamid-treated, mice but not in cortisone-treated mice. Cryptococcosis did not respond to G-CSF therapy. Combined treatment using G-CSF and conventional antimycotics (Amph B, 5FC, Flu, Itra) shows a significant beneficial effect in candidosis, pulmonary aspergillosis, and systemic aspergillosis, but not in cryptococcosis [483, 528]. G-CSF showed no synergistic effect with SCH 56592, a new triazole, in a model of pulmonary aspergillosis in neutropenic (cyclophosphamide-treated) mice when the fungal burden of the lung was measured. However, the combination increased the survival in another model of aspergillosis; the mice were then pre-treated with hydrocortisone [529]. These findings are in contrast to the results of Polak [528], who found no efficacy in animals pre-treated with cortisone. M-CSF exerts effects broadly similar to those of G-CSF. Addition of M-GSF to Amph B or Flu potentiated the antifungal effect in various *Candida* models [483, 530]. The immunomodulator M-GSF also shows synergistic effect with Amph B in murine histoplasmosis [531]. Lactoferrin peptide potentiated the effect of Amph B plus GM-CSF in murine candidosis [532].

Thus, the role of cytokines alone or in combination is now better understood, and the confidence in using cytokines in human chemotherapy for fungal infections has grown significantly. Large clinical trials are not available, but case reports on the use of cytokines alone (as prevention) or combined with an antifungal (as an adjunct to therapy) are accumulating. No guidelines concerning the appropriate doses and duration of therapy are yet available, but the adjunct therapy has found a niche in the fungal infection field, despite the costs of the immunomodulators.

Clinical experience [483]: The data from preliminary human studies combining cytokines with traditional antifungal therapy generally suggest that augmentation of the immune system complements the effect of antifungal therapy. For example, reversal of immunodeficiency is essential for successful recovery from invasive aspergillosis. The depth and duration of granulocytopenia can be decreased by addition of G-CSF or GM-CSF to conventional antifungal therapy, leading to more rapid and complete recovery.

IFNγ proved to be of benefit in the treatment of CNS aspergillosis in a patient with chronic granulomatous disease. The patient recovered after combination therapy with IFNγ + Itra. A case of *Aspergillus sinusitis* refractory to conventional therapy was successfully cured with a combination therapy of IFNγ plus Amph B, Itra, and 5FC. IFNγ in combination with oral Amph B and nystatin drastically improved the symptoms of a Flu-refractory oropharyngeal candidosis in an AIDS patient [533]. IFNγ was successfully used as adjuvant therapy to L-Amph B in a case of hepatosplenic *Blastoschizomyces capitus* infection [534]. The triple combination of IFNγ + L-Amph B + GM-CSF led to a successful resolution of a hepatosplenic *Candidosis* after chemotherapy for acute myeloid leukemia in a young woman and a middle-aged man.

Most clinical work has been done with the various colony-stimulating factors (G-CSF, GM-CSF, M-CSF). Several encouraging reports exist describing the use of G-CSF in patients with fungal infections and underlying conditions that cause neutrophilic deficiency, such as aplastic anaemia or chronic granulomatous disease [483]. Promising results have been seen in Japan by combining miconazole and G-CSF for the treatment of deep-seated mycoses in patients with gynecological cancers. The beneficial role of G-CSF in the management of two cases of unusual fungal infections caused by *Fusarium* and

Trichosporon also has been described. Both patients died from the underlying disease, but the fungal infections had been cured. Invasive aspergillosis due to *Aspergillus nidulans* in a child with chronic granulomatous disease did not respond to IFNγ + Amph B. However, the child was successfully cured after a bone marrow transplantation and concomitant therapy with L-Amph B + G-CSF. The combination of Flu + G-CSF was also successfully used to treat fungemia in patients with hematological malignancies. Two poorly controlled diabetic patients with rhinocerebral mucormycosis responded well to a combination therapy with G-CSF + lipid complex Amph B.

GM-CSF has been used successfully as adjuvant therapy for various fungal infections in cancer patients [483]. A case of massive intracerebral aspergillosis responded to a combination of high-dose L-Amph B and GM-CSF therapy without surgery. The potential role of GM-CSF in the treatment of HIV-associated cryptococcal meningitis also has been discussed. The authors suggest that addition of GM-CSF expedites eradication of live fungus but also specifically reduces raised intracranial pressure. They support this hypothesis with two case reports: both patients only poorly responded to Amph B therapy, whereas the symptoms and the fungus rapidly disappeared under the addition of GM-CSF. The combination GM-CSF + L-Amph B was efficacious in the treatment of pediatric AIDS-related cryptococcosis. GM-CSF should also be considered as adjuvant therapy in patients with rhinocerebral zygomycosis [535]. A case of disseminated *Fusarium* infection has been described that was successfully treated with a concomitant therapy of GM-CSF and Amph B.

Bone marrow transplant recipients treated with M-CSF for proven aspergillosis fared better than did historical controls. M-CSF was evaluated in a phase II study as adjuvant therapy in 15 transplant and 10 cancer patients with *Candida* or *Aspergillus* infections. The patients treated with the combination of Amph B + M-CSF survived longer than those with Amph B alone. Long-term mortality was reduced by 19%.

In conclusion, even though the clinical data accumulated to date are still limited, in the future these modulators will become important adjuncts to conventional antifungal therapy of established fungal infections in severely immunosuppresssed patients. These cytokines as single therapy have already found their place in the prevention of fungal infections. The success in reducing the rate of infections in immunosuppressed patients has in some cases been remarkable and awakens real hope for the future. The costs of cytokines are unfortunately still rather high, preventing widespread use in patients at risk of developing fungal infections.

4.4 The methodology: empirical and prophylactic therapy

In recent years both epidemiological studies and autopsy surveys have documented an inexorable rise in the incidence of yeast and mould infections, a significant proportion of which are diagnosed only post-mortem [536, 537]. This phenomen is partially explained by AIDS, the increased frequency of bone marrow and organ transplants, aggressive antineoplastic therapy, and better control of complications such as bacterial infections and hemorrhages. All these changes and improvements have led to an increase in the number of patients at risk for invasive fungal infections. The high associated mortality rate results partially from difficulties in obtaining a reliable diagnosis at an early stage of the disease, often leading to a fatal delay in adequate therapy. Therefore, clinicians are interested in other strategies to fight against invasive fungal diseases.

Four strategies exist today: the normal therapy of proven infections, described on the preceding pages, the empirical therapy, the pre-empiric therapy and the prevention. Efficient antifungal prophylaxis and preemptive therapy are based on the early recognition of groups of patients at high risk and on the elimination of both exogenous and colonizing organisms. Preemptive therapy is frequently given in patients who have some evidence of infection but who do not meet the usual criteria for definite diagnosis or for initiating empirical therapy. The discussion about when and which antifungal should be used for prevention or empiric therapy is still ongoing, and no clear guidelines exist.

Polyene antifungals have been used as prophylactic agents in the management of neutropenic patients for more than two decades, but there was and still is considerable debate about their use. As long as only one, rather toxic, drug existed, the use for prevention was limited; nowadays, however, with a bigger assortment of safe antifungals, the discussion arose whether prevention should be applied for all neutropenic patients or only for specific groups highly at risk to acquire fungal infections. The borders between risk-adapted prophylactic, preemptive, and early empirical use of antifungals become elusive and clinical decision-making depends on local epidemiology-resistant patterns, good definitions of patient risk factors, and calculation of cost-benefit ratios. Empiric and preemptive strategies target a subset of high-risk population that can be identified by serial screening of fungal metabolites or antigens or by early implementation of sensitive imaging techniques. Such a tactic could reduce toxicity, drug resistance development, and costs and exert less epidemiological pressure.

Patients with high suspected fungal infections, without definite diagnosis, are treated empirically. These patients at risk have a high probability (20–40%) of developing invasive fungal infections, and the mortality of established fungal disease remains high (ca. 40–80%) despite chemotherapy. In the past, Amph B has been used as the "gold standard" for empirical therapy.

The environment in which empirical Amph B therapy is practiced has changed. First the azoles appeared, with their potential to be used as empiric antifungal therapy; later the use of hematopoietic factors had an important impact on the use of empirical therapy. Immunostimulators such as G-CSF are able to reduce the duration of neutropenia, and, as a consequence, fewer patients may be at risk to acquire invasive aspergillosis or candidosis. Furthermore, reasonably effective antifungal prophylactic regimens exist nowadays.

The place of empirical antifungal therapy in patients already benefiting from the new treatments mentioned above has to be investigated, and the criteria to initiate empirical therapy have to be defined. The use and choice of antifungals for empiric therapy most probably depends on the local experiences. If aspergillosis is the main problem, an aggressive approach with an early start of empirical Amph B is imperative; however, in centers where aspergillosis is a minor problem, a more liberal approach appears to be appropriate, with a longer period under antibiotic therapy [538]. In 1993, J.S. Faser and D.W. Denning [539] reappraised the empirical use of Amph B, considering all new developments, and they have suggested that use of empirical Amph B be based on risk factors and prophylaxis. The choice of the appropriate antifungal should also be adapted to the epidemiological settings: Flu, the drug with better safety but narrower spectrum, should only be used in those clinics where the risk to acquire aspergillosis is minimal.

The strategic problems are not discussed in full detail in this section, but the clinical experiences with various antifungals in this developing field are presented.

4.4.1 Empirical therapy

Empirical treatment is initiated in immunocompromised patients with persistent fever of unknown origin (4–7 days) that is unresponsive to broad-spectrum antibiotics or when pulmonary infiltrates or cavities are detected by computer tomography scan. Generally, empirical treatment reduces the hospital stay and the duration of treatment and, therefore, the costs; it also reduces the use of aggressive antifungal therapy for established fungal infections and the relapse rates due to therapy failures, as well as reducing mortality and therefore increasing the chances of survival. Unfortunately, no guidelines exist yet about the optimal duration of therapy; the dose; or the ideal antifungal in relation to toxicity and efficacy, the risk factors, and the costs.

For several years, Amph B has been the only drug used to treat febrile neutropenia, and it is still the standard that all new antifungals have to be compared to.

The value of conventional Amph B for empirical treatment was documented in the 1980s in two randomized clinical trials [540, 541]. These studies proved that the use of empirical Amph B in persistently or recurrently febrile neutropenic patients decreased the frequency, morbidity, and mortality of invasive fungal infections. However, in these thorough studies, questions regarding the optimal dose, the length of treatment, and the toxicity remained unanswered. Empirical Amph B clearly reduces the occurrence of a broad spectrum of fungal infections, including aspergillosis, but it does not have the capacity to completely prevent the development of invasive infections. Under empirical Amph B, a breakthrough due to non-*Candida albicans*, *Aspergillus*, *Trichosporon*, *Fusarium*, and *Blastoschizomyces* has been observed [2].

The efficacy of the three new Amph B formulations have been investigated in comparison to conventional Amph B in several studies. All three showed efficacy in this clinical setting [542–545]. Most data exist for L-Amph B [182, 183]: in non-comparative studies, the empirical use of L-Amph B produced clinical improvement in 50–87% of the patients [182]. In two large comparative studies including patients with febrile neutropenia undergoing bone marrow transplantation, L-Amph B showed improved safety and efficacy over conventional Amph B. In the first study [542], the side effects were significantly lower with L-Amph B than with Amph B (36–43% vs. 64%). Nephrotoxic effects were observed in 10-12% of the patients receiving L-Amph and in 24% of the patients treated with Amph B ($p < 0.01$). Additionally, a slight trend toward enhanced efficacy of L-Amph B was seen. In the second large study [546], L-Amph B was again better tolerated, and the overall clinical success (measured as survival, defervescence, resolution of preexisting fungal infections, prevention of breakthrough, and no discontinuation due to toxic side effects) was similar in both groups, but there were significantly fewer breakthrough infections with L-Amph B [180, 183 264a]. Thus, L Amph B has proven to be the better choice than Amph B for empirical therapy and has FDA approval for this indication. Given the higher cost of L-Amph B, the subsequent challenge for therapeutic decision-making will have less to do with efficacy than with costs. ABCD compared with Amph B showed equivalency in the clinical result, while the safety data were rather variable; the nephrotoxicity was lower, but infusion-related side effects were more frequent under ABCD than under Amph B [180, 183, 206, 541]. The empirical use of ABLC was not compared with conventional Amph B but with L-Amph B; the study was mainly focused on the safety issue and not on the efficacy. The outcome of the study clearly favored L-Amph B [541, 547].

The triazoles clearly have potential to be used for empirical therapy, as they are better tolerated and easier to handle than conventional Amph B. Unfortunately, Flu covers no mould infections, and oral Itra (capsule) had bioavailability problems. Flu proved its activity in several clinical studies including bone marrow transplant patients as well as febrile neutropenia patients with cancer [541, 548–551]. In comparative trials, Flu showed equivalency to conventional Amph B when the clinical outcome was studied: the mortality rates and the overall outcome were similar. However, the safety issue clearly favored Flu [548–550]. Itra (intravenous and oral solution) also proved its efficacy for the treatment of febrile neutropenia [395, 396, 541]. Itra was assessed in a comparative trial using the following strategy: the empirical treatment started with intravenous Itra for 2 days followed by oral Itra for 5–14 days. The results showed that Itra was at least as effective as Amph B for the treatment of persistent fever of unknown origin. A secondary analysis revealed a trend towards statistical superiority compared with Amph B. Naturally, Itra was safer than Amph B [451, 552]. Vori, the newest triazole on the market, also showed high efficacy in the treatment of febrile neutropenia [469, 541, 553]. In comparison to L-Amph B, the overall success rates were similar (26–30%), and there were substantially fewer breakthrough fungal infections seen under Vori compared to L-Amph B (8 vs. 21 cases). In comparison to L-Amph B, the Vori group had significantly less infusion-related and nephrotoxic adverse events, and the incidence of hepatotoxicity was similar; however, more visual changes (22% vs. 1%) and more hallucinations (4.3% vs. 0.5%) occurred in the Vori group [553].

In conclusion, the armamentarium of antifungal drugs effective for the treatment of febrile neutropenia is steadily increasing, giving a chance for all patients at risk.

4.4.2 Prophylaxis and preemptive therapy

The success of prophylaxis depends on both the host and the pathogenicity of the fungus. Different measures have to be used to prevent an airborne *Aspergillus* infection compared with an endogenous *Candida* infection preceded by colonization of mucosal surfaces. The literature describing the usefulness and the danger of widely applied prevention is impressive; recently the field has been reviewed by Groll and colleagues; additionally, guidelines are given regarding both technical and chemotherapy-related prevention [554].

Generally, antifungal prophylaxis has been found to be effective in reducing fungal colonization, in empirical antifungal therapy, and in cases of invasive candidosis; however, there has been no proven successful prevention of invasive aspergillosis, and the data on overall mortality are not highly convincing. Effective chemoprophylaxis of invasive *Candida* infections with a long-term benefit of overall survival has been demonstrated in patients with allogeneic bone marrow transplants [554, 555]. The oldest technique used in prevention was topical decontamination with oral polyenes or non-absorbable azoles. Oral polyenes were beneficial against superficial candidosis by *Candida*, but the results in prevention of invasive fungal infections were not overwhelming [554, 556]. Moreover, oral polyenes are not well-tolerated and do not prevent invasive aspergillosis.

Technical measures are useful to avoid exposure of high-risk patients to aerosolized spores of *Aspergillus*. Isolation in laminar air-flow rooms equipped with high-efficiency particulate air filters (HEPA) have reduced the incidence of aspergillosis. This technique is mandatory for all bone marrow transplant recipients.

Nasal administration of Amph B aerosol may be another prophylactic technique against infections by *Aspergillus*. Amph B aerosols have shown high effectiveness in preventing pulmonary aspergillosis in animal models. Based on positive animal data, prophylaxis with aerosolized Amph B has been proposed for human chemotherapy as well. This technique remains, however, controversial; in some papers the aerosolized Amph B showed a high potential for prevention, while in other studies the efficacy and tolerability were disappointing [1, 2, 554, 555, 557]. Long-term inhalation of Amph B, however, resulted in preventing invasive aspergillosis in all lung transplant patients.

Parenteral Amph B has clearly shown activity in prevention, but its wide use has been hampered by its high rate of side effects and its complicated handling [558–560]. Combining conventional Amph B in its oral, parenteral, and aerosol formulations was highly effective in preventing invasive fungal infections in high-risk patients [561]. The use of conventional Amph B home infusion proved to be efficacious and well tolerated [562]. The potential of the new lipid formulations of Amph B for prophylaxis has also been investigated in some clinical studies: L-Amph B is probably the only form that can be used for prophylactic therapy because toxicity is reduced in all measures [183, 562a]. ABCD shows too many infusion-related side effects, and ABLC is indeed associated with a reduction in nephrotoxicity, but less in other parameters. L-Amph B showed high efficacy in reducing colonization and in preventing invasive fungal infections [180, 183, 563, 563a]. L-Amph B is therefore a clear step forward in the field of prevention and is a positive alternative to conventional Amph B.

The advent of the absorbable, well-tolerated triazoles Flu and Itra has revolutionized prevention against fungal infections. For the first time, absorbable agents are available that are well tolerated and easy to handle. They can be more widely applied and therefore are predestined to replace parenteral Amph B in prevention. Most clinical studies have been done with Flu, which is intensively used for therapy of oral candidosis and secondary prevention of recurrent oral candidosis and meningeal cryptococcosis in AIDS patients. Itra (in the form of oral solution), on the other hand, with the broader spectrum including aspergillosis, holds promise for treatment and prophylaxis of aspergillosis.

In a large multi-center study with AIDS patients in an advanced state of the disease, Flu given prophylactically reduced the frequency of cryptococcosis, mucosal candidosis, and superficial fungal infections but did not influence the overall mortality rate [564]. Unfortunately, the study did not investigate the rates of Flu resistance. Thus, the central question remains whether the benefits of primary prevention outweight the risk of drug resistance. The same positive results were seen in other studies [565, 566]. Before the HAART era, weekly prevention with Flu was successfully and widely used in patients with AIDS. In countries using the highly effective antiviral therapy (HAART), secondary prophylaxis can be discontinued [567].

Primary prophylaxis with Flu has been investigated in a variety of patient groups, including bone marrow transplant recipients, patients undergoing intensive chemotherapy for hematological neoplasia, liver transplant patients, surgical patients, and pediatric patients with cancer [2, 554]. All clinical data confirm that Flu is better tolerated than oral Amph B or nystatin and that Flu has a good safety profile in all patient groups. In all clinical studies, Flu significantly reduced the incidence of fungal colonization, in particular with respect to *C. albicans*. In connection with this vital reduction, Flu was found to prevent intraabdominal candidosis in high-risk surgical patients [568]. Colonization of non-*albicans* species (*C. glabrata* or *tropicalis*) seems, however, to be increased under Flu prophylaxis [554, 569]. Effective chemoprophylaxis with Flu of invasive candidosis with a long-term benefit for overall survival has been clearly demonstrated in the patient group with allogeneic bone marrow transplantation. In comparison to placebo, Flu significantly reduced superficial candidosis (7 vs. 0%), invasive fungal infections (18 vs. 7%), empirical Amph B (55 vs. 38%), fungal-related mortality (21 vs. 17%), and overall mortality (34 vs. 20%). Eight years later, the patients with Flu prophylaxis showed a significantly higher survival rate (44.7 vs. 27.7%, $p = 0.0001$) [554, 570].

The beneficial value of Flu prophylaxis in other patient groups is variable, i.e., it is dependent on specific risk factors. Flu reduces the incidence of invasive fungal infection and fungal related mortality in some subgroups of patients, but in others only the incidence of superficial candidosis is reduced [554, 560, 571–575].

In a meta-analysis of 16 randomized trials including 3734 patients with neutropenia, Flu did not show an overwhelming beneficial effect: Flu reduced superficial fungal infections but not fungal-related death or invasive fungal infections. The authors of this analysis concluded that the widespread use of Flu prophylaxis in neutropenic patients is not supported by clinical data [576]. One study performed in a center where aspergillosis is known to be the predominant opportunistic infection should be mentioned: in none of the patients treated prophylactically with Flu was invasive candidosis diagnosed, but this advantage was offset by an increased number of infections caused by moulds [577]. Finally, the hidden danger of widespread prevention with Flu has to be mentioned. Continuous long-term Flu prophylaxis can lead to cryptococcal meningitis with Flu-resistant strains and to invasive *Candida* infections due to non-*albicans* species [554, 578, 579]. On the other hand, the widely used secondary prophylaxis with Flu for oropharyngeal candidosis in patients with AIDS significantly reduced the incidence of cryptococcosis in AIDS patients.

Itra, the triazole with a broader activity against aspergilli, represents an alternative to Flu in prevention. The use of Itra in prophylaxis – compared to placebo, oral Amph B or Flu – has been intensively studied in the last few years (reviewed in [416, 554, 555, 580, 581]). Itra is recommended as primary prophylaxis in AIDS patients who live in developing countries, where the highly active combination antiretroviral therapy is not available [582]. The capsule form showed variable results due to gastrointestinal resorption problems in different patient populations; it seems that a correlation exists between serum levels and prophylactic efficacy of the drug [560]. Itra in its oral or intravenous form may be a step forward in preventing invasive aspergillosis. Oral solution has proven its value in the field of chemoprophylaxis: Itra significantly reduced superficial candidosis and proven or suspected systemic fungal infections [416]. The patients with the longest duration of neutropenia and the highest proportion of bone marrow transplant patients showed the greatest advantage [579]. Itra showed similar or even better efficacy than Flu; in one trial Itra reduced proven fungal infections and fungal-related mortality to a greater degree than Flu. Itra clearly has a superiority to prevent aspergillosis but it is less well tolerated than Flu, probably due to its carrier, showing osmotic effects in the gastrointestinal tract [416, 554, 583]. Itra also showed better efficacy than oral Amph B [416, 584]. Intravenous Itra has not yet been studied in the field of prevention.

Chemoprophylaxis unfortunately does not prevent all invasive fungal infections. For example, six cases of breakthrough *C. tropicalis* fungemia were reported during Keto prophylaxis [585]. Nosocomial breakthrough fungemia due to *C. albicans* and non-*albicans Candida* as well as *Trichosporon* were diagnosed in 41 cancer patients treated prophylactically with Flu, Itra, Keto, and/or empirically with Amph B [586]. The risk factors have been investigated; breakthrough infections are more frequent in patients with acute leukemia, quinolone prophylaxis, mucositis, and catheter-associated infections. Most of these breakthrough infections respond well to the combination of 5FC + Amph B.

An open question that is not yet solved is: to which costs is a broad prevention allowed? For example, chemoprophylaxis in neutropenic patients with Flu is more expensive than with other drugs used for prevention. The good efficacy of prophylactic Itra – in post cardiac transplant patients – however, seems to balance the additional cost of the antifungal [587].

An alternative to widespread chemoprophylaxis is surely preemptive treatment in well-defined groups of patients at high risk. Preemptive therapy with ABLC, Flu, or Itra has a beneficial effect in highly immunosuppressed patients. Preemptive ABLC was a clinically effective, cost-effective, and non-invasive therapy that allowed scheduled chemotherapy to be continued but prevented the morbidity and mortality associated with recurrent pulmonary fungal infection [588]. Preemptive ABLC in 10 high-risk liver transplant recipients cleared fungal colonization [589]. Preemptive Flu or Itra after lung transplantation led to a lower incidence of invasive fungal infections [590].

5 The near future in research and clinics

In recent years, biochemists and molecular biologists have intensively studied fungal cells and have identified several potential targets for antifungal chemotherapy, including cell wall synthesis, membrane function barriers, sterol biosynthesis, nucleic acid synthesis, metabolic inhibition, amino acid synthesis, transport systems, macromolecular biosynthesis, adhesion, and dimorphism. Three research lines on the established proven side are being worked on: several scientific groups are still looking for a new cloth of Amph B. Scientific knowledge about the sterol biosynthesis pathway has increased enormously since the first synthesis of a sterol biosynthesis inhibitor more than 30 years ago; the skill of chemists in synthesizing fungus-specific sterol biosynthesis inhibitors has also increased. Finally, extensive clinical experience has guided both biochemists and chemists in designing specific, safer inhibitors. The last newcomer is Vori, with its particular activity against moulds and other triazole molecules with individual properties in clinical trials. The inhibition of cell wall constituents, a fungal-specific target, is another attractive field for research. After enormous efforts in research and many drawbacks, the breakthrough in 2001 with the candin group was successful, and other derivatives may soon follow.

Intensive interest in innovative, specific new approaches to antifungal chemotherapy is evident in universities and pharmaceutical industries [591–597]; but compared with the three targets mentioned above, the practical use of these new targets is still in its adolescence. The most cutting-edge scientists study the areas of genome manipulation and inhibition of virulence factors.

5.1 Polyenes

After the success of the three lipid formulations of Amph B, further formulations of Amph B, the antifungal with the broadest spectrum, have been investigated. Additionally, nystatin, the highly active but also highly toxic polyene, has been developed in its lipid formulation for systemic application.

Attenuation of nephrotoxicity is achieved by incorporating Amph B into lipid nanospheres (NS-718) or into intralipids containing 10-20% soybean oil. These new formulations were active *in vitro* and *in vivo* against yeasts. Additionally, immunoliposomal Amph B-formulations (the liposome is modified by monoclonal antibodies for active targeting to specific sites) are being investigated [164, 596, 597]. For years, the name of Borowski has been associated with the study of new Amph B derivatives, since his group synthesized less toxic and more soluble derivatives. Amph B-methyl ester even reached the clinic, but the development had to be discontinued due to neurotoxic side effects. One of the newer publications describes a N-methyl-N-fructosyl Amph B-methyl ester, a derivative aggregating in different forms in various solutions [2, 598]. A derivative of patricin, N-demethylaminoacetyl-patricin, is still in preclinical development in Japan [599, 600]. The most advanced polyene in clinical development is Nyotran, the liposomal formulation of nystatin. Nyotran has a broad spectrum *in vitro* and is highly active in various animal models. It is, in contrast to the mother compound, well tolerated and exerts no toxicity toward human erythrocytes [195]. Equal doses of Nyotran were more efficacious and safer than traditional Amph B in animal models. In humans Nyotran is safely tolerated and revealed a pharmacokinetic profile with a rapid initial clearance from blood and a terminal-phase half-life of 207 ± 79 min. Nyotran is far advanced in its clinical development.

It showed the same efficacy as Amph B in empirical therapy. Nyotran was also efficacious in treatment of invasive candidosis, meningeal cryptococcosis, and aspergillosis, but in cryptococcal meningitis Nyotran was not equivalent to Amph B. Interestingly, Nyotran has been shown to have antiviral activity and inhibits proliferation of two different HIV-1 strains [2, 164, 195, 490a, 601–603].

Additionally, new macrolide structures have been isolated from nature, and new derivatives are being synthesized in laboratories of the industry, such as spongistatin, cryptosporin, galbonide, erythromycin derivatives, or SPK-843. The state of development is, however, uncertain [591, 604, 605].

5.2 Sterol biosynthesis inhibitors

The class of lanosterol $C_{14}\alpha$-demethylase inhibitors, specifically the triazoles, is still the most intensively studied field. In the near future, at least two molecules will reach the market after having finished the phase III studies: posoconazole (SCH56592; Pos) is a close relative to Itra with a broad antifungal spectrum. Its *in vitro* activity proved to be superior to Flu and Amph B against a variety of primary pathogens and opportunistic fungi, including Flu-resistant strains. It also showed high activity against dermatophytes [591, 592]. Some fungicidal activity was also demonstrated [2]. Pos was highly active in animal models of opportunistic and true pathogen fungi. It seems to be the first triazole with *in vivo* activity in murine fusariosis, a real hope for the medical world; additionally, it shows activity in murine chagas infection, leishmaniasis, and pseudallescheriosis [2, 490a, 591]. Pos may have the advantage over Itra of penetrating into the brain [164]; as with Itra, an oral suspension showed a significantly better bioavailability than the tablet forms. The terminal elimination half-life is 25 h; therefore, a once-daily dosing is possible, as Pos has an interaction profile with cyclosporin A similar to that of the other azoles [164, 490a]. Pos suspension is an equally well tolerated and effective alternative to Flu in the treatment of oropharyngeal candidosis in HIV-positive patients. Pos was efficacious as salvage treatment of serious invasive fungal infections and it was well tolerated. Additionally, Pos merits further evaluation in coccidioidomycosis [591].

Ravuconazole (BMS 207147, formerly ER 30346; Rav) shows the same broad antifungal spectrum as Vori or Pos, including Flu-resistant *Candida* sp.

Rav was minimally affected by overexpression of the gene encoding efflux pump MDR1, thus it may show minimal cross-resistance [169]. Rav showed *in vivo* activity in various animal models of opportunistic and true pathogenic fungi [164, 196, 490a, 591, 593]. Rav is well tolerated with no dose-limiting adverse reactions: the most frequent adverse event was headache. Rav has a long elimination half-life, between 29–53 h, and modest inter-subject variability. Rav seems to be a less potent inhibitor of CYP3A4 compared to other azoles; therefore, a lower rate of interactions with other drugs may be anticipated [490a, 591]. Rav also showed activity in oropharyngeal candidosis [490a].

There is still intensive research going on in the triazole field; 24 new azole derivatives are in the pipeline, and some derivatives are already on the way to be clinically tested. Whether they will be able to overcome the ever-increasing hurdle of market introduction is not yet clear. Some of the new molecules are: Tak-456, R120758 (CS-758); UR 9825, syn 2836/2869/2903/2921; and SS750 and CS758 [2, 490a, 591, 604]. Janssen recently discovered lead structures based on 4-substituted imidazoles [606]; most azoles with antifungal activity have N-substitution.

Ergosterol biosynthesis remains an interesting field for research: several researchers are looking for non-azole inhibitors of the lanosterol $C_{14}\alpha$-demethylase. Roche and Merck discovered by microbiological screening restrictin, a tetrahydropyran derivative with an alkenyl side chain, which inhibits the demethylase of *Candida* and also shows some *in vitro* and *in vivo* activity [2, 607]. Abott has put considerable effort into research to develop non-azole inhibitors of lanosterol $C_{14}\alpha$-demethylase. A-39806, the most potent compound, showed good activity on the level of the enzyme and also exerts *in vitro* activity [608]. Derivatives inhibiting the essential C_4-demethylation have been characterized [2], e.g., 6-amino-22-n-phenylthiobenzathiazole inhibits the C_4-demethylation step and also interferes with C_{14}-demethylation and squalene epoxidase [609]. The inhibitory activity of 2,2, diamino-4,4-dithiazol derivatives most probably is also based on interference with the lanosterol $C_{14}\alpha$-demethylase [610]. Besides the above-mentioned lanosterol $C_{14}\alpha$-demethylase, other enzymes in the long cascade of enzymatic steps to ergosterol are targeted; CJ-15183 [611] and bisabosquals [612] inhibiting the squalene synthase have been isolated and characterized. The 4-pyrrolidinoyridines are a new family of highly potent inhibitors of the oxido-squalene cyclase [591].

5.3 Antifungal targeting fungal cell wall

Fungal cell walls are composed of some unique components, such as 1,3-β-glucan, mannan, and chitin. Unlike sterols, these components have no mammalian counterpart. Highly specific antifungals can be detected In this field.

5.3.1 Target: glucan

The first inhibitor of 1,3-β-glucan synthase, caspofungin, has recently reached the market. Two derivatives also belonging to the class of candins are far advanced in their development.

Micafungin (FK-463, MICA) is just filing for approval. MICA has the same antifungal spectrum as CAS, including *Candida* and *Aspergillus*; it is fungicidal against *Candida* but exerts no activity against *Cr. neoformans*, *Fusarium*, and *Trichosporon*. MICA, similar to all echinocandins, significantly inhibits the adherence of *C. albicans* to epithelial cells [490a, 591, 613, 614]. MICA showed high efficacy in various animal models in immunocompetent and immunosuppressed animals [591, 615–617]. MICA in combination with nikkomycin, but not with Itra or Amph B, showed synergism in murine aspergillosis [490a]. However, in another model of aspergillosis, MICA and Amph B were synergistic [591]. Intravenous MICA is well tolerated in adults and in children, the maximal tolerated dose being clearly above 4 mg/kg/day, and its elimination half-life lies between 11.6 and 15.2 h [490a, 618]. The full phase III studies are not yet published, but some preliminary clinical reports show that MICA is clearing oropharyngeal candidosis in AIDS patients [591]. MICA is of beneficial value for candidemia in cancer patients and for invasive candidosis and aspergillosis [490a]. The third candin candidate far advanced in its development is anidulafungin (V-echinocandin, Ly-303366, VECH). This compound was first developed as an oral drug; however, the bioavailability was too low to show high efficacy in the clinic [2]. The molecule is now developed as parenteral formulation and is in the late phase III studies. VECH is also a potent inhibitor of the 1,3-β-glucan synthase and has the well-known antifungal spectrum of echinocandins, with fungicidal activity against yeasts and aspergilli. It showed high efficacy in murine candidosis due to Flu-sensitive or Flu-resistant strains; it was active in invasive and pulmonary aspergillosis in neutropenic animals and showed beneficial effect in infections due to *Pneumocystis carinii* [490a, 591, 615]. VEC was well tolerated up to 70–100 mg over 10 days [591], the maximal tolerated dose being estimated as 100–140 mg [490a, 591]. The elimination half-life is dependent on the liver function and lies, dependent on hepatic impairment, between 30–40 h [490a, 619]. Common adverse events are dizziness, nausea, headache, facial flushing, dyspnea, and increased aspartat aminotransferase [615]. VECH does not influence the *in vitro* metabolism of cyclosporin A by pooled human hepatic microsomal fraction [490a]. The extensive phase II/III studies are not yet published, but preliminary studies showed clinical efficacy in candidosis and aspergillosis. VECH is safe and efficacious in treating esophageal candidosis [591]. Other echinocandin analogues in preclinical development have been reported by Roche, Lilly Fujisawa, and Aventis; some of them show improved water solubility. All are highly active *in vitro* and show efficacy in animal models, but it is questionable whether they will reach the market, given the size of the injectable market and the very limited solubility of natural Echinocandins [490a, 615, 620, 621]. Abott synthesized, *via* combinatorial chemistry, cyclopeptamines, echinocandin-type compounds. One such compound, A19421129, has *in vitro* activity comparable to Amph B and Flu.

Recently a non-echinocandin-type lipopeptide, FR 901469, has been isolated. This compound also inhibits glucan synthase, has a good *in vitro* activity against yeasts and aspergilli, and is active in murine candidosis and aspergillosis [615, 622].

5.3.2 Target: chitin

Chitin synthesis is inhibited competitively by the naturally occurring nucleoside-peptides polyoxin and nikkomycin Z. Polyoxin is used as fungicide in agriculture, but nikkomycin has languished in the development process for decades and has never reached the full development stage. Initially nikkomycin Z was found to be highly effective against murine coccidioidomycosis, histoplasmosis, and pulmonary blastomycosis, but the spectrum of the drug was considered to be too narrow to warrant expanded development [2, 623]. Nikkomycin Z inhibits the chitin synthase of *C. albicans*, but its antifungal activity against this yeast is only moderate. The reason that interest in nikkomycin has never died is that this drug potentiates the effect of 5FC, azoles, and echinocandins. Nikkomycin Z showed synergistic or additive effects against the majority of opportunistic fungi when combined with Itra. The already high susceptibility of dimorphic fungi to nikkomycin Z could be significantly increased by combining nikkomycin with Flu [2]. An impressive synergy was also seen between nikkomycin and VECH/MICA/CAS in *Aspergillus fumigatus* and *Coccidioides* immitis [2, 624–626]. Nikkomycin Z combinations also have a synergistic potential in various animal models [164]. Clinicians are in favor of developing nikkomycin as a combination partner for the clinic; however, the problems in developing a drug for combination therapy without the drug's showing efficacy in monotherapy are enormous.

Other inhibitors of the chitin synthases Chs1 or Chs2 have been preclinically characterized: lufenuron was *in vitro* but not *in vivo* active against *Coccidioides immitis* [2]. The aromatic natural product xanthofulvin selectively inhibits the enzyme Chs2 of *C. albicans* and other aromatic natural products. RO 9-3143 or RO 41-0986 specifically inhibited Chs1, leading to cell growth inhibition in wild-type *Candida* strains; simultaneous inhibition of Chs2 is fungicidal [615, 627, 628]. A novel, semi-synthetic protoberberine exhibited the most significant activity against *Candida* by inhibiting two different targets, namely, chitin synthase and sterol Δ-24-methyltransferase [629].

Chitinase, whose action is opposite from chitin synthase, i.e., it lyses the chains of chitin, may become an interesting approach to antifungal therapy. Human chitinase acts synergistically with various antifungals like Amph B, Itra, Flu, nikkomycin Z, and VECH [630].

Researchers at universities are still investigating the nature of cell wall synthesis. They are isolating genes governing the synthesis of chitin and are trying to understand the mechanisms involved in glucan or mannan synthesis. They synthesize various inhibitors of enzymes involved in cell wall synthesis, such as derivatives of bacilysin, inhibitors of L-glutamin-fructose amidotransferase or new azasaccharides, inhibitors of β-1,4-glycosyltransferase [631, 632]. Thus, it may be possible that, based on the new knowledge, better and more specific inhibitors of cell wall synthesis may be discovered for human chemotherapy.

5.4 Natural products and new targets

The literature is full of new antibiotics, and a good proportion of them are antifungals. Every week one can spend a couple of hours in the library reading inhibition zones and MICs of new substances. Some of the antibiotics mentioned stay with us a while, while some disappear very fast, and few are actually new leads for antifungal chemotherapy. It is encouraging to be constantly reminded of the diversity of active substances that nature presents us, and it has happened, and will hopefully happen again, that the next significant advance in antifungal chemotherapy will have had its basis in the *Journal of Antibiotics*.

On the other hand, ancient – nearly lost – knowledge about herbal therapy and medicinal plants has experienced an incredible revival [633, 634]. Extracts from exotic plants are being tested for antifungal activity *in vitro*, and old recipes are detected for the treatment of fungal infections in dermatology. Tea tree oil and garlic are used for fungal infections, and garlic (*Allium sativum*) is highly efficacious against *Cr. neoformans* [635] and is even used for human chemotherapy in China. Benzoic acid derivatives from *Piper lanceaefolium* show weak antifungal activity [636], whereas thyme oil is highly efficacious against *C. albicans* [637]. Mungin, a novel cyclopholin-like antifungal from the mung bean, shows activity against *Fusarium oxysporum* [638]. Crude extracts of dry cayenne pepper were purified, and a new fungicidal saponin has been detected recently [591]. The venom of the snake *Crotalus duriisus* shows *in vitro* efficacy against a variety of *Candida* species, *Sporotrix schenckii*, *Mucor indicus*, and *Rhizopus* spp. [639]. It may be that the industry will use one of these known compounds to lead to totally new developments; at any rate, the literature is full of natural products with antifungal activity [604, 633, 634].

The isolation and structure elucidation of the antibiotic azoxybacilin, an unusual amino acid structure with an azoxy moiety, have led researchers toward a new antifungal target: azoxybacilin exerts its antifungal activity through inhibition of the regulation of the genes for fungal-specific sulfate assimilation. It inhibits the enhancement of transcription of the MET4 gene, which in turn would result in partial repression of the genes required for sulfate assimilation. This was the first time that an antifungal has been detected that interferes with the regulation of gene expression, and thus isolation of new natural products provides an approach for identifying an antifungal with a totally new mode of action [640].

Peptides and protein derivatives are a new class of antifungal agents that are drawing high interest. Besides the echinocandin class, which is far advanced in development, several polypeptides with partially unidentified modes of action but clear antifungal properties have been patented and are under investigation by various pharmaceutical companies, e.g., a cyclic hexapeptide, A175800.0, shows *in vitro* and *in vivo* activity against *C. albicans*, and a lipoprotein (WF 11899A) exerts good *in vitro* activity [195, 604, 641].

Other new targets used in screening for antifungals are:

- proton-pumping ATPase (complex carbohydrates and conjugated steryl ketones inhibit this enzyme and show antifungal activity *in vitro* [591, 642, 643]);
- fatty acid synthetase (in microbiological screening, eight related compounds were identified by Dorlin Pharmaceuticals [591]);
- Zn-chelation, an essential element for fungal growth;
- *Candida*: yeast transcription factor IIB; protein kinase, phenotypc switching protein Cg51n etc. [604];
- a new family of DNA-targeting compounds has been detected with activity against moulds and yeasts [490a];
- the target elongation factor 2 has lead to a new class of antifungals intensively studied, namely, the sordarins.

5.4.1 Sordarins

Sordarin derivatives, a new class of antifungals, are selective inhibitors of the protein synthesis specifically impairing elongation factor 2 function [644–646]. Sordarin derivatives have a broad antifungal spectrum that includes opportunistic fungi and true pathogen fungi. The degree of activity varies from derivative to derivative, azasordarins showing a slightly different spectrum than the traditional sordarins, e.g., they have potential against dermatophytes. Sordarins are always highly sensitive against azole-sensitive or -resistant *C. albicans*; the sensitivity of the other *Candidas* varies from derivative to derivative. The same is true for aspergilli. Sordarins are also active against true pathogenic fungi such as *H. capsulatum*, *P. brasiliensis*, *B. dermatitidis* (yeast form), and *Cocc. immitis* (mycelium form). They also influence the growth of some rare moulds and dermatophytes [195, 591, 647–649]. Combinations of sordarins plus Amph B or Itra were synergistic or additive against *Candida*, *Aspergillus*, and *Scedosporium*; Flu plus sordarins was additive against Candida [195]. Sordarins are also efficacious in several animal models such as systemic candidosis, oral or vaginal candidosis, coccidioidomycosis, histoplasmosis, and pneumocystosis [195, 591, 650–653]. Preliminary toxicological data show that sordarins are rather safe [591]. Human data are not yet available, but sordarins appear promising based on their favorable activity on pathogenic yeasts and *P. carinii*. We will surely hear more about this class of compounds in the near future.

5.5 Virulence

So far all antifungals have been targeted to inhibit metabolic pathways of the fungi; none of the available drugs interfere directly with the virulence of the fungus. In the past, because basic research mainly tried to understand cell structure and to evaluate the biochemical functioning of a fungal cell, less interest was invested in understanding the process of pathogenicity.

Interest in better understanding the pathogenicity and virulence of fungal cells has continuously increased in the past few years. Several virulence factors or virulence genes have been identified. The group of Kwong Chung has studied the virulence and pathogenicity of *Cr. neoformans* [2]. They identified at least three virulence factors: the fungus has to (1) be able to grow at 37 °C, (2) produce polysaccharide capsules, and (3) have an active phenol oxydase in order to synthesize melanin from dopa. These three factors are located in three different alleles and are easily and independently changed by appropriate genetic manipulation. A single mutation at any one of these three characteristics leads to a significant reduction in virulence. Glyphosphate inhibits melanization of *Cr. neoformans* and decreases the survival following systemic infection in mice [654]. Melanin also plays an important role in the pathogenicity of dematiaceous fungi. Mutants unable to synthesize melanin, which is located in the cell wall of this black fungi, lose their virulence [2, 655]. The virulence of *C. albicans* has been found to be strongly dependent on phosphate lipase and proteinase production [2]. These two virulence factors are being intensively investigated at various universities [655]. In 1994, F. Odds [656] profoundly discussed various putative virulence factors of *Candida*, including the rapid switching of the surface, hydrophobicity, and other properties of this yeast. The state of the art regarding fungal virulence genes as targets for antifungal chemotherapy was summarized in 1996 [657]. In this review all of the above-mentioned factors are included and several others are mentioned, such as the chitin synthesis genes CHS2 and CHS3 [658], the elastase gene AFA7P, the purin metabolism gene ADE2, and the multiple drug resistance gene CaMDR1, among others.

Some available antifungals have the ability to decrease the virulence of the fungal cell in addition to their primary mechanism of action. For example, fungal cells pre-treated with subinhibitory concentrations of Amph B or azoles lose some of their virulence. Some *Candida* isolates resistant to 5FC have decreased virulence in comparison to wild-type isolates. Echinocandins significantly interfere with the adherence of *Candida* cells to epithelial cells, the first step toward penetration and pathogenicity [613]. Exposure to subinhibitory concentration of Flu can result in enhanced extracellular production of aspartyl proteinase [659]. Induction of Flu resistance in *C. albicans* also may induce changes of virulence factors; a Flu-resistant mutant was superior in all the virulence traits examined, including germination, adherence ability, secreted proteinase, and phospholipase production [660]. On the other hand, some Flu-resistant strains show decreased virulence. Thus, the relationship of Flu *versus Candida* is rather complex if virulence is taken as a marker [661].

Most studies attempting to understand pathogenicity of fungi have been conducted at universities, but in recent years several pharmaceutical companies have risked studying virulence factors and initiating chemical programs in this field [662]. Two virulence factors of *C. albicans* have been intensively studied, namely, phospholipase and proteinase.

C. albicans secretes phospholipases, which are considered to be one of the mediators of cell penetration and consequently one of the main factors in pathogenicity. Up to present, many different groups and subgroups of phospholipases have been detected; the known phospolipases have been recently described under clinical aspects [663]. It is known that other phospolipases from mammalian cells can be inhibited by lipophilic beta-blocking structures. Aventis had a chemical synthesis program in the field of beta-blocking, and, as a result of this effort, several structures with antifungal activity deriving from the structure of β-hydroxyethylamine have been detected. These compounds inhibit the secretion of phospholipase and fungal growth *in vitro*. Histological examination confirmed the inhibitory effect of the beta-blocker-like structures on tissue penetration. Most of these compounds showed only weak efficacy in animal models when given alone, but in combination with Flu they were able to prevent death in mice infected with lethal inocula of *C. albicans* [664]. These β-hydroxyethylamine derivatives are the lead structures for new antifungals with a totally new attack on the fungal cells.

The aspartate proteinases (SAP) of *C. albicans* are the most thoroughly studied virulence factor. Their role in the pathogenicity of *Candida* species has been established in various studies and today is undisputed [2, 655]. The relationship between SAP gene(s) expression and pathogenicity has been intensively studied: some SAP-deleted strains suffered a substantial loss of virulence, and, more interestingly, this was specifically associated with selected gene products and selected experimental pathologies. There is now initial evidence that distinct SAPs are produced differently in various *Candida* illnesses or stages of them [665]. One of the genes has been sequenced [666], and proteinase A has been crystallized [667].

It has been known for a long time that pepstatin A inhibits the production of proteinases and reduces the adherence of *Candida* cells to epithelial cells. Pepstatin A was also found to be moderately efficacious in a model of murine candidosis [668]. Also, some of the antifungals on the market have been found to be potent inhibitors of the *Candida* proteinases [669]. Meanwhile, new natural products with pepstatin-like structures have been isolated that significantly impaired the *in vitro* activity of some *Candida* proteases. Additionally, new peptidomimetic aspartic protease inhibitors derived from pepstatin showed excellent activity in the range of 0.1–1 nM against four *Candida* proteases [670].

Based on the positive results with pepstatin and the existing chemical programs for inhibitors of the HIV proteases, several institutions started innovative programs to detect new *Candida*-specific protease inhibitors with higher activity at the enzyme level combined with *in vivo* activity. Abbott and Yamanouchi have a long-standing chemical program and have detected compounds with good inhibitory activity on the level of the enzyme, but the *in vitro* activity of these compounds is not yet overwhelming [671].

Remarkable knowledge regarding the interaction of inhibitors with the *Candida* proteases can be accumulated since the introduction of the potent HIV-protease inhibitors. Ritonavir, saquinavir, and indinavir inhibit the proteases SAP1, SAP2, and SAP3 but not the proteases SAP4, SAP5, and SAP6. These HIV protease inhibitors react on the level of the enzyme, decrease the production of enzyme, and reduce the adherence of yeast cells to epithelial cells, ritonavir being the most potent of the three agents [672–675]. Furthermore, viability and growth of *C. albicans* were markedly reduced by indinavir [676]. These inhibitory effects explain how the antiviral protease inhibitors may help to resolve mucosal candidosis and suggest that future derivatives could constitute alternatives to current treatments in refractory cases. The HIV inhibitors additionally have a clear influence on the epidemiology of oropharyngeal candidosis in AIDS patients. A marked reduction in oral candidosis following the initiation of combination antiretroviral therapy including a protease inhibitor was noted in the UK and also in other western countries [677]. This phenomenon is explainable by the better immune status of the patients but also may be explained by a direct influence of the drugs on the yeast cells.

Pepstatin and the four HIV protease inhibitors indinavir, ritonavir, nelfinavir, and saquinavir additionally exerted strong growth-inhibitory effects on *P. cariinii* trophozoites [678].

Bioassay-guided fractionation of the active chloroform fraction from the roots of *Tovomita krukovii* using *Candida* protease assay led to the isolation of four new xanthones and 10 known compounds. Four of these compounds not only showed activity on the enzyme level but also displayed *in vitro* activity against *C. albicans* and *Cr. neoformans* [679].

Fluphenazine is known to antagonize azole activity and to up-regulate gene expression of the drug efflux pump in Flu-sensitive isolates. This compound increases in azole-susceptible strains the production of the virulence factor aspartyl proteinase; this double interaction may adversely influence the clinical outcome of patients infected with a azole-susceptible *Candida* strains and treated with fluphenazine plus azole [490a].

6 Conclusions

Instead of a summary of the data presented in the chapter, several tables summarize the options the medical world has today to treat fungal infections caused by dermatophytes or opportunistic or true pathogenic fungi (see Tables 1–4).

Table 1.
Management options for superficial fungal infections

Dermatomycoses	*Oral*: terbinafine, itraconazole, fluconazole; *topical*: azoles, allylamines, morpholines etc. (oral therapy is essential for tinea capitis)
Onychomycoses mild	*Oral*: terbinafine, itraconazole, fluconazole; *topical*; nail lacquer: ciclopyrox or amorolfine
Onychomycoses severe	Combination of topical and short oral treatment
Vaginal candidosis	*Oral*: fluconazole, itraconazole; *topical*: azoles, polyenes
Pityriasis	Azoles: oral or topical
Seborrhoeic eczema	Ketoconazole shampoo, terbinafine solution, ciclopyrox shampoo, selsun (selenium sulfide) shampoo

Table 2.
Management options for invasive fungal infections caused by opportunistic yeasts

Fungal disease	First choice	Second choice	Future
Candidosis			
Oral candidosis	Fluconazole	Itraconazole, oral Amph B	Caspofungin
Candidaemia	Conventional or liposomal amphotericin B, fluconazole	Itraconazole intravenous	Caspofungin
Acute single site or disseminated candidosis ± fungemia	Conventional or liposomal amphotericin B, amphotericin B (conventional or liposomal) + flucytosine	Fluconazole	New combinations Second generation triazoles Echinocandins
Cryptococcosis			
CNS in HIV-negative patients: initial therapy	Amphotericin B ± flucytosine	Amphoterin B (conventional or liposomal)	
Pulmonary on HIV patients	Fluconazole	Amphotericin B (conventional or liposomal)	
CNS on HIV patients: initial therapy	Amphotericin B + flucytosine; 5FC + Flu + Amph B	Liposomal Amph B; flucytosine + fluconazole; amphotericin B + itraconazole; 5FC + Amph B + Itra	
Consolidation and maintenance	Fluconazole	Itraconazole	Amphotericin B
Trichosporon and blastoschizomyces infections	Fluconazole	Second generation triazoles	
Other rare yeast infections			
Rodotorula rubra infection *Hansenula anomala* etc.	Amphotericin B + flucytosine	Fluconazole	
Empiric therapy			
Fever and neutropenia	Amphotericin B (conventional or liposomal), i.v. itraconazole	Fluconazole	
Intensive care	Fluconazole		

Table 3.
Management options for invasive fungal infections caused by opportunistic moulds

Fungal disease	First choice	Second choice	Future
Aspergillosis			
Initial therapy	Conventional or liposomal amphotericin B, voriconazole	Itraconazole (i.v.); voriconazole caspafungin	New combinations
Consolidation or maintenance therapy	Amphotericin B (conventional or liposomal)	Caspofungin, voriconazole	Second generation triazoles
Aspergillom	Itraconazole		Voriconazole
Allergic aspergillosis	Itraconazole		
Zygomycosis	Amphotericin B (conventional or liposomal)		
Fusariosis	Conventional amphotericin	Voriconazole	Combinations
Phaeohyphomycosis	Itraconazole ± flucytosine	Amphotericin B	Combinations
Penicillium marneffeiinfection	Amphotericn B followed by itraconazole		
Scedosporiosis	Voriconazole		

Table 4.
Management options for invasive fungal infections caused by endemic fungi

Fungal disease	First choice	Second choice	Future
Histoplasmosis			
Life-threatening CNS	Amphotericin B	Fluconazole	
Mild	Itraconazole		
Maintenance in AIDS patients	Itraconazole		
Blastomycosis			
Mild	Itraconazole	Amphotericin B	
Life threatening	Amphotericin B		
Paracoccidiodomycosis			
Mild	Itraconazole	Amphotericin B	
Severe	Amphotericin B	Itraconazole	
Coccidioidomycosis			
Life threatening	Amphotericin B		
Immunocompetent and non-meningeal	Itraconazole		
Immunocompetent and meningeal	Fluconazole		
Maintenance	Fluconazole, itraconazole		
Madura feet	Triazoles		
Chromomycosis	Itraconazole	Itraconazole + flucytosine	
Sporotrichosis			
Lymphocutan, bone, pulmonal	Itraconazole	Fluconazole	Terbinafine (for lymphocutan)
CNS, disseminated	Amphotericin B (conventional or liposomal)		

References

1 A. Polak and P.G. Hartman, in: E. Jucker (ed.): Progress in Drug Research, Vol. 37, Birkhäuser Verlag, Basel 1991, 181–269.

2 A. Polak, in: E. Jucker (ed.): Progress in Drug Research, Vol. 49, Birkhäuser Verlag, Basel 1997, 219–297.

3 P.D. Hoeprich, in: E. Jucker (ed.): Progress in Drug Research, Vol. 44, Birkhäuser Verlag, Basel 1995, 87–127.

4 A.K. Gupta, T.R. Einarson, R.C. Summerbell and N.H. Shear: Drugs *55*, 645–674 (1998).

5 V. Havu, H. Heikkila, K. Kuokkanen, M. Nutinem, T. Rantanen et al.: Br. J. Dermatol. *142*, 97–102 (2000).

6 S. Rand: J. Am. Acad. Dermatol. *43*, 104–112 (2000).

7 J.F.G.M. Meis, and P.E. Verweij: Drugs *61*, 13–25 (2001).

8 M. Abdel Rahman, D.A. Powell, M.C. Nahata: Pharmacotherapy *17*, 1103 (1997).

9 A.K. Gupta, M. E. Alexis, N. Raboobee, S.L.R. Hofstader, C.W. Lynde et al.: Br. J. Dermatol. 137, 251–254 (1997).

10 L.C. Fuller, C.H. Smith, R. Cerio, R.A. Marsden, G.Midgley, A.L. Beard, E.M. Higgins and R.J. Hay: Br. J. Dermatol. *144*, 321–327 (2001).

11 S. U. Budimulja, K. Kuswadji, S. Bramano, J. Basuki, L.S. Judanarso and S. Untung: Br. J. Dermatology. *130* (Suppl. 43), 29 (1994).

12 G.F. Altomare, G.L. Capella, V. Boneschi and M.A. Viviani: Br. J. Dermatol. *142*, 840–841 (2000).

13 A.K. Gupta, P. de Doncker, A. Heremans, P. Stofels, G. E. Piérard, J. Decroix, M. Heenen, H. Degreef.: J. Amer. Academy Dermatol *36*, 789–792 (1997).

14 J. Remme, F.H.J. Rampen, F.C.J. Van Neer: Mycoses *41*, 515–520 (1998).

15 F. Baudraz Rosselet, M. Monod, S. Laccoud, E. Frenk: Br. J. Dermatol *135*, 1011–1012 (1996).

16 H. Hamm, A. Schwinn, M. Bräutigam: Br. J. Dermatol. *140*, 480–482 (1999).

17 G. Baleviciene, O.Ceburkovas and D. Maciuliene: Acta Derm. Venereol. *82*, 61 (2001).

18 J. McClellan, L.R. Wisemann and A. Markham: Drugs *58*, 179–202 (1999).

19 J. Sanjeev and S. Viendra: Int. J. Dermatol. *39*, 4412–423 (2000).

20 ISHAM 14th Congress, 8–12 May 2000, in Argentina, Abstract book.

21 B.H.C. Stricker, M.M. van Riemsdijk, M.C.J.M. Sturkenboom and J.P. Ottervanger: Br. J. Pharmacol *42*, 313 (1996).

22 M. Hall, C. Monka, P. Krupp, D. O'Sullivan: Arch. Dermatol. *133*, 1213–1219 (1997).

23 A.K. Gupta, C.W. Lynde, G.J. Lauzon, M.-A. Mehlmauer, S.W. Braddock et al.: Br. J. Dermatol. *138*, 529–532 (1998).

24 S.M. Abdel-Rahman and M.C. Nahata: Annales Pharmacother. *31*, 445–456 (1997).

24a B. Amichai and M.H. Grunwald: Intern. J. Dermatol. *37*, 410 (1998).

25 D.P. O'Sullivan: Br. J. Dermatol. *141* (Suppl. 56), 21–25 (1999).

26 M. Murphy and L. Barnes: Br. J. Dermatol. *138*, 708–709 (1998).

27 M. Shapiro, I.J. Li and J. Miller: Br. J. Dermatol. *140*, 1196–1197 (1999).

28 C. Rogalski, A. Hürlimann, G. Burg et al.: Hautarzt *52*, 444–448 (2001).

29 N.F. Fernandez, S.A. Geller and T.L. Fong: J. Gastroenterol. *93*, 459–460 (1998).

30 K. Agarwal, D.M. Manas and M. Hudson: N. Engl. J. Med. *340*, 1292–1293 (1999).

31 H.I. Katz: J. Am. Podiatric Med. Assoc. *87*, 571–574 (1997).

32 H.I. Katz: Br. J. Dermatol. *141* (Suppl. 56), 26–32 (1999).

33 E. Schatz, M. Bräutigam, E. Obrowolski, L. Effendy, H. Haberl et al.: Clin. Exp. Dermatol. *20*, 377 (1995).
34 N.H. Shear and A.K. Gupta: Arch. Dermatol. *131*, 937 (1995).
35 M. Bräutigam, S. Nolting, R.E. Schöpf and G. Weidinger: Br. Med. J. *311*, 919 (1995).
36 A.K. Gupta, R.K. Scher and P. de Doncker: Dermatol. Clinics *15*, 121–135 (1997).
37 M. Feuilhade de Chauvin, R. Baran and D. Chabasse: J. Mycol. Med. *11*, 205–215 (2001).
38 A.K. Gupta, N. Konnikov and C.W. Lynde: J. Amer. Acad. Dermatol. *44*, 479–484 (2001).
39 A. Tosti, B.M. Piraccini, C. Stinchi, M.D. Colombo: Dermatology *197*, 162–166 (1998).
39a E.M. Reisberger and R.M. Szeimies: Medizinische Klinik *95*, 618 (2000).
40 L. Molin, M. Tarstedt and C. Engman: Br. J. Dermatol. *143*, 682–683 (2000).
41 E.K.A. van Doorslaer, G. Tormans, A.K. Gupta, K. Van Rossem, A. Eggleston, D.J. Dubois, P. De Doncker, E. Haneke: Dermatology *193*, 239–244 (1996).
42 W. Bergman and F.F.H. Rutten: Ned. Tijdschr. Geneeskd. *138*, 2346 (1994).
43 A. Perez: Mycoses *42* (Suppl. 2), 111–114 (1999).
44 G.E. Schiraldi, S. Lo Cicero, M.D. Colombo, D. Rossato, M. Ferrarese and E. Soresi: Br. J. Dermatol. *134* (Suppl. 46), 25 (1996).
45 R.J. Hay: Br. J. Dermatol. *141* (Suppl. 56), 36–40 (1999).
46 J. Gonzalez Ruperez, M. de Javaloyas de Morlius, A. Moreno Carazo: Dermatology *194*, 85–86 (1997).
47 N.M. Clark: Clin. Infect. Dis. *28* (5), 1169–1170 (1999).
48 M. Rotoli, G. Sascaro and S. Cavalieri: Dermatology *202*, 143 (2001).
49 J.M. Ollague, A.M. Zurita and G. de Calero : Br. J. Dermatol. *143*, 188–191 (2000).
50 P. De Doncker, J. Decroix, G.E. Pidrard, D. Roelant, R. Woestenborghs et al.: Arch. Dermatol. *132*, 34 (1996).
51 K. De Beule and J. Van Gestel: Drugs *61* (Suppl. 1), 27–37 (2001).
52 A.K. Gupta and T.G. Novak: Dermatology *202*, 235–238 (2001).
52a A. Ingber: Med. Mycology *39*, 471 (2001).
53 H. Heikkila and S. Stubb: Acta Derm. Venereol. *77*, 70–71 (1997).
54 W. Bergman and E.R.H. Rutten: Ned. Tijdschr. Geneeskd. *138*, 2346 (1994).
55 D.T. Roberts: Br. J. Dermatol. *141* (Suppl. 56), 1–4 (1999).
56 B. Sigurgeirsson, S. Billstein, T. Rantanen, T. Ruzicka, E. Di Fonzos et al.: Br. J. Dermatol. *141* (Suppl. 56), 5–14 (1999).
57 A.K. Gupta, N. Konnikov, C.W. Lynde: J. Dermatol. Treatment *11*, 151–154 (2000) .
58 A.K. Gupta, Ch. K. Lynde and N. Konnikov: J. Am. Acad. Dermatol. *44*, 485–491 (2001).
58a J. Am. Acad. Dermatol. *38*, S73, S77, S87, S95, S101, S110 (1998).
58b K. Halmy and J. Serfoezoe: Mycoses *44*, 219 (2001).
59 A. Polak: J. Eur. Acad. Dermatol. Venerol. *4* (Suppl. 1), SI 1 (1995).
60 M. Haria and H.M. Bryson: Drugs *49*, 103 (1995).
61 Y. Clayton: Poster at the Dermatology 2000, Vienna (1993).
62 J.W Rippon and R. Fromtling (eds.): Cutaneous Antifungal Agents 1, Marcel Dekker, New York 1993.
63 W. Melchinger, A. Polak and J. Müller: Mycoses *33*, 393 (1988).
64 E.G.V. Evans: Br. J. Dermatol. *145* (Suppl. 60), 9–11 (2001).
65 A. Polak: Mycoses *36*, 101 (1993).
66 M. Zaug: J. Eur. Acad. Dermat. Venerol. *4* (Suppl. 1), S23 (1995).
67 G.G. Lestringant, H. Nszane, M. Nada, M.A. Usmani, R.A. Micallef, A. Montague, P.M. Frossard: J. Dermatol. Treatment *7*, 89–92 (1996).

68 T.R. Einarsen, P.L. Oh, A.K. Gupta, N.H. Shear: J. Dermatol. Treatment *8*, 229–235 (1997).
69 K.M. Humphry, M.J. Cork, A. Haycox: Br. J. Dermatol. *139*, 660–664 (1998).
70 M. Bohn and K. Th. Krämer: J. Am. Acad. Dermatol. *43*, S57–S69 (2000).
71 A.K. Gupta, Ph. Fleckman and R. Baran: J. Am. Acad. Dermatol. *43*, S70–S80 (2000).
72 A.K. Gupta: J. Am. Acad. Dermatol. *43*, S81–S95 (2000).
73 A.K. Gupta and R. Baran: J. Am. Acad. Dermatol. *43*, S96–102 (2000).
74 A. Polak: Mycoses *36*, 43 (1993).
75 J. Laurahanta, M. Zaug, A. Polak and D. Reine: JAMA Southeast Asia *9* (Suppl. 4), 23 (1993).
76 R. Baran, M. Feuilhade, A. Datry, S. Goetmann, P. Pietrini et al.: Br. J. Dermatol. *142*, 1177–1183 (2000).
77 Swiss study, presented by Prof. Burg Zürich in München, Juli 2000.
78 S. Dole, C. Larnier and A. Chicoye: Clinical Dermatology 2000 Vancouver, Abstract 309 (1996).
78a M. Lecha: Br. J. Dermatol. *145* (Suppl. 60), 21 (2001).
78b K.S. Nolting and H. Ulbricht: Mycoses *44*, 247 (2001).
79 G.E. Pierard, C. Pierard-Franchimont and J.E. Arrese: Med. Mycol. *38*, 391–392 (2000).
80 R. Savin: J. Familiy Practice *43*, 127–132 (1996).
81 D.S. Lang, H.M. Richards, J. Guarneri, J.M. Humeniuk, R.C. Savin et al.: J. Am. Acad. Dermatol. *39*, 944–950 (1998).
82 R.T. Borelli, S. Patel, J.S. Venglarcik, D. Moses, D. Gemmel: Pediatric Dermatol. *15*, 406–407 (1998).
83 S. Georgiou, A. Monastirli, E. Pasmatzi, C. Zografakis and D. Tsambaos: J. Eur Acad. Dermatol. Venereol. *8*, 203–207 (1997).
84 M.A. Amer: Int. J. Dermatol. *36*, 940–942 (1997).
85 E. Scaparro, G. Quadri, G. Virno, C. Orfici and M. Dilani: Br. J. Dermatol. *144*, 854–857 (2001).
86 B.J. Vermeer and C.G.C. Staats: Dermatology *194* (Suppl. 1), 22–24 (1997).
87 J. Faergemann, K. Hersle, P. Nordin: Dermatology *194* (Suppl. 1), 19–21 (1997).
88 M. Pazzaglia, E. Ghetti, F. Stacul and A. Tosti: Giornale Italiano di Dermatologia e Venerologia *135*, 247–251 (2000).
89 P. Dupuy, C. Maurette, J.C. Amoric and O. Chosidow: Br. J. Dermatol. *144*, 1033–1037 (2001).
90 S.E. Reef, M.M. McNeil, J.D. Sobel and R. Pinner: Infect. Dis. Clin. Practice *4*, 36 (1995).
91 S. Faro: Infect. Dis. Obstetrics Gyn. *4*, 247–254 (1996).
92 I.W. Fong: Pharmacoeconomics *9*, 497–505 (1996).
93 A. Stary: Dermatologic Therapy *3*, 37–42 (1997).
94 C.M. Perry, R. Whittington and D. McTavish: Drugs *49*, 984 (1995).
95 M. Ramam, G. Taru, P. D'Souza, K. Verma, B.K. Khattan et al.: Acta Dermatol. Venereol. 80, 378–380 (2000).
96 E.S. Mahgoub, in: G.L. Mandell, R.G. Douglas and J.E.J. Bennett (eds.): Agents of mycetoma in principles and practice of infectious diseases, Springer, New York 1990, 197.
97 B. Degavre, J.M. Joujoux, M. Dour and B. Guillot: J. Am. Acad. Dermatol. *37*, 318–320 (1997).
98 G. Sanjiv, R. Partho and S. Gurbir: Med. J. Armed Forces India *57*, 163–164 (2001).
99 D. Borelli: Rev. Infect. Dis. *9* (Suppl. 1), S57 (1987).

100 R. Minotto, C.V.D. Bernardi, L.F. Mallmann, M.I.A. Edelweiss and M.L. Scroferneker: J. Am. Acad. Dermatol. *44*, 589–592 (2001).
101 K. Tintelnot: Mycoses *40* (Suppl. 1), 91–96 (1997).
102 J.P. Silva, W. de Souza and S. Rozental: Mycopathologia *143*, 171–175 (1999).
103 A. Bonifaz, E. Carrasco-Gerard and A. Saul: Mycoses *444*, 1–7 (2001).
104 H.C. Gugnani, N. Sood, B. Singh and R. Makkar: Mycoses *43*, 85–86 (2000).
105 M. Pérez-Blanco, G. Fernez-Zeppenfeldt, V.R. Hernez, F. Yegres and D. Borelli: Revista Iberoamericano Microbiologica *15*, 51–54 (1998).
106 P. Mayser, K. Gründer, S. Quadripur, E.M. Koehn, W.B. Schill and G.S. de Hoog: Hautarzt *47*, 693 (1996).
107 P. Esterre, C.K. Inzan, E.R. Ramarcel, A. Andriantsimahavandy, M. Ratsiohalana et al.: Br. J. Dermatol. *134* (Suppl. 46), 33 (1996).
108 C. Czabezas, B. Bustamante, W. Holgado and R.E. Begue: Ped. Infect. Dis. J. *15*, 352–354 (1996).
109 C.A. Kaufman: Clin. Infect. Dis. *33* (Suppl. 2), S 148–153 (1996).
110 S. Conias and P. Wilson: Austr. J. Dermatology *39*, 34–37 (1998).
111 G. Karalayali, N. Lenk, N. Alli, E. Güngör, F. Artüz et al.: Cutis *61*, 106–107 (1998).
112 C.A. Kaufman, R. Hajjeh and S.W. Chapman: Clin. Infect. Dis. *30*, 684–687 (2000).
113 A.D. Badley and R.E. van Scoy: Clin. Infect. Dis. *23*, 394–395 (1996).
114 A.J. Ware, C.J. Cockerell, D.J. Skiest and H.M. Kussman: J. Am. Acas. Dermatol *40*, 350–355 (1999).
115 C. Edwards, W.L. Reuther and D.L. Greer: Southern Medical J. *93*, 803–806 (2000).
116 C.A. Kaufman, P.G. Pappas, D.S. McKinsey, R.A. Grenfield, J. Perfect et al.: Clin. Infect. Dis. *22*, 46 (1996).
117 A.H. Groll and T.J. Walsh: Clin. Microbiol. Infect. *7* (Suppl. 2), 8–24 (2001).
118 O.H. Gyaurgeva, T.S. Bogomolova and G.I. Gorishkova: J. Med. Vet. Mycol. *34*, 357–359 (1996).
119 E. Anaissie, P. Nelson, M. Beremand, D. Kontoyiannis and M.G. Rinaldi: Curr. Top. Med. Mycol. *4*, 231 (1992).
120 C. Hennequin, V. Lavarde, J.L. Poirot, M. Rabodonirina, A. Datry et al.: J. Med. Vet. Micol. *35*, 107–114 (1997).
121 S.T. Yildiran, S. Kömurcü, M.A. Sarach, A. Gönlüm, H. Gün et al.: Mycoses *41*, 467–469 (1998).
122 D.J. Fisher, C. Christy, P. Spafford, M. Maniscalco, D.J. Hardy and P.S. Graman: Ped. Infect. Dis. J. *12*, 151 (1993).
123 P. Kamberi, H. Atsuro, T.Takayoshi and N. Masaru: Chemotherapy *44*, 55–62 (1998).
124 T.J. Walsh, B. de Pauw, E. Anaissie and P. Martino: J. Med. Vet. Mycol. *32* (Suppl. 1), 33 (1994).
125 T Sirisantha: Japanese J. Med. Mycol. *37*, 5 (1996).
126 V. Sirisantha and T. Sirisantha: Pediatr. Infect. Dis. J. *14*, 935 (1995).
127 Hsueh PoRen, Teng LeeJene, Hung ChienChing et al.: J. Infect. Dis. *81*, 1706–1712 (2000).
128 W.M. Tsui, K.E. Ma and D.N.C. Tsang: Histopathology *20*, 287 (1992).
129 S. Remadi, C. Lotfi, V. Finci, A. Ismail, D. Rogiano et al.: Acta Cytol. *39*, 798 (1995).
130 K.H. Keddy and K.P. Klugman: Southern African J. Epidemiol. Infect . *9*, 51 (1994).
131 S. Yamada, T. Maruaka, K. Nagai, N. Tsumura, T. Yamada et al.: Scan. J. Infect. Dis. *27*, 85 (1995).

132 L.C.S. Thuler, S. Faivichenco, E. Velasco, C.A. Martins, C.R.G. Nascimento et al.: Mycoses *40*, 193–196 (1997).
133 A. Kunova, S. Spanik, T. Klar, J. Trupl and V. Kremery: Chemotherapy *42*, 157 (1996).
134 O. Masure, A. Minoui, P. le Gall, M. Cornen, A.M. Le Flohic: J. Mycol. Médicale *7*, 33–36 (1997).
135 S.E. Welbel, M.M. McNeil, A. Pramanik, R. Silberman, A.D. Oberle et al.: Pediatr. Infect. Dis. J. *13*, 104 (1994).
136 T.A. Ruxin, W.D. Steck, T.N. Helm, W.E Bergfeld and B.J. Bolwell: Arch. Dermatol. *132*, 382 (1996).
137 G. Poza, J. Montoya, C. Ridondo, J. Ruiz, N. Vila et al.: Clin. Infect. Dis. *30*, 981 (2000).
138 M.A. Nesky, E.C. McDougal and J.E. Peacock: Clin. Infect. Dis. *31*, 673–677 (2000).
139 J. Gene, A. Masoliver, J. Guardo, G. de Febrer, A. Martinez et al.: J. Clin. Microbiol. *39*, 1134–1136 (2001).
140 J. Guarro, W. Gams, I. Pujol and J. Gene: Clin Infect. Dis. *25*, 1222 (1997).
141 M. Martin, P. Tornero, P.M. Rabadan and M. Rodrigues Creixems: Clin. Infect. Dis. *31*, 1499 (2000).
142 W. Wanachiwanawin, M. Thianprasit, S. Fucharoen, A. Chaiprasert, N.S.N. Ayudhya et al.: Trans. Roy. Soc. Trop. Med. Hyg. *87*, 296 (1993).
143 S.M. Mathews and S. Sen: Mycoses *41*, 427–428 (1998).
144 W. Mohl, M.M. Lerch, M. Klotz, H. Freidank, M. Zeitz: Mycoses *41*, 425–426 (1998).
145 G. Kac, P. Piriou, E. Gueho, P. Roux, J. Trémoulet, M. Denis, T. Judet: Med. Mycol. *37*, 213–217 (1999).
146 S.M. Singh, J. Naidu, S. Jain, S.R. Nawange, M.K. Dhindsa: J. Med. Vet. Mycol. *34*, 215–218 (1996).
147 K.M. Chan Tack, C.L. Thio, N.S. Miller, C.L. Kapp, C. Ho and W.G. Merz: Med. Mycol. *37*, 57–60 (1999).
148 I.U. Scott, H.W. Flynn, D. Miller, J.W. Speights, R.C. Snip et al.: Arch. Ophthalmol. 119, 916 (2001).
149 I. Hilmarsdottir, S. Thorsteinsson, P. Asmundsson, M. Bodvarsson and M. Arnadottir: Scand. J. Infect. Dis. *32*, 331 (2000).
150 S. Hood and D.W. Denning: J. Antimicrob. Chemother. *37* (Suppl. B), 71 (1996).
151 ECMM Survey : Mycoses *44*, 345 (2001).
151a R. Manfredi, F. Pieri, St.A. Pileri and F. Chiodo: Mycopathologia *148*, 73 (1999).
152 M. Petoello-Montovani, A. Casadevall, T.R. Kollmann, A. Rubinstein and H. Goldstein: Lancet *339*, 21 (1992).
153 P.D. Hoeprich, in: E. Jucker (ed.): Progress in Drug Research, Vol. 44, Birkhäuser Verlag, Basel 1995, 87–100.
154 E.K. Manavathu, G.J. Alangaden, P.H. Chandrasekar: J. Antimicrob. Chemother. *41*, 615–619 (1998).
155 K. Seo, H. Akiiyoshi and Y. Ohnishi: Microbiol. Immunol. *43*, 1017–1025 (1999).
156 T.R. Sterling and G. Merz: Drug Resistance Updates *1*, 161–165 (1998).
157 B.K. Carroll, S. Cohen, J. Whisenant, D. Riley, and P. Beatty: Ninety-fourth Meeting of the American Society of Microbiology, Abstract 606 (1994).
158 S.L. Kelly, D.C. Lamb, D. Kelly, N.J. Manning, J. Loeffler, H. Hebart, U. Schuhmacher and H. Einsele: FEBS Lett. *400*, 80 (1997).
159 R.M. Singh and B.E. Perdue: Formulary *33*, 424–447 (1998).

160 F.S. Nolte, T. Parkinson, D.J. Falconer, S. Dix, J. Williams et al.: Antimicrob. Agents Chemother. *41*, 196 (1997).

161 D.A. Sutton, S.E. Sanche, S.G. Revankar, A.W. Fothergill and M.G. Rinaldi: J. Clin. Microbiol. *37*, 2343–2345 (1999).

162 A. Polak, in: J.F. Ryley (ed.): Handbook of Experimental Pharmacology, vol. 96. Chemotherapy of Fungal Diseases, Springer Verlag, 1990, 153–182.

163 B.E. Cohen: Int. J. Pharm. *162*, 95–106 (1998).

164 M.A. Hossein and M.A. Ghannoum: Exp. Opin. Invest. Drugs *9*, 1797 (2000).

165 J.S. Conklin, M. Kwing and W.M. Wasan: Pharm Res. *13* (9 Suppl.), S 117 (1996).

166 M.M. Zaman, S. Burney, D. Landman and I.M. Quale: Clin. Infect. Dis. *22*, 378 (1996).

167 R. Patel: Mayo Clin. Proc. *73*, 1205–1225 (1998).

168 A. Pathak, F.D. Pien and L. Carvalho: Clin. Infect. Dis. *26*, 334–338 (1998).

169 G.E. White, D.T. Jayaweera, K. Hobdy Henderson and K. Marshall: Pharmacotherapy *18*, 426 (1998).

170 J.R. Wingrad, P. Kubilis, L. Lee, G. Yee, M. White et al.: Blood *92* (10, pt. 1 Suppl. 1), 518a–519a (1998).

171 M.E. Fernandez-Miera, M. Farinas, M.J. Del C Hazas Feo and P. Sanroma Mendizabal: Medicina Clinica *102*, 434 (1994).

172 M.P. Nagata, C.A. Gentry and E.M. Hampton: Ann. Pharmacother. *30*, 811 (1996).

173 V.R. Singh, D.K. Smith, J. Lawrence, P.C. Kelly, A.R.Thomas et al.: Clin. Infect. Dis. *23*, 563 (1996).

174 B. Dupont, D.W. Denning, D. Marriot, A. Sugar, M.A. Viviani and T. Sirisanthana: J. Med. Vet. Mycol. *32* (Suppl. 1), 65 (1994).

175 E. de Lalla, G. Pellizer, A. Vaglia, V. Manfrin, M. Franzetti, P. Fabris and C. Stecca: Clin. Infect. Dis. *20*, 263 (1995).

176 A. Polak: Mycoses *42*, 355–370 (1999).

177 K.A. Kostiuk, R.A. Jacobs, M.L. Stoller and B.J. Guglielmo: Pharmacotherapy *19*, 488–489 (1999).

178 D. Benoit, J. Decruyenaere, K. Vendewoude, C. Roosens, E. Hoste, J. Poelaert, F. Vermassen and F. Colardyn: Clin. Infect. Dis. *26*, 393–397 (1998).

179 D.W. Denning: Clin. Infect. Dis. *23*, 608 (1996).

180 J.W. Hiemenz and T.J. Walsh: J Liposome Res. *8*, 443–467 (1998).

181 G.W. Boswell, D. Buell, I. Bekersky: J. Clin. Pharmacol. *38*, 583–592 (1998).

181a Review on L-Amph B: J. Antimicrob. Chemother. *49* (Suppl. 1), (2002).

182 A.J. Coukell and R.N. Brogden: Drugs *55*, 585–612 (1998).

183 I.M. Hann and H.G. Prentic: Int. J. Antimicrob. Agents *17*, 161–169 (2001).

184 B.G. Yu, T. Okano, K. Katakoa, S. Sardari, G.S. Kwon: J. Controlled Release *56*, 285–291 (1998).

185 Y. Shadkam, E. Segal, A. Bor, Y. Gov, M. Rubin and D. Lichtenberg: J. Antimicrob. Agents *39*, 655–658 (1997).

186 R. Manfredi and F. Chiodo: Pharmacotherapy *18*, 1087–92 (1998).

187 S. Kohno, M. Ashraf Hossain, S. Maesaki, F. Sasaki, H. Kakeya, K. Tomono and Y. Tashiro: Clin. Infect Dis. *25*, 489 (1997).

188 R. Santangelo, P. Paderu, G. Delmas, Z. Chen, R. Mannino et al.: Antimicrob. Agents Chemother. *44*, 2356–2360 (2000).

189 O. Ericsson: Ann. Pharmacother. *30*, 298 (1996).

190 S. Saxenam, P.K. Bhatnagar, P.C. Goshm, P. Usha Sarma: Int J. Pharm. *188*, 19–30 (1999).

191 M. Nucci, M. Loureiro, F. Silveira, A.R. Casali, L.F. Bouzas, E. Velasco, N. Spector, W. Pulcheri: Antimicrob. Agents Chemother. *43*, 1445–1448 (1999).
192 C.E. Nath, P.J. Shaw, R. Gunning, A.J. Mclachlan and J.W. Earl: Antimicrob. Agents Chemother. *43*, 1417–1423 (1999).
193 D. Torre, G. Banfi, R. Speranza, C. Zeroli, R. Martegani, M. Airoldi and F. Fiori: I. Infect. *37*, 36–38 (1998).
194 M.S. Razzaque, M.A. Hossain, N. Ahsan and T. Taguchi: Nephron *89*, 251 (2001).
195 S. Arikan and J.H. Rex: Emerging Drugs *51*, 135–160 (2000).
196 M.A. Hossain, H.G. Reyes and M.A. Ghannoum: Rev. Med. Microbiol. *12* (Suppl. 19), S3–S12 (2001).
197 J. Adler-Moore and R.T. Proffilt: J. Liposome Res. *3*, 429 (1993).
198 J. Adler-Moore: Bone Marrow Transplantation *14* (Suppl. 5), S3 (1994).
199 R.W. Finberg, A. Cross, J. Reinhardt, G. Donowitz and M. Wong: Blood *90* (10, Suppl. 1, Pt. 1), 72A (1997).
200 R. Hebrecht, V. Letscher and A. Cavalier: Chemotherapy *45* (Suppl. 1), 67–76 (1999).
201 A. Wong-Behringer, P.M. Behringer and J.P Rho: Forrnulary *31*, 169 (1996).
202 M. White, R.A. Bowden, E.S. Sandler, M.L. Graham, G.A. Noskin et al.: Infect. Dis. *27*, 296–302 (1998).
203 V. Heinemann, B. Kähny, A. Debus, K. Wachholz and U. Jehn: Bone Marrow Transplantation *14* (Suppl. 5), S8 (1994).
204 E. Spath Schwalbe, A. Koschuth, A. Dietzmann, J. Schanz, K. Possinger: Clin. Infect. Dis. *28*, 680–681 (1999).
205 M.D. Johnson, R.H. Drew and J.R. Perfect: Pharmacotherapy *18*, 1053–1061 (1998).
206 R.N. Brogden, K.L. Goa and A.J. Coukell: Drugs *56*, 365–368 (1998).
207 R.A. Bowden, M. Cays, T. Gooley, R.D. Mamelok and J.A. Van Burik: J. Infect. Dis. *17*, 1208 (1996).
208 J. Strickland, G. Yee, J. Lister, L. Lee and J. Wingard: Pharmacotherapy *19*, 504 (1999).
209 J.A. Boyle and E.J. Anaissie: Blood *88*, 89b (1996).
210 I.W. Blau and A.A. Fauser: Mycoses *43*, 325–332 (2000).
211 A.R. Craig, C.V. Holden, I.J. Lewis and S.E. Kinsey: Blood *90* (10, Suppl. 1, Pt. 2), 240 B (1997).
212 J.H. Weitkamp, C.F. Poets, R. Sievers, E. Mussessels, P. Groneck et al.: Infection *26*, 11–15 (1998).
213 H. Schneemann: Krankenhausphamazie *4*, 161–171 (1992).
214 M. Ellis, D. Spence, B. de Pauw. F. Meunier, A. Marinus et al.: Clin. Infect. Dis. *27*, 1406–1412 (1998).
215 A.V. Leenders, S. Daenen, R.L. Jansen, W.C.J. Hop, B. Lowenberg et al.: Br. J. Haematol. *103*, 205–212 (1998).
216 S. Maury, M. Leblanc, M. Feuilhalde, J.M. Molina and G. Schaison: Clin. Infect. Dis. *26*, 200–202 (1998).
217 D.D. Sweet and M. Reich: J. Infect. *36*, 120–121 (1998).
218 A.R. Craig, C.V. Holden, I.J. Lewis and S.E. Kinsey: Blood *90*, 240 B (1997).
219 A. Meyerhof: Clin. Infect. Dis. *28*, 42–28 (1999).
220 U. Schuler: 4th International Janssen-Cilag Symposium, Abstract book, p. 20 (2000).
221 R.A. Bowden, M. Cays, T. Gooley, R.D. Mamelok and J.A. van Burik: J. Infect. Dis. *173*, 1208–1215 (1996).

222 W.H. White, E.J. Anaissie, S. Kusne, J.R. Wingard, J.W. Hiemenz et al : Clin. Infect. Dis. *24*, 635–42 (1997).

223 G.A. Noskin, L. Pietrelli, G. Coffey, M. Gurwith and L.J. Liang: Clin. Infect. Dis. *26*, 461–467 (1998).

224 R. Hebrecht, V. Letscher, E. Andres, S. Kusne and M. Gurwith: Blood *88* (10, Suppl. 1, Pt. 1), 502a (1996).

225 A.E. Moses, G. Rahav, Y. Barenholz, J. Elidan, B. Azaz et al.: Clin. Infect. Dis. *26*, 1430–1433 (1998).

226 R. Dietze, V.G. Fowler Jr., T.S. Steiner, P.M. Pecanha and G.R. Corey: Am. J. Trop. Med. Hyg. *60*, 837–839 (1999).

227 P. Linden, L. Lee and T.J. Walsh: Pharamcotherapy *19*, 1261–1268 (1999).

228 W.S. Velasquez, F. Dunphy and G. Horwith: Proc. Am. Aoc. Clin. Oncol. *16*, 33 Meet 84a (1997).

229 L.M. Baddour: Clin. Infect. Dis. *29*, 1013 (1999).

230 J.A. Larkin, M.C. Targino and H. Waskin: Clin. Infect. Dis. *29*, 999 (1999).

231 E.J. Anaissie, R. Ramphal and G. Horwith: Blood 88 (10, Suppl. 1, Pt. 1), 426a (1996).

232 A.P. Koehler, A.F.B. Cheng, K.C. Chu, C.H.S. Chan and A.S.S. Ho: J. Infect. *36*, 113–115 (1998).

233 P.P. Cook: South. Med. J. *94*, 548 (2001).

234 J. Nolla Sallas, J.M. Torres Roderiguez, S. Grau, F. Isbert, T. Torella et al.: Scand. J. Infect. Dis. *32*, 560 (2000).

235 S.R. Virata, J.A. Kylstra, J.C. Brown, D.A. Wohl and M.S. Cohen: Clin. Infect. Dis. 28, 1177–1778 (1999).

236 S. de Marie, R. Janknegt and I.A.J.M. Bakker Woudenberg: J. Antimicrob. Chem. *33*, 907 (1994).

237 A. Clark, R. Chopra, S. McKendrick, P. Tansey and J.M. Franklin: Blood *90* (10, Suppl. 1, Pt. 1), 544–545 A (1997).

238 J.R. Johnson, P.J. Kangas and M. West: Clin. Infect. Dis. *27*, 1342–1343 (1998).

239 S.P. Gelone: Blood *96* (11, Pt. 29), 389b (2000).

240 L. Annemans: 4th International Janssen-Cilag Symposium, Abstract book, p. 22 (2000).

241 A. Polak and H. Scholer: Rev. Inst. Pasteur *13*, 233 (1980).

242 A. Polak: J. Antimicrob. Chemother. *26*, 465 (1990).

243 J.P. Greenstein, C.E. Carter, H.W. Chalkley and F.M. Lezuthaidt: J. Nati. Cancer Inst. *7*, 9 (1946).

244 B.E. Harris, R.B. Diasio, B.W. Manning and T.W. Federle: Antimicrob. Agents Chemother. *29*, 44 (1986).

245 H.J. Scholer and A. Polak, in: Antimicrob. Drug Resistance, Academic Press, New York 1984, 393–460.

246 S. Weber and A. Polak: Mycoses *35*, 16–3 (1992).

247 W.L. Whelan and P. Magee: J. Bacteriol. *145*, 896 (1981).

248 M.O. Fasoli, D. Kerridge and J.F. Ryley: J. Med. Vet. Mycol. *28*, 27 (1990).

249 A. Polak: Mycoses *35*, 9 (1992).

250 C.A. Kaufmann and P.T. Frame: Antimicrob. Agents Chemother. *11*, 244 (1997).

251 A.M. Stamm, R.B. Diasio, W.E. Dismuskes, S. Shadomy, C.A. Cloud, C.A. Bowles, G.H. Karam and A. Espinel-Ingroff: Am. J. Med. *83*, 236 (1987).

252 T.J. Walsh: Clin. Infect. Dis. *15*, 1003–1018 (1992).

253 M. White, C. Cirrinicione, A. Blevins and D. Armstrong: J. Infect. Dis. *165*, 960 (1992).

253a A. Vernes, H.J. Guchelaar and J. Dankert: Chemotherapy *46*, 335 (2000).
254 H. Vanden Bosche and P. Marichal, in: H. Yamaguchi, G.S. Kobayashi and H. Takahashim (eds.): Recent Progress in Antifungal Chemotherapy, Marcel Dekker, New York 1991, 25–40.
255 C.A. Hitchcock and R.J. Wittle, in: J.W. Rippon and R. Fromtling (eds.): Cutaneous Antifungal Agents, Marcel Dekker, New York 1993, 183–197.
256 C.A. Lyman and T.J. Walsh: Drugs *44*, 9 (1992).
257 J.A. Como and W.E. Dismuskes: N. Eng. J. Med. *330*, 263 (1993).
258 A. Datry, M. Thellier, B. Traoré, O. Alfa Cissé and M. Danis: Ann. Fr. Anesth. Réanim. *20*, 389 (2001) .
259 J.A. Bronstein, P. Gros, E. Hernandez. P. Larroque and C. Molinie: Clin. Infect. Dis. *25*, 1266–1267 (1997).
260 M.A. Pfaller, M. Bale, B. Buschelman, M. Lancaster, A. Espinel-Ingroff et al.: J. Clin. Microbiol. *33*, 1104–1107 (1995).
261 M.A. Ghannoum, J.H. Rex and J.N. Galgiani: J. Clin. Microbiol. *34*, 489–495 (1996).
261a L. SaiCheong, F. ChangPhone, H. JenSeng, T. ChiJen, C. KuoSu et al.: Antimicrob. Agents Chemother. *44*, 2715–2718 (2000).
262 B.F. Dupont, E. Dromer and L. Improvisi: J. Mycol. Med. *6* (Suppl. 2), 12 (1996).
263 B.S. Zingman: J. Mycol. Med. *6* (Suppl. 2), 3 (1996).
264 M.H. Nguyen, J.E. Peacock, A.J. Morris, D.C. Tanner, M.L. Nguyen et al.: Am. J. Med. *100*, 617–623 (1996).
264a T.R. Rogers: Current Opinion in Critical Care *7*, 238 (2001).
264b R. Rüchel, S. Keller and M. Schaffrinski: Mycoses *45*, 109 (2002).
265 J.R. Maenza, W.G. Merz, M.J. Romagnoli, J.C. Keruly, R.D. Moore and J.E. Gallant: Clin. Infect. Dis. *24*, 28–34 (1997).
266 S. Metzger and H. Hofmann: Mycoses *40*, 56–63 (1997).
266a M. Masia Canuto, F. Gutierrez Rodero, V. de la Ortiz, V. Tabla Ducasse, I. Hernandez Aguado et al.: Eur. J Clin. Microbiol. Infect. Dis. *19*, 593 (2000).
267 M. Ruhnke, A. Eigler, L. Teenegen, B. Geisler, E. Engelmann and M. Traulmann: J. Clin. Microbiol. *32*, 2093 (1994).
268 E.M. Johnson and D.W Warnock: J. Antimicrob. Chemother. *36*, 751 (1995).
269 M. McCullough and S. Hume: J. Med. Vet. Mycol. *33*, 33 (1995).
270 F. Barchiesi, R.J. Hollis, D.A. McGough, G. Scalise, M.G. Rinaldi and M.A. Pfaller: Clin. Infect. Dis. *20*, 634 (1995).
271 J. Berenguer, T.M. Diaz-Guerra, B. Ruiz Diez, J.C.L.B. de Quiros, J.L. Rodriguez Tudela and J.V. Martinez-Suarez: J. Clin. Microbiol. *34*, 1542 (1996).
272 F. Barchiesi, R.J. Hollis, M. Del Poeta, D.A. McGough, G. Scalise, M.G. Rinaldi and M.A. Pfaller: Clin. Infect. Dis. *27*, 561 (1995).
273 X. JianPing, C. Onyewu, H.J. Yoel, R.Y. All, R.J. Vilgalys et al.: Antimicrob. Agents Chemother. *45*, 420 (2001).
274 D.A. Goff, S.L. Koletar, W.J. Buesching, J. Barnishan and R.J. Fass: Clin. Infect. Dis. *20*, 77 (1995).
275 A. Kunova, J. Trupl, S. Spanik, L. Drgona, J. Sufliarsky et al.: Chemotherapy *41*, 39 (1995).
276 M.E Price, M.T. LaRocco and L.O. Gentry: Antimicrob. Agents Chemother. *38*, 1422 (1994).
277 K. Venkateswarlu, M. Taylor, N.J. Manning, M.G. Rinaldi and S.L. Kelly: Antimicrob. Agents Chemother. *41*, 748–751 (1997).

278 J. Wheat, P. Marchial, H. VanddenBosche, A. Le Monte and P. Connolly: Antimicrob. Agents Chemother. *41*, 410–414 (1997).
279 A.S. Orozco, M. Higgenbotham, C.A. Hitchcock, T. Parkinson, D. Falconer, A.S. Ibrahim et al.: Antimicrob. Agents Chemother. *42*, 2645–2649 (1998).
280 S.L. Kelly, D.C. Lamb and D.E. Kelly: FEMS Microbiol. Lett. *180*, 171 (1999).
281 D.C. Lamb, A. Corran, B.C. Baldwin, J. Kwong-Chung and S.L. Kelly: FEBS Lett. *368*, 326 (1995).
282 D. Sanglard, K. Kuchler, F. Ischer, J. Pagani, M. Monod and J. Bille: Antimicrob. Agents Chemother. *39*, 2378 (1995).
283 T. Parkinson, D.J. Falconer and C.A. Hitchcock: Antimicrob. Agents Chemother. *39*, 1696 (1995).
284 D.G. Albertson, M. Nimi, R.D. Cannon and H.F. Jenkinson: Antimicrob. Agents Chemother. *40*, 2835–2841 (1996).
285 K.W. Henry, J.T. Nickels and T.D. Edlind: Antimicrob. Agents Chemother. *44*, 2693 (2000).
286 A. Defontaine, J.P. Bouchara, P. Declerk, C. Planchenault, D. Chabasse and J.N. Hallet: J. Med. Microbiol. *48*, 663–670 (1999).
287 H.M. Kasai, A. Francesconi, D. Landsman and S.J. Chanock: J. Med. Vet. Myc. *35*, 133–137 (1997).
288 S. Wirsching, S. Michel, G. Köhler and J. Morschhäuser: J. Bacteriol. *182*, 499 (2000).
289 C.N. Lyons and T.C. White: Antimicrob. Agents Chemother. *44*, 2296 (2000).
290 S. Wirsching, S. Michel and J. Morschhäuser: Molecular Microbiol. *36*, 856 (2000).
291 S.K. Katiyar and T.D. Edlind: Medical Mycology *39*, 109 (2001).
292 X. He, R.N. Tiballi, L.T. Zarins, S.F. Bradley, J.A. Sangeorzan and C.A. Kauffman: Antimicrob. Agents Chemother. *38*, 2495 (1994).
293 E.M. Johnson, G.D. Kathleen, A.Azeleey and D.W. Warnock: J. Antimicrob. Chemother. *36*, 787 (1995).
294 T.P. Le, C.U. Tuzon, M. Levine, M. Borum and C. Rollhaiser: Clin. Infect. Dis. *23*, 649–650 (1996).
295 M. Ruhnke, A. Adler and F.M. Müller: Clin. Microbiol. Infect. *6*, 220 (2000).
296 K. Fekete Forgas, L. Gyüre and B. Lenkey: Mycoses *43*, 273 (2000).
297 V. Novelli and H. Holzel: Antimicrob. Agents Chemother. *43*, 1955–1960 (1999).
298 V. Krcmery Jr.: J. Antimicrob. Chemother. *44* (Suppl. A), 49 (1999).
299 D.A. Stevens, M. Diaz, R. Negroni, F. Montero-Gei, L.G. Castro et al.: Chemotherapy *43*, 372 (1997).
300 C.A. Lawson, J.A. Karlowsky and G.G. Zhanel: Can. J. Hosp. Pharm. *51*, 61–63 (1998).
301 M.O. Gearthart: Ann. Pharmacother. *28*, 1177 (1994).
302 C.A. Lawson, J.A. Karlowsky, and G.G. Zhanel: Can. J. Hosp. Pharm. *51*, 61 (1998).
303 W. Inman, G. Pearce and L. Wilton: Eur. J. Clin. Pharmacol. *46*, 115 (1994).
304 S.S. Jick: Pharmacotherapy *19*, 221–222 (1999).
305 P. Mastroiacovo, T. Mazzone, L.D. Botto, M.A. Serafini, A. Finardi et al.: Am. J. Obstet. Gynecol. *175*, 1645–1650 (1996).
306 T.J. Pursley, J.K. Blomquist, J. Abraham, H.F. Andersen and J.A. Bartley: Clin. Infect. Dis. 22, 336 (1996).
307 K.A. Aleck and D.I. Bartley: Am J. Med. Genetics: *72*, 253–256 (1997).
308 D.P. Niclau, H.M. Crowe, C.H. Nightingale and R. Quintiliani: Ann. Pharmacother. *29*, 994 (1995).

309 R.M. Cadle, G.J. Zenon, M.C. Rodriguez Barradas and R.J. Hamill: Ann. Pharmacother. *29*, 191 (1994).
310 V.J. Palkama, M.H. Isohanni, P.J. Neuvonen and K.T. Olkkola: Anesth. Analg. *87*, 190–194 (1998).
311 P. Czyborra, B. Kremens, E. Brendel, M. Bald and M.C. Michel: Arch. Pharmacol. *357* (Suppl.), R165 (1998).
312 K.M. Kaukonen, K.T. Olkkola and P.J. Neuvonen: Clin. Pharm. Ther. *63*, 151 (1998).
313 S. de Wit, M. Debier, M. de Smet, J. McCrea, J. Stone et al.: Antimicrob. Agents Chemother. *42*, 223 (1998).
314 M.T. Borin, S.R. Coy, B.D. Herman, B.J. Carel, R.D. Anderson and W.W. Freimuth: Antimicrob. Agents Chemother. *41*, 1892–1897 (1997).
315 S. De Wit, E. O'Doherty, C. De Vroey and N. Clumeck: J. Int. Med. Res. *26*, 159–170 (1998).
316 A. Plettenberg, A. Stoehr, G. Hoeffken, C. Bergs, B. Tschechne and M. Ruhnke: Infection *22*, 118 (1994).
317 G. Barbaro, G. Barbarini, W. Calderon, B. Grisiorio, P. Alcini and G. Di Lorenz: Gastroenterology *111*, 1169 (1996).
318 M. Akova, H.E. Akalm, O. Uzum, M. Hyran, G. Tekuman and E. Kansu: Clin. Infect. Dis. *18*, 298 (1994).
319 D.E. Lake, J. Kunzweiler, M. Beer, D.N. Buell and M.Z. Islam: Chemotherapy *42*, 308 (1996).
320 G. Barbaro, G. Barbarini, W. Calderon, B. Griserio, P. Alcini and G. Di Lorenzo: *Gut* 39 (Suppl. 3), A35 (1996).
321 F. Parente, S. Ardizzone, M. Cernuschi, S. Antinori, R. Esposito and M. Moroni: Am. J. Gastroenterol. *89*, 416 (1994).
322 L. Rabeneck and L. Laine: Arch. Intern. Med. *154*, 2705 (1994).
323 S.G. Revankar, W.R. Kirkpatrick, R.K. McAtee, O.P. Dib, A.W. Fothergill et al.: Am. J. Med. *105*, 7–11 (1998).
324 J. Hendel, E. Svejgaard, E. Hage and I. Hendel: Scan. J. Gastroenterol. *32*, 65 (1997).
325 B.M. Gripshover, H. Veldez, R.A. Salata and M.M. Lederman: AIDS *12*, 2513–2514 (1998).
326 S.G. Revankar, S.E. Sanche, O.P. Dib, M. Caceres and T.F. Patterson: AIDS *12*, 2511–2513 (1998).
327 J.L. Pagani, J.P. Chave, A. Iten, C. Durussel, J. Bille and M.P Glauser: Schweiz. Med. Wochenschr. *126* (9, Suppl. 74, Pt. 2), 49S (1996).
328 L. Bernstein, W. Hsu, J. Schliozberg and S. Iqbal: *76*, 83 (1996).
329 S.G. Revankar, W. Kirkpatrick, R.K. McAtee, O.P. Dib, A.W. Fothergill et al.: J. Infect. Dis. *174*, 821 (1996).
330 C. Domenge, J.L. Lefebvre and Y. Esnault: Eur. J. Cancer *35* (Suppl. 4), S161 (1999).
331 A. Wildfeuer, H. Laufen, R.A. Yeates and T. Zimmermann: Mycoses *39*, 123 (1996).
332 M.D. Martins and J.H. Rex: Ann. Intern. Med. *126*, 332–333 (1997).
333 A. Plattenberg, A. Stöhr, W. Heise, F. Schlote, E. Sarnow and M. Migdal: Mycoses *42*, 269–272 (1999).
334 J.H. Rex, J.E. Bennettt, A.M. Sugar, P.G. Pappas, C.M. van der Horst et al.: N. Eng. J. Med. *331*, 1325 (1994).
335 K.M. Kramer, D.J. Skaar and B.H. Ackerman: Pharmacotherapy *17*, 538–548 (1997).
336 J. Baran, B. Muckatira and R. Khatib: Scand. Infect. Dis. *33*, 137 (2001).
337 D.L. Gibbs: Curr. Ther. Res. *59*, 197–202 (1998).

338 P. Kujath, K. Lerch, P. Kochendorfer and C. Boos: Infection *21*, 376 (1993).

339 B.E. de Pauw, J.M.M. Raemaekers, J.P. Donnelly, B.J. Kullberg and EG.M. Meis: Annals of Hematology *70*, 83 (1995).

340 E. Anaissie, R.O. Darouiche, D. Abi Said, O. Uzon, J. Mera et al.: Clin. Infect. Dis. *23*, 964 (1996).

341 D. Armstrong: Clin. Infect. Dis. *16*, 1–10 (1993).

342 E. Presterl and W. Graninger: Eur. J. Clin. Microbiol. Infect. Dis. *13*, 347 (1994).

343 C. Fasano, J. O'Keeffe and D. Gibbs: Eur. J. Clin. Microbiol. Infect. Dis. *13*, 351 (1994).

344 H. Bilgen, E. Ozek, V. Korten, B. Ener and D. Molbay: Infection *23*, 394 (1995).

345 A.N. Gurpinar, E. Balkan, N. Kilcik, I. Kiristioglu, I. Avsar and H. Dogruyol: J. Int. Med. Res. *25*, 214–218 (1997).

346 R. Schwarze, A. Penk and L. Pittrow: Mycoses *41* (Suppl. 1), 61–70 (1998).

347 N. Gurses and A.G. Kalayci: Clin. Infect. Dis. *23*, 645 (1996).

347a M.K. Hostetter: Seminars Pediat. Infect. Dis. *12*, 296–300 (2001).

348 J. Walsh, P.O. Whitcomber, S.G. Revankar and P.A. Pizzo: Cancer *76*, 2357 (1995).

349 A. del Palacio, M.S. Cuetera, M. Ferro, E. Perez Blazquez, J.A. Lopez Sana and M.P. Roiz: Mycoses *36*, 193 (1993).

350 M.E. Akler, H. Vellend, D.M. McNeely, S.L. Walmsley and W.L. Gold: Clin. Infect. Dis. *20*, 657 (1995).

351 A. Penk: J. Antimicrob. Chemother. *44* (Suppl. A), 48–49 (1999).

352 Z. Trizna, S.H. Chen, S. Lockart, K.F. Lundquist, E.B. Schmith et al.: Arch Dermatol. *136*, 804 (2000).

353 P. Rossel, H.C. Schonheyder and H. Nielsen: Scan. J. Infect. Dis. *30*, 527–530 (1998).

354 D.L. Turner, S.A. Johnson and S.A. Rule: J. Infect. *38*, 51–53 (1999).

355 A. Penk and L.A. Pittrow: J. Antimicrob. Agents *44* (Suppl. A), 49 (1999).

356 M. Zervos and F. Meunier: J. Antimicrob. Agents Chemother. 3, 147 (1994).

357 L.G. Jacobs, E.A. Skidmore, K. Freeman, D. Lipschultz and N. Fox: Clin. Infect. Dis. *22*, 30 (1996).

358 E.N. Vergis, I. Memel, M.H. Nguyen, E.S. Wong, A. Goetz and R.R. Muder: Clin. Infect. Dis. *25*, 381 (1997).

359 J.D. Sobel, D. McKinsey, C. Kauffman, M. Zervos, J.A. Vezquez and J. Lee: Clin. Infect. Dis. *25*, 357 (1997).

360 J.D. Sobel, C.A. Kauffman, C.A. McKinsey, M. Zervos, J.A. Vazquez et al.: Clin. Infect. Dis. *30*, 19 (2000).

361 H.S. Leu and C.T. Huang: Clin. Infect. Dis. *20*, 1152 (1995).

362 S.H. Ansari, M.H. Levin and S. Lipshitz: J. Urol. *154*, 1870 (1995).

363 R.B. Corales, J.O. Tavee, G. Hall, G. Procop, T.R. Prasad et al.: Clin. Infect. Dis. *29*, 1004 (1999).

364 E. Menichetti, M.Fiorio, A. Tosti, G. Gatti, M.B. Pasticci et al.: Clin. Infect. Dis. *22*, 838 (1996).

365 S.D. Nightingale: Arch. Intern. Med. *155*, 538 (1995).

366 R. Manfredi and F. Chiodo: Chemotherapy *44*, 206–214 (1998).

367 M.C. Meyohas, J.L. Meynard, D. Bollens, P. Roux, A.M. Deluol et al.: J. Infect. *33*, 7 (1996).

368 A.B. Clark, B.L. Lobo and M.S.Gelfand: Ann. Pharmacother. *30*, 1408–1410 (1996).

369 F. Dromer, S. Mathoulin, B. Dupont, O. Burgiere, L. Letenneur and the French Cryptococcosis Group: Clin. Infect. Dis. *22* (Suppl. 2), S154 (1996).

370 W.W. Yew, P.C. Wong, C.E. Wong, J. Lee and C.H. Chau: Drugs. Exp. Clin. Res. *22*, 25 (1996).

370a E. Martinez, M.A. Garcia-Viejo, M.A. Marcos, J.B. Pérez-Cuevas, J.L. Blanco et al.: AIDS *14*, 2615 (2000).

371 J.A. Newton, P. Olson, S.A. Tasker, W.D. Bone, M.T. Nguyen and E.C. Oldfield: Clin. Infect. Dis. *17*, 563 (1993).

372 J.P. Viard, C. Hennequin, N. Fortineau, N. Pertuiset, C. Rothschild and H. Zylberberg: Lancet *346*, 118 (1995).

373 A. Armengou, C. Porcar, J. Mascaro and F. Garcia Bragado: Clin. Infect. Dis. *23*, 1337–1338 (1996).

374 K. Tintelnot, G. Schär and A. Polak: Mycoses *44*, 345 (2001).

375 E.J. Anaissie, D.P. Kontoyiannis, V. Huls, S.E. Vartvarian, C. Karl, R. Prince, J. Bosso and G.P. Bodey: J. Infect. Dis. *172*, 599 (1995).

376 D.A. Stevens: N. Engl. J. Med. *332*, 1077 (1996).

377 C.A. Kauffman: Clin. Infect. Dis. *22* (Suppl. 2), S148 (1996).

378 C.A. Kauffman: Curr. Treatment Opinions Infect. Dis. *2*, 487 (2001).

379 C.A. Kauffman: Curr. Treatment Opinions Infect. Dis. *2*, 481 (2001).

380 St.W. Chapman, R.W. Bradsher, G. Douglas Campell, P.G. Pappas and C.A. Kauffman: Clin. Infect. Dis. *30*, 679 (2000).

381 G.P. Pappas, R.W. Bradsher, S.W. Chapman, C.A. Kauffman, A. Dine, G.A. Cloud and W.A. Dismuskes: Clin. Infect. Dis. *20*, 267 (1995).

382 P.G. Pappas, R.W. Bradsher, C.A. Kauffman, G.A. Cloud, C.J. Thomas et al.: Clin. Infect. Dis. *25*, 200–205 (1997).

383 J. Wheat, S. MacWhinney, R. Hafner, D. McKinsey, D. Chen et al.: Am. J. Med. *103*, 223–232 (1997).

384 J.F.G.M. Meis and P.E. Verweij: Drugs *61* (Suppl. l), 13 (2001).

385 J. N. Galgiani, A.G. Cloud, A. Catanzaro, R.H. Johnson, L.F. Mirels et al.: Clin. Infect. Dis. *27*, 939 (1998).

386 J.N. Galgiani, A. Catanzaro, G.A. Cloud, R.H. Johnson, P.L. Williams et al.: Ann. Intern. Medicine *133*, 676 (2000).

387 S. Norris, J. Wheat, D. McKinsey, D. Lancaster, B. Katz and J. Black: Am. J. Med. *96* (6), 504 (1994).

388 H. Vanden Bossche, D.WR. Mackenzie, G. Cauwenbourg (eds.): Aspergillus and Aspergillosis, Plenum Press, New York 1988.

389 Mycoses *37* (Suppl. 2) (1994).

390 J.M. Poirier, E. Berlioz, E. Isnard and G. Cheymol: Therapy *50* (Suppl.), 492 (1995).

391 J.M. Poirier, S. Hardy, F. Isnard, G. Cheymol and P. Jaillon: Fundam. Clin. Pharmacol. *12*, 356 (1998).

392 V.J.S. van der Velde, AP. Van Peer, J.J.P. Heykants, R.J.H. Woestenborghs, P. Van Rooy et al.: Pharmacotherapy *16*, 424–428 (1996).

393 A. Barone, B.I. Moskoitz, J. Guarnieri, A.E. Hassel, J.L. Colaizzi et al.: Pharmacotherapy *18*, 295–301 (1998).

394 K. Vandewoude, D. Vogelaers, J. Decruyenaere, P. Jaqmin, K. de Beule et al.: Antimicrob. Agents Chemother. *41*, 2714–2718 (1997).

395 L. Willems, R. van der Geest and K. de Beule: J. Clin. Pharmacy Therapeut. *26*, 159 (2001).

396 D. Slain, P.D. Rogers, J.D. Clearly and St.W. Chapman: Ann. Pharmacother. *35*, 720 (2001).

397 M. Schaffner-Korting, H. Korting, W. Rittler and W. Obermüller: Infection *23*, 292 (1995).
398 K. Ventkateswarlu, D.W. Denning, N.J. Manning and S.L. Kelly: Antimicrob. Agents Chemother. *40*, 2443–2446 (1996).
399 M. Pfaller, R.N. Jones, G.V. Doern, H.S. Sader, R.J. Hollis and S.A. Messer: J. Clin. Microbiol. *36*, 1886–1889 (1998).
400 R.M. Tucker, Y. Haq, D.W. Denning et al.: J. Antimicrob. Chemother. *26*, 561–66 (1990).
401 F. Queiroz Telles, K.S. Purim, C.L. Boguszewski, F.C.S. Alfonso and H. Graf: J. Antimicrob. Chemother. *40*, 899–901 (1997).
402 J.A. Talwalkar, R.E. Soetikno, D. Carr Locke and C.L. Berg: Am. J. Gastroenterol. *94*, 3632–3633 (1999).
403 F. Persat, P.E. Schwartzbrod, J. Troncy, Q. Timour, A. Maul et al.: Therapie *54*, 294 (1999).
403a S.R. Ahmad, S.J. Singer and B.G. Leissa: Lancet *357*, 1766 (2001).
403b B. Bar Oz, M.F. Moretti, R. Bishai, G. Mareels, T. van Tittelboom et al.: J. Obstet. Gynaecol. *183*, 617 (2000).
404 A.B.M. Foot, P.A. Veys and B.E.S. Gibson: Br. J. Haematol. *102*, 211 (1998).
405 J. Drayton, G. Dickinson and M.G. Rinaldi: Clin. Infect. Dis. *18*, 266 (1994).
406 D.J. Greenblatt, L.L. Von Moltke, J.S. Harmatz, M. Counihan, J.A. Graf et al.: J. Clin. Pharmacol. *38*, 865 (1998).
407 J. Ahonen, K.T. Alkkola and R.J. Neuvonen: Therapie *50* (Suppl.), 190 and 421 (1995).
408 J.M. Poirier and G. Cheymol: Clin. Pharnacokinet. *35*, 461–73 (1998).
409 T.F. Patterson, J. Peters, S.M. Levine, A. Anzueto, C. Bryan et al.: Antimicrob. Agents Chemother. *40*, 2217–2220 (1996).
410 K.M. Jalava, K. Olkkola, P.J. Neuvonen: Clin. Pharmacol. Ther. *61*, 410–415 (1997).
411 C.H.W. Koks, R.P.G. Van Heerswijk, A.I. Veldkamp, P.L. Meenhorst, J.W. van der Meer et al.: AIDS *14*, 89–90 (2000).
412 J.C. Levron, Y. Mouton, C. Bazin, J.P. Moing, E. Chwetzoff et al : Fundam. Clin. Pharmacol. *13*, 400 (1999).
413 A.R. MacKenzie Wood, M.J. Whitefield and J.E. Ray: Med. J. Austr. *170*, 46–47 (1999).
414 J. Verspeelt, G. Marynissen, A.K. Gupta and P. De Doncker: Dermatology *198*, 382–384 (1999).
415 P. Philipps, K. de Beule, G. Frechette, S. Tchamouroff, B. Vendercam et al.: Clin. Infect. Dis. *26*, 1368–1373 (1998).
416 M. Boogaerts and J. Maertens: Drugs *61* (Suppl.), 39 (2001).
417 E. Peters, A. Pitie and M. Richardson: AIDS *12* (Suppl. 4), S 30 (1998).
418 J.R. Graybill, J. Vazquez, R.O. Darouiche, R. Morhart, G. Greenspan et al.: Am. J. Med. *104*, 33–39 (1998).
419 C.M. Wilcox, R.O. Darouiche, L. Laine, B.L. Moskovitz, I. Mallegol et al.: J. Infect. Dis. *176*, 227–232 (1997).
420 A. Urabe, Y. Mutoh, H. Mizoguchi, T. Miyazaki, A. Miura et al.: Jpn. J. Chemother. *47*, 80–88 (1999).
421 J. de Gans, P. Portegies, G. Tiessens, J.K. Eeftinck-Schattenkerk and C.J. van Boxtel Patton: AIDS *6*, 185 (1992).
422 M.A. Viviani, A.M. Tortorano, R. Woenstenberghs and R. Cauwenbergh: Mykosen *30*, 233 (1988).
423 M.A. Viviani, A.M. Tortorano, A. Pagano, G.M. Vigevani, G. Gubertini, S. Cristina, M.L. Assaisso, E. Suter, C. Farina, B. Minetti et al.: J. Am. Acad. Dermatol. *23*, 587 (1990).

424 M. Saag, R.J. Graybill, R.A. Larsen, P.G. Pappas, J.R. Perfect et al.: Clin. Infect. Dis. *30*, 710 (2000).
425 M.S. Saag, G.A. Cloud, J.R. Graybill, J.D. Sobel, C.U. Tuzon et al.: Clin. Infect. Dis. *28*, 291–296 (1999).
426 D.W. Dismuskes and D.A. Stevens: Rev. Infect. Dis. *12*, 1147 (1990).
427 J.J. Keating, T. Rogers, M. Petrou, J.D. Cartledge, D. Woodrow and M. Nelson: J. Clin. Pathol. *47*, 805 (1994).
428 D.W. Denning, J.Y. Lee, J.S. Hodtetler, R. Pappas, C.A. Kauffman, D.H. Dewsnup, J.N. Galgiani, J.R. Graybill, A.M. Sugar, A. Catanzaro et al.: Am. J. Med. *97*, 135 (1994).
429 D.A. Stevens and J.Y. Lee: Arch. Intern. Med. *16*, 1857–1862 (1997).
430 D.W. Denning, A. Marinus, J. Cohen, D. Spence, R. Herbrecht et al.: J. Infect. *37*, 173–180 (1998).
430a D. Caillot, H. Bassaris, A. McGeer, C. Arthur, H.G. Prentice et al.: Clin. Infect. Dis. *33*, 83 (2001).
431 S. Lankron, C. Bachier, J. Lowder, C. Berkowitz and C.F. Le Maistre: Blood *96*, 340b (2000).
432 S.M. Hakim, L.J.R. Milne, C. Fox, L.M. Nawroz, G. Webb and G.T. Vaugham: Br. J. Clin. Pract. *47*, 312 (1993).
433 J.A.H. Van Burik, R. Colven and D.H. Spach: Clin. Infect. Dis. *27*, 643–344 (1998).
434 S. Tasci, H. Schäfer, S. Ewig, G. Layer and A. Gillesen: Dtsch. Med. Wochenschr. *124*, 1419–1422 (1999).
435 V. Le Moing, O. Lortholary, J.F. Timsit, A. Couvelard, C. Bouges Michel et al.: Clin. Infect. Dis. *26*, 451–460 (1998).
436 F. Salez, A. Brichet, B. Wallaert and A.B. Tonnel: Eur. Resp. J. *12* (Suppl. 28), 97s (1998).
437 H.J. Schwartz, D.A. Stevens, J.Y. Lee, D. Jerome and A. Catanzaro: J. Allergy Clin. Immunol. *103*, S198 (1999).
438 I.B. Nepomuceno, S. Erig and S.R. Moss: Chest *115*, 364–370 (1999).
439 M.L. Belli, B. Tubino, M.C. Diana, G. Manno, E. Ugolotti et al : Eur. Res. J. *10* (Suppl. 1), 335S (1997).
440 M.A. Canales, J. Sevilla, E.O. Gutierrez and F.H. Navarro: Clin. Infect. Dis. *26*, 999–1000 (1998).
441 S.L. Goldberg, D.J. Geha, W.F. Marshall, D.J. Inwards and H.C. Hoagland: Clin. Infect. Dis. 16, 803–805 (1993).
442 K. Parthiban, S. Gnanaguruvelan, C. Janaki, G. Sentamilselvi and J.M. Boopalraj: Mycoses *41*, 51–53 (1998).
443 W. Shaoxi, G. Ningru, L. Guixiz, X. Zhuin and S.Y. Nain: J. Mycol. Med. *7*, 40–42 (1997).
444 S.K. Kabra, Y. Jain, T. Sudhin, K.V. Iyer, S. Ninan and V. Seith: Indian Pediatrics *35*, 163–166 (1998).
445 L. Sigler, S. Estrada, N.A. Montealegre, M. Arango, C. de Bedout and A. Restrepo: J. Med. Vet. Mycol. *35*, 365–370 (1997).
446 K.L. Jacobson, E.A. Whimbey and D.P. Kontoyiannis: Clin. Infect. Dis. *31*, 251 (2000).
447 J.R. Graybill, in: J.E Ryley (ed.): Chemotherapy of Fungal Therapy, Springer Verlag, Berlin 1990, 455–482.
448 A. del Palacio, C. Gomez-Hernando, E. Revenga, E. Carabias, A. Gonzalez et al.: Clin. Exp. Dermatol. *21*, 241 (1996).
449 K.M. Acland, R.J. Hay and R. Groves: Br. J. Dermatol. *138*, 354–356 (1998).
450 D.I. Wittle and S. Kominos: Clin. Infect. Dis. *21*, 1068 (1995).

451 T.J. Babinchak, E.B. Rotheram and M. Slifkin: Clin. Infect. Dis. *21*, 772 (1995).
452 K.C. Mouzner, S. Rhoades and J.E. Blank : Clin. Infect. Dis. *29*, 1380 and 1559 (1999).
453 S.M. Kralovic and J.C. Rhodes: J. Infect. *31*, 107 (1995).
454 U.M. Tendolkar, P. Kerkar, A. Gogate and A.A. Padhye: J. Infection 36, 122–125 (1998).
455 D.A. Sutton, W.D. Timm, G. Morgan-Jones and M.G. Rinaldi: J. Clin. Microbiol. *37*, 807–811 (1999).
456 M.R. Vieria, A. Milheiro and F.A. Pacheco: Med. Mycol. *39*, 135 (2001).
457 C.A. Kauffman: Clin. Infect. Dis. *22* (Suppl. 2), S148 (1996).
458 A.M. Tobon, L. Franco, D. Espinal, I. Gomez, M. Arango et al.: Pediatric Infect. Dis. J. *15*, 1002–1008 (1996.
459 K. Bodily, J.R. Perfect, G. Procop, M.K. Washington and J. Affronti: Gastrointest. Ebdoscopy *43*, 518–521 (1996).
460 G.C. Velho, J.M. Babral, A. Massa: J. Eur. Acad. Dermatol. Venerol. 10, 77–80 (1998).
461 J. Wheat, R. Hafner, A.H. Korzun, M.T. Limjoco, P. Spencer, R.A. Larsen, E.M. Hecht and W. Powderly: Am. J. Med. *98*, 336 (1995).
462 F.M. Hecht, J. Wheat, A.H. Korzun, R. Hafner, K.J. Skahan et al.: J. AIDS and Human Retrovirology: *16*, 100–107 (1997).
463 W.E. Dismuskes, R.W Bradsher, G.C. Cloud, C.A. Kauffman, R.B. George, D et al.: Am. J. Med. *93*, 489 (1992).
464 R. Negroni, O. Palmierei, F. Koren, L.N. Tiraboschi and R.L. Galimberti: Rev. Infect Dis. *9* (Suppl.), S47 (1987).
465 L.F. Mirels and D.A. Stevens: Western. J. Med. *166*, 58–59 (1997).
466 J.N. Galgiani, A. Catanzaro, G.A. Cloud, R.H. Johnson, P.L. Williams et al.: Ann. Intern. Med. *133*, 676 (2000).
467 A.D. Badley and R.E. van Scoy: Clin. Infect. Dis. *23*, 384–95 (1996).
468 P.K. Sharkey-Mathis, C.A. Kauffman, J.R. Graybill, D.A. Stevens, J.S. Hostetler et al.: Am. J. Med. *95*, 279 (1993).
469 P.H. Chandrasekar and E. Manavathu: Drugs of Today *37*, 135 (2001).
470 J.A. Sabo and S.A. Abdel-Rahman: Ann. Pharmacother. *34*, 1032 (2000).
471 FDA Briefing Document for Voriconazole (2001).
472 Pfizer: Drug of the Future *21*, 266–271 (1996).
473 H. Sanati, P. Belanger, R. Fratti and M. Ghonnoum: Antimicrob. Agents Chemother. *41*, 2492–2496 (1997).
474 R. Ally, D. Schürmann, W. Kreisel, G. Carosi, K. Auirrrebengoa et al.: Clin. Infect. Dis. *33*, 1447 (2001).
475 B. Dupont, D. Denning, H. Lode, S. Yonren, P. Troke et al.: 35th ICAAC San Francisco, Abstract book (1995).
476 D. Denning, A. del Favara, B. Glackman, D. Norfolk, M. Ruhnke et al.: 35th ICAAC San Francisco, Abstract book (1995).
477 D.W. Denning, P. Ribaud, N. Milpied, D. Caillot, R. Hebrecht et al : Clin. Infect. Dis. *34* in print (2002).
478 A.H. Groll and T.J. Walsh: Expert Opinion Investig. Drugs *10*, 1545 (2001).
479 FDA Briefing Document for Candidas® (2001).
480 G.M. Keating and B. Javis: Drugs *61*, 1121 (2001).
481 T. Chiller, K. Farrokhshad, E. Brummer and D.A. Stevens: Antimicrob. Agents Chemother. *44*, 3302 (2000).

482 G. Medoff, M. Comfort and G.S. Kobayashi: Proc. Assoc. Exp. Biol. Med. *138*, 571–574 (1971).
483 A. Polak: Mycoses *42*, 355–370 (1999) .
483a P.P. Cook: South. Med: J. *94*, 936 (2001).
484 L. Rodero, S. Cordoba, P. Cahn, F. Hochenfellner, G. Davel et al.: J. Antimicrob. Chemother. *45*, 239 (2000).
485 A. Louie, P. Kaw, P. Banerjee, W. Liu, G. Chen and M.H. Miller: Antimicrob. Agents Chemother. *45*, 485 (2001).
486 S. Velasquez, E. Bailey and A. Jandourek: Clin. Infect. Dis. *31*, 266 (2000).
487 D.P. Kontoyiannis, R.E. Lewis, N. Sager, G. May, R.A. Pronce et al.: Antimicrob. Agents Chemother. *44*, 2915 (2000). .
488 N.S. Ryder and I. Leitner: Medical Mycology *39*, 91 (2001).
488a S. Arikan, M. Lozano-Chiu, V. Pathnick and J.H. Rex: Antimicrob. Agents Chemother. *46*, 245 (2002).
489 F. Barchiesi, D. Gallo, F. Caselli, L. Falconi Do Francesco, D. Arzeni, A. Giacometti and G. Scalise: J. Antimicrob. Chemother. *44*, 65–70 (1999).
489a F. Barchiesi, A.M. Schimizzi, L.K. Najvar, R. Bocanegra, F. Caselli et al.: Antimicrob. Agents Chemother. *45*, 1355 (2001).
490 M. Weig and F.M.C. Müller: Antimicrob. Agents Chemother. *45*, 966 (2001).
490a 41th Interscience Confecrence on Abtimicrobial Agents and Chemotherapy (ICAAC), Abstract book (2001).
491 A.T. Hoang: Am. J. Health Syst. Pharm. *58*, 1206 (2001).
491a A. Wasson, M.E. Klepser, R.E. Lewis, E.J. Ernst and M.A. Pfaller: Pharmacotherapy *19*, 489 (1999).
492 O. Marchetti, P. Moreillon, M.P. Glauser, J. Bille and D. Sanglard: Antimicrob. Agents Chemother. *44*, 2373–2381 (2000).
493 C. Pina Vaz, F. Sansonetty, A.G. Roderigues, M.J. Martinez de Olivera, A.F. Fonseca et al.: J. Med. Microbiol. *49*, 831 (2000).
494 A. Louie, W. Liu, D.A. Miller, A.C. Sucke, Q.F.F. Liu, G.L. Drusano, M. Mayers and M.H. Miller: Antimicrob. Agents Chemother *43*, 2831–2840 (1999).
495 A.M. Lemonte: Abstr. Gen. Meet. Am. Soc. Microbiol. *99*, 320 (1999).
496 A.M. LeMonte, K.E. Washum, M.L. Smedana, C. Schnizlein Bick, S.M. Kohler et al.: J. Infect. Dis. *182*, 545 (2000).
497 A. Louie, P. Banerjee, G.L. Drusano, M. Shayegani and M.H. Miller: Antimicrob. Agents Chemother *43*, 2841–2847 (1999).
498 O. Marchetti, D. Sanglard, J. Bille and M.P. Glauser: Antimicrob. Agents Chemother. *44*, 2932 (2000).
499 J.E. Bennett, W.E. Dismuskes, R.J. Duma, G. Medoff, M.A. Sande et al.: J. N. Engl. J. Med. *301*, 127 (1979).
500 W.E. Dismuskes, G. Cloud, H.A. Gallis, I.M. Kerkering, G. Medoff et al.: N. Engl. J. Med. *317*, 334 (1987).
501 M. White, C. Cirrincione, A. Blevins and D. Armstrong: J. Infect. Dis. *165*, 960 (1992).
502 Ch.M. Van der Horst, M.S. Saag, G.A. Cloud, R.J. Hamill, R.J. Graybill et al.: New. Eng. J. Med. *337*, 15–21 (1997).
503 R.A. Larsen, S.A. Bozzette, B.E. Jones, D. Haghighat, M.A. Leal et al.: Clin. Infect. Dis. *19*, 741 (1994).

504 M.D. Witt, R.J. Lewis, R.A. Larsen, E.N. Milefchik, A.F. Leal et al.: Clin. Infect. Dis. *22*, 322–328 (1996).
505 Z. Yao, W. Liao and H. Wen: Chin. Med. J *113*, 178 (2000).
506 R.E. Verweij, J.P. Donnelly, B.J. Kullberg, J.F.G.M. Meis and P.E. de Pauw: Infection *22*, 81 (1994).
507 M. Fernandez, E.H. Moylett, D. Noyola and C.J. Barker: Clin. Infect. Dis. *31*, 458 (2000).
508 J.L. Casado, C. Quereda, J. Oliva et al.: Clin. Infect. Dis. *2*, 673 (1997).
509 I.K.P Cheng, G.X. Fang, T.M. Chan and M.K. Chan: Quart. J. Med. *71*, 265, 407 (1989).
510 A. Slingeneyer, B. Laroche, E. Stec, B. Canaud, J.J. Beraud and C. Mion: Perit. Dial. Bulletin *4* (Suppl. 1), 60 (1984).
511 P.A. Burch, J.E. Karp and J. Merz: J. Clin. Oncol. *5*, 1985 (1987).
512 B. Zimmermann, D. Hobusch, C. Hain, U. Kaben and C. Plath: Klein. Paediatr. *212*, S120 (2000).
513 I.E. Bajjoka, E.M. Bailey, J.A. Vazquez and M.S. Abouljoud: Pharmacothetrapy *19*, 118 (1999).
514 R. Negroni, A.M. Robles and A. Arechiavala: Rev. Argentina de Micologia *18*, 2 (1995).
515 T.J. Walsh, J. Van Cutsem, A. Polak and J.R. Graybill: J. Med.Vet. Mycol. *30* (Suppl. 1), 225 (1992).
516 D. Metcalf: Blood *74*, 1673–1677 (1989).
517 S. Schelenz, D.A. Schmith and G.J. Bancroft: Medical Mycology *37*, 183–194 (1999).
518 M. Egerton, S.E. Koshlukova, M.W. B. Araujo, R.C. Patel, J. Dong et al.: Antimicrob. Agents Chemother. *44*, 3310 (2000).
519 E. Roilides, A. Anastasiou-Katsiardani, A. Dimitradou Georgiadou, I. Kadilsoglou, S. Tsaparidou et al.: J. Infect. Dis. *178*, 1734–1742 (1998).
520 N. Vazquez, T.J. Walsh, D. Friedman, S. Chanok and C.A. Lyman: Infect. Immun. *66*, 145–150 (1998).
521 J.E. Lutz, K.V. Clemons, W.C. Darbonne, J.T. Curnutte and D.A. Stevens: Clin. Infect. Dis. *23*, 899 (1996).
522 E. Sasaki, T. Tashiro, M. Kuroki, M. Seki, Y. Miyazaki et al.: Clin. Ex. Infect. *119*, 293 (2000).
523 J.L. Herrmann, N. Dubois, M. Fourgeaud, D. Bassei and P.H. Lagrange: J. Antimicrob. Chemother. *34*, 1051 (1994).
524 A.L. Baltch, R.P. Smith, M. Franke, W. Ritz, P. Michelsen et al.: Antimicrob. Agents Chemother. *45*, 96 (2001).
525 A.L. Baltch, R.P. Smith, M. Franke, P. Michelsen and W. Ritz: Clin. Infect. Dis. *27*, 984 (1998).
526 S.M. Vora, S. Chauhan, E. Brummer and D.A. Stevens: Antimicrob. Agents Chemother. *42*, 2299 (1998).
527 K.V. Clemons, J.E. Lutz and D.A. Stevens: Antimicrob. Agents Chemother. *45*, 686 (2001).
528 A. Polak: Mycoses *34*, 109 and 205 (1991).
529 J.R. Graybill, R. Bocanegra, L.K. Loebenberg and M.F. Luther: Antimicrob. Agents Chemother. *42*, 3467 (1998).
530 T. Kuhara, K .Uccida and H. Yamaguchi: Antimicrob. Agents Chemother. *44*, 19 (2000).
531 G.S. Deepe and R. Gibbons: Antimicrob. Agents Chemother. *44*, 3328 (2000).
532 T. Tanica, F. Rao, T. Hamada, E. Ueta and T. Osaki: Infect. Immun. *69*, 3883 (2001).
533 N. Bodasing, R.A. Seaton, G. Shankland and A. Pithie: AIDS *14*, S128 (2000).

534 J. DeMaio and I. Colman: Clin. Infect. Dis. 31, 822 (2000).

535 J.B. Garcia Diaz, L. Palau and G.A. Pankey: Clin. Infect. Dis. *32,* 166 (2001).

536 M. Boogaerts: 4th International Janssen-Cilag Symposium, Abstract book, p. 18 (2000).

537 H.J. Tietz, H. Martin and S. Koch: Mycoses *44,* 450 (2001).

538 A. Schaffner: Baillieres Clin. Infect. Dis. *1,* 449 (1994).

539 I.S. Faser and D.W. Denning: Blood Rev. *7,* 208 (1993).

540 EORTC International Antimicrob.Therapy Cooperative Group: Am. J. Med. *86,* 668 (1989).

541 K.A. Marr: N. Engl. J. Med. *346,* 278 (2002).

542 H.G. Prentice, I.M. Hann, R. Herbrecht, M. Auon, S. Kvaloy et al.: Bt. J. Haematol. *98,* 711–718 (1997).

543 M.H. White, R.A. Bowden, E.S. Sandler, M.L. Graham, G.A. Noskin et al.: Clin. Infect. Dis. *27,* 296–302 (1998).

544 R. Martino, A. Domingo Albos, A. Sureda, S. Brunet and J. Sierra: Chemotherapy *45,* 205 (1999).

545 J. Mehta, R. Powles, B. Sirohi, J. Treleaven, S. Kulkarni et al : Blood *96,* 24a (2000).

546 T.J. Walsh, R.W. Finberg, C. Arndt, J. Hiemenz, C. Schwarz et al.: N. Engl. J. Med. *340,* 764–771 (1999).

547 J.R. Wingard, M.H. White, E. Anaissie et al : Clin. Infect. Dis. *31,* 1155 (2000).

548 S.M. Stemmer and I. Hardan: Proc. Am. Soc. Clin. Oncol. *15* (32 Meet.), 544 (1996).

549 I.A. Malik, I. Moid, Z. Aziz, S. Khan, M. Suleman: Am. J. Med. *105,* 478–483 (1998).

550 D.J. Winston, J.W. Hathorn, M.G. Schuster, G.J. Schiller, M.C. Trerrito et al.: Am. J. Med. *108,* 282–289 (2000).

551 R.K. Pelz, C.W. Hendrix, S.M. Swoboda, M. Diener-West, W.G. Merz et al.: Ann. Surgery, *233,* 542 (2001).

552 M. Boogaerts, D.J. Winston, E.J. Bow, G. Garber, A.C. Reboli et al.: Ann. Intern. Med. *135,* 412 (2001).

553 T.J. Walsh, P. Pappas, D.J. Winston, M. Hillard, M.D. Lazarus et al.: N. Eng. J. Med. *346,* 225 (2002).

554 A.H. Groll, J. Ritter and F.M.C. Müller: Klein. Pädiatr. *213* (Suppl. 1), A50 (2001).

555 A. Böhme, M. Karthaus and D. Hoelzer: Chemotherapy *45,* 224–232 (1999).

556 Working Party of the British Society for Antimicrob. Chemotherapy: J. Antimicrob. Chemother. *32,* 5 (1993).

557 E. Devigili, M. Casini, V. Casiba, G. Amaddii, M. Fabris and P. Coser: Blood *94* (10, Suppl. 1, Pt.), 219b (1999).

558 M. Karthus, T. Döllmann, T. Klimasch, C. Elser, C. Rosenthal et al.: Chemotherapy *46,* 293–302 (2000).

559 A. Böhme and D. Hölzer: Blood *94* (10, Suppl. 1, Pt. 2), 47b (1999).

560 P.O. Gubbins, J.L. Bowman and S.R. Penzak : Pharmacotherapy *18,* 549 (1998).

561 A. de Laurenzi, A. Matteocci, A. Lanti, L. Pescador, F. Blandino et al.: Infection *24,* 361 (1996).

562 S.B. Mossad, D.L. Longworth, R.K. Avery, S.K. Schmitt, K.A. Adal et al.: Clin. Infect. Dis. *31,* 265 (2000).

562a S. Uhlenbrock, M. Zimmermann, W. Fegeler, H. Jürgens and J. Ritter: Mycoses *44,* 455 (2001).

563 T. Pühler, H. Böttker, S.W. Möller, B. Bewig and J. Cremer: Pneumologie *54,* S71 (2000).

563a A. Pession, C. Castellini, G. Giorgiani, S. Cesaro, A. Prete et al.: Blood *96,* 786a (2000).

564 W.G. Powderly, D.M. Finkelstein, J. Feinberg, P. Frame, W. He, Ch. van der Horst, S.L. Koletar, M.E. Eyster, S.A. Spector and S.A. Bozette: N. Engl. J. Med. *332*, 700 (1995).
565 P. Schuman, L. Capps, G. Peng, J. Vazquez, W. El Sadr et al.: Ann. Intern. Med. *126*, 689–696 (1997).
566 D.V. Havlir, M.P. Dube, J.A. McCutchan, D.N. Forthal, C.A. Kemper et al.: Clin. Infect. Dis. *27*, 1369–1375 (1998).
567 V. Soriano, C. Dona, R. Rodriguez Rosado, P. Barreiro and J. Gonzalez Lahoz: AIDS *14*, 383–386 (2000).
568 A.H. Groll, G. Just Nübling, M. Kurz, C. Müller, U. Nowak Göttl et al.: J. Antimicrob. Chemother. *40*, 855–862 (1997).
569 M.E. Ellis, S.M. Hussein Quadri, D. Spence, M.A. Halim, P. Ernst and H. Clink: J. Antimicrob. Chemother. *33*, 1223 (1994).
570 K.A. Marr, K. Seidel, M.A. Slavin, R.A.Bowden, H.G. Schoch et al.: Blood *96*, 2055 (2000).
571 K.A. Marr, K. Seidel, M.A. Slavin, R.A. Bowden, H.G. Schoch et al.: Blood *94* (10, Suppl. 1), 394a (1999).
572 R. Powles, D. Cunningham, B. Jameson, C. Tiley, J. Mehta et al.: Blood *92* (10, Suppl. 1) 337b (1998).
573 K. Violaris, B. Doraiswamy, O. Olawepo, D. Risucci and M. Gulrajani LaCorte: Pediatrics *102*, 775 (1998).
574 J. Garbino, P. Lew, J. Romand, J.C. Chevrolet, R. Auckenthaler and F.D. Pittet: Schweiz. Med. Wochenschr. *129* (Suppl. 105, Pt 2), 10s (1999).
575 W.T. Spula, P.B. Kale Pradhan: Ann Pharmacother. *36*, 155 (2002).
576 Y. Kanada, R. Yamamoto, A. Chizuka, T. Suguro, C. Arai et al.: Cancer *89*, 1611 (2000).
577 A. Schaffner and M. Schaffner: J. Infect. Dis. *172*, 1035 (1995).
578 K.A. Marr, K. Seidel, T.C. White and R.A. Bowden: J. Infect. Dis. *181*, 308–316 (2000).
579 J. Berg, C.J. Clancy and M.H. Nguyen: Clin Infect. Dis. *26*, 186–187 (1998).
580 C.C. Kibbler: Mycoses *42* (Suppl. 2), 121–124 (1999).
581 N. Singh: J. Antimicrob. Chemother. *45*, 749 (2000).
582 S. Chariyalertsak, K. Supparatpinyo, T. Sirisanthana and K.E. Nelson: Clin. Infect. Dis. *34*, 277 (2002).
583 F. Morgenstern, A.G. Prentice, H.G. Prentice, J.E. Ropner, S.A Schey et al.: Br. J. Haematol. *105*, 901 (1999).
584 J.L. Harousseau, A.W. Dekker, A. Stamatoullas. H. Bassaris, W. Linkesch et al.: Antimicrob. Agents Chemother. *44*, 1887 (2000).
585 G. Kovacicova, V. Krcmery, A. Roidova, J. Trupl, D. Sejnova et al.: J. Antimicrob. Chemother. *44* (Suppl. A), 49–50 (1999).
586 V. Krcmery, E. Oravcova, S. Spanik, M. Mrazova Studena, J. Trupl et al.: J. Antimicrob. Chemother. *41*, 373–380 (1998).
587 M.G. Crespo, J.A. Rodriguez, F. Portela, J.J. Cuenca, A. Juffe et al.: Eur. Heart J. *18* (Abstr Suppl.) 180 (1997).
588 H. Myint, R. Hall, S. Bolam, A.A. Kyi and R. Winn: Blood *92* (10, Suppl. 1, Pt. 2), 336b (1998).
589 R.W. Ellis, S. Singhai, D.J. Mutimer, J.G.M. Hastings: J. Infect. *36*, A16 (1998).
590 J. Hamacher, A. Spiliopoulos, A.M. Kurt and L.P. Nocod: Schweiz. Med. Wochenschr. *128* (Suppl. 100), 12 S (1998).
591 40th Interscience Conference on Antimicrobial Agents and Chemotherapy (ICAAC), Abstract book (2000).

592 F. Barchiesi, D. Arzeni, V. Cmiletti, O. Simonetti, A. Cellini et al.: J. Clin. Microbiol. *39*, 4208 (2001).
593 C. Lurigados, I. Izquierdo, I. Perez and E. Nieto: Mycoses *44* (Suppl. 1), 46 (2001).
594 S.M. Salama, H. Atwal, A. Gandhi, J. Simon, M. Poglod et al.: Antimicrob. Agents Chemother. *45*, 2420 (2001).
595 T. Konosu, S. Oida, Y, Nakamura, S. Seki, T. Uchida et al.: Chem. Pharm. Bull. *49*, 1649 (2001).
596 M.A. Hossain, S. Maesaki, M.S. Razzaque, K. Tomono, T. Taguchi et al.: J. Antimicrob. Chemother. *46*, 263 (2000).
597 S. Kohno, M.A. Hossain, S. Sasaki, H. Kakeya, K. Tomono et al.: Clin. Infect. Dis. *25*, 489 (1997).
598 J. Szlinder Richert, J. Mazerski, B. Cybulska, J. Grzybowska, E. Borowski: Biochem. Biophys. Acta Gen. Subj. *1528*, 15 (2001).
599 C. Rimaroli and T. Bruzzese: Chemotherapy *46*, 28–35 (2000).
600 V. Strippoli, F.D. D'Auria, G. Simonetti, T. Bruzzese, N. Simonetty: J. Chemother. *45*, 235–237 (2000).
601 R. Powles, S. Kulkarni, J. Treleavan, K. Hobbs, B. Sirohi et al.: Blood *94* (10 Suppl. 1, Pt.). 342 a (1999).
602 D. Gordon, K. Baird, R. Darouiche, V. Fainstein, L. Juaregui et al.: Clin. Infect. Dis. *25*, 382 (1997).
603 D.R. Graham, O.H. Wesly, V.L. Molnar, D.C. Crabtree and S.H. Jennison: Abstr. Gen. Meet. Am. Soc. Microbiol. *98*, 48–49 (1998).
604 E.T. Burt: Exp. Opin. Ther. Patents *11*, 269 (2001).
605 C. Rimorali and T. Bruzzese: Chemotherapy *46*, 28 (2000).
606 A. Saha, L. Liu, R.l. Simoneaux, M.J. Kukla, F.C. Odds et al.: Abstr. Pap. Am. Chem. Soc. 219, 158 (2000).
607 T. Tsukuda, Y. Shiratori, M. Watanabe, H. Ontsuka, K. Hattori et al.: Bioorg. Med. Chem. Lett. *8*, 1819/1825 (1998).
608 D. Zakula, J.O. Capobianco and R.C. Goldman: J. Antimicrob. Chemother. *39*, 261–264 (1997).
609 T. Kuchta, H. Bujdakova and E. Sidoova: Folia Microbiol. *34*, 504 (1998).
610 A. Scozzafava, A. Nicolae, O. Maior, F. Briganti and C.T. Supuran: J. Enzym. Inhib. *14*, 49–68 (1998).
611 S. Watanabe, H. Hirai, M. Ishiguro, T. Kambara, T. Matsunaga et al.: J. Antibiot. *54*, 904 (2001).
612 K. Minagawa, S. Kouzuki, K. Nomura, T. Yamaguchi, T. Kawamura et al.: J. Antibiot. *54*, 890/896 (2001).
613 M. Borg, V. Zeppelin, K. Zazchke, U. Gross and F.M. Müller: Mycoses *44*, 209 (2001).
614 R.J. Graybill: Int. J. Clin. Oract. *55*, 633 (2001).
615 N.H. Georgopapadakou: Exp. Opin. Invest. Drugs *10*, 269 (2001).
616 S. Tawara, F. Ikeda, K. Maki, Y. Morishita, K. Otomo et al.: Antimicrob. Agents Chemother. *44*, 57/614 (2000).
617 S. Matsumoto, Y. Wakai, T. Nakai, K. Hatano, T. Ushitani et al.: Antimicrob. Agents Chemother. *44*, 619 (2000).
618 38th ICAAC Abstract Book F141, F143, F144, F146 (1998).
619 38th ICAAC Abstract Book, F 50, J 134 (1998).
620 J. Onishi, M. Meinz, J. Thompson, J. Currotto, S. Dreikorn et al.: Antimicrob. Agents Chemother. *44*, 368 (2000).

621 A. Fujie, T. Wamoto, B. Sato, H. Muramatsu, C. Kasakara: Bioorg. Med. Chem. Lett. *11*, 399 (2001).
622 D. Barrett, A. Tanaka, K. Harada, E. Watabe, K. Maki et al.: Bioorg. Med. Chem. Lett. *11*, 1843 (2001).
623 J. Goldberg, P. Connolly, C. Schnizlein Bick, M. Durkin, S. Kohler et al.: Antimicrob. Agents Chemother. *44*, 1624 (2000).
624 L.T. Ganesan, E.K. Manavathu, J.L. Cutright and P. Chandrasekar: Clin. Infect. Dis. *22*, 1199 (2001).
625 C.C. Chiou, N. Mavrogiorgos, E. Tillem, R. Hector and T. Walsh: Antimicrob. Agents Chemother. *45*, 3310 (2001).
626 D.A. Stevens: Antimicrob. Agents Chemother. *44*, 2547 (2000).
627 K. Masubuchi, M. Taniguchi, K. Hattori, H. Suda, Y. Kohchi et al.: Bioorg. Med. Chem. Lett. *10*, 1459 (2000).
628 M. Sudoh, T. Yamazaki, K. Masubuchi, M. Taniguchi, N. Shimma et al.: J. Biol. Chem. 275, 32901 (2000). .
629 Kang Sik Park, Kap Chul Kang, Ki Young Kim et al.: J. Antimicrob. Chemother. *47*, 513 (2001).
630 D.A. Stevens, H.A. Brammer, D.W. Meyer and B.H. Steiner: Clin. Infect. Dis. *27*, 987 (1998).
631 A.M. Janiak, S. Milewsi: Med. Mycol. *39*, 401 (2001).
632 I. Gautier Lefebvre, J.B. Behr, G. Guillerm and N.S. Ryder: Bioorg. Med. Chem. Lett *10*, 1483 (2000).
633 J. Leclerque: J. Pharm. Belg. *56*, 95 (2001).
634 M.K. Bedi and P.D. Sheenefelt: Arch. Dermatol. *138*, 232 (2002).
635 Z.F. Khana and R. Katiyar: Pharm Biol. *38*, 87 (2000).
636 A. Lopez, D.S. Ming and G.H.N. Towets: J. Nat. Prod. *65*, 62 (2002).
637 C. Pina Vaz, A. Goncalves Rodrigues, E. Pinot, S. Costa de Oliviera, A. Martinez de Oliviera et al.: Mycoses *44* (Suppl. 1), 59 (2001).
638 X.Y. Ye and T.B. Ng: Biochem. Biophys. Res. Commun. *273*, 111 (2000).
639 S. Magaldi, M.E. Giron and A. Rodriguez-Acosta: Mycoses *45*, 19 (2002).
640 Y. Aoki, M. Yamamoto, S.M. Hosseini-Mazinani, N. Koshikawa, K. Sugimoto and M. Arisawa: Antimicrob. Agents Chemother. *40*, 127 (1996).
641 A.I. de Lucca and T.J. Walsh: Antimicrob. Agents Chemother. *43*, 1(1999).
642 A.M. Ben Josef, E.K. Manavathu, D. Platt and J.D. Sobel: Int. J. Antimicrob. Agents *13*, 287 (2000).
643 E. Manavathu, J.R. Dimmok, S.C. Vashishta and P.H. Chandrasekar: Antimoicrob. Agents Chemother. *43*, 2950 (1999).
644 M.C. Justice, M.J. Hsu, T. Ku, J. Balkovecs, D. Schmatz et al.: J. Biol. Chem. *273*, 3148 (1998).
645 J.M. Dominguez, M.G. Gomez-Lorenzo and J.J. Martin: J. Biol. Chem. *274*, 22423 (1999).
646 M. Skastry, J. Nielsen, T. Ku, M.J. Hsu, P. Liberator et al.: Microbiology *147*, 393 (2001).
647 E. Herreros, C.M. Martinez, M.J. Almela, M.S. Marriott, F.G. de las Heras et al.: Antimicrob. Agents Chemother. *42*, 283 (1998).
648 E. Herreros, M.J. Almela, S. Lozano, F.G. de las Heras and D. Gargallo Viola: Antimicrob. Agents Chemother. *45*, 3132 (2001).
649 M. Cuenca-Estrella, E. Mellado, T.M. Diaz-Guerra, A. Monzon and J.L. Rodriguez-Tudela: Antimicrob. Agents Chemother. *45*, 905 (2001).

650 A. Martinez, P. Aviles, E. Jimenez, J. Caballero and D. Gargallo-Viola : Antimicrob. Agents Chemother. *44*, 3389 (2000).
651 K.V. Clemons and D.A. Stevens. Antimicrob. Agents Chemother. *44*, 1874 (2000).
652 A. Martinez, J. Regardera, E. Jimenez, I. Santos and D. Gargallo-Viola. Antimicrob. Agents Chemother. *45*, 1008 (2001).
653 A. Martinez, S. Ferrer, I. Santos, E. Jimenez, J. Sparrowe et al.: Antimicrob. Agents Chemother. *45*, 3304 (2001).
654 J.D. Nosanchuk, R. Ovalle and A. Casadevall: J. Infect. Dis. *183*, 1093 (2001).
655 34th Tagung der DMyk: Mycoses 43, pages 217, 222, 233, 240, 248, 250 (2000).
656 F.C. Odds: ASM News *60*, 313 (1994).
657 J.R. Perfect: Antimicrob. Agents Chemother. *40*, 1577 (1996).
658 Ch. Bulawa, D.W. Miller, L.K. Henry and J.M. Becker: Proc. Natl. Acad. Sci. USA *92*, 10579 (1995).
659 T. Wu, K. Wright, S.F. Hurst and C.J. Morrison: Antimicrob. Agents Chemother. *44*, 1200 (2000).
660 K. Fekere Forgacs, L. Gyure and B. Lenkey: Mycoses *43*, 273 (2000).
661 J.R. Graybill, E. Montalbo, W.R. Kircpatrick, M.F. Luther, S.G. Revankar et al.: Antimicrob. Agents Chemother. *42*, 2938 (1998).
662 S. Rupp: Bio World *3*, 21 (2000).
663 M. Niewerth and H.C. Korting: Mycoses *44*, 361 (2001).
664 H. Hänel, R. Kirsch, H.L. Schmidts and K. Kottmann: Mycoses *38*, 251 (1995).
665 F. de Bernardis, P. Sullivan and A. Cassone: Medical Mycology *39*, 303 (2001).
666 B. Hube, C.J. Turver, F.C. Odds, H. Eifert, G.J. Boulnois et al.: J. Med. Vet. Mycol. *29*, 129 (1991).
667 M. Badasso, S.P. Wood, C. Anuiler, J.B. Cooper, T.L. Blundell and T. Dreyer: J. Mol. Biol. *232*, 701 (1992).
668 R. Rüchel, B. Ritter and M. Schaffrinski: Zbl. Bakt. *273*, 391 (1990).
669 L. Angiolella, E. De Bernardis, C. Bromuro, E. Mondollo, T. Ceddia and A. Cassone: J. Chemother. *2*, 55 (1990).
670 O. Hruskova Heidingsfeldova, J. Dostal, L. Pavlickova, M. Soucek and V. Pichova: Mycoses *44*, 252 (2001).
671 H. Matayuki, I. Masoto, A. Kenji: Jpn. Kokai Tokkyo Koho, 8 pp (1993).
672 H.C. Korting, M. Schaller, G. Eder, G. Hamm, U. Böhmer and B. Hube: Antimicrob. Agents Chemother. *43*, 2038–2042 (1999).
673 M. Monond, A. Telenti and D. Sanglard: Dermatoloy *197*, 209 (1998).
674 M. Monod, M. Borg-von Zepelin, A. Telenti and D. Samglard: Dermatology *198*, 412–414 (1999).
675 R. Wurzner, J. Bektic, M. Borg-Von Zeppelin and M.P. Dietrich: Mycoses *44*, 249 (2001).
676 A. Gruber, C. Speth, E. Lukasser-Vogel, R. Zangerle, M. Borg-von Zepelin et al.: Immunopharmacology *41*, 227–234 (1999).
677 S. Hood, A. Bonington, J. Evans and D. Denning: AIDS *12*, 447–448 (1998).
678 C. Atzori, E. Angelli, A. Macinini, F. Agostani, V. Michell and A. Cargnell: J. Infect. Dis. *181*, 1629 (2000).
679 Z. Thang, H.N. El Sohly, M.R. Jacob, D.S. Walker and A.M. Clark: Planta Med. *68*, 49 (2002).

Antifungal Agents – Advances and Problems (E. Jucker, Ed.)

Susceptibility testing of fungi – current status and open questions

By Michael Seibold and Kathrin Tintelnot

Robert Koch-Institut, Mykologie, Nordufer 20, 13353 Berlin, Germany

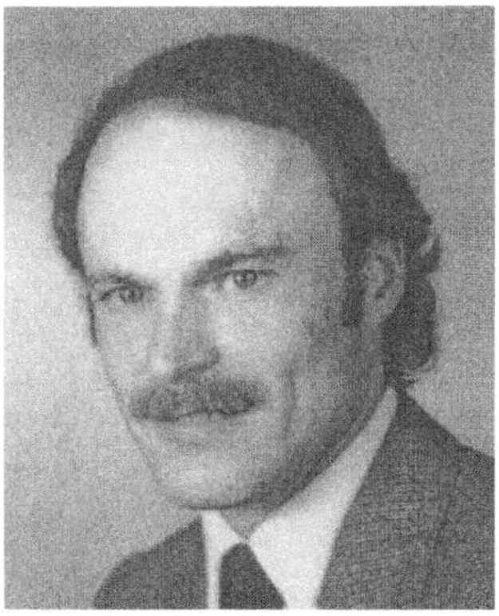

Michael Seibold

studied microbiology and received his diploma at the University of Tübingen, Germany. From 1980 to 1984 he was assistant at the Technical University of Berlin and was involved in technical mycology and training of students. Thereafter he joined the medical mycology group of F. Staib (since 1992 led by K. Tintelnot) at the Robert Koch-Institut and worked as a specialist in the diagnosis of mycoses, advising clinicians, antifungal susceptibility testing, and the physiology of fungi.

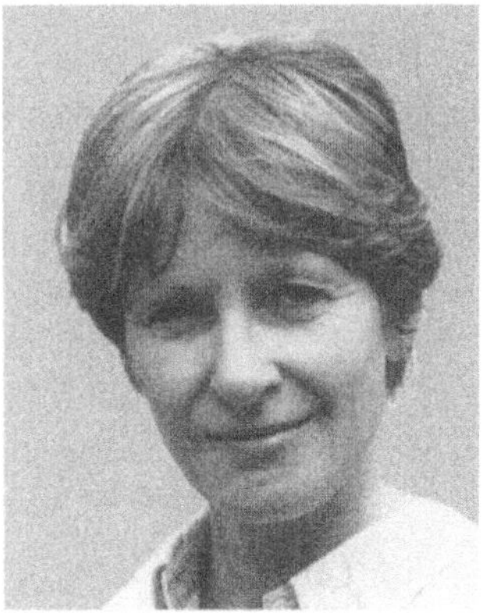

Kathrin Tintelnot

studied Human Medicine and received her MD at the Free University of Berlin, Germany. She worked at the Institut für Pathologie and the Institut für Hygiene & Mikrobiologie at the University of Würzburg. She specialized in microbiology and the epidemiology of infectious diseases with a particular emphasis on the diagnosis of fungal infections under the guidiance of H.P.R. Seeliger. Since 1992 she has been head of the project "Mycology" at the Robert Koch-Institut, Berlin. Her fields of special interests are imported systemic mycoses, cryptococcosis, and diagnosis and therapy of fungal infections due to uncommon pathogens as well as their histopathology.

Summary

The increase of fungal infections and the improvement of therapeutical options demand reliable antifungal susceptibility testing. *In vitro* susceptibility testing of fungi – in contrast to bacteria – is not yet established as a routine method. The NCCLS (National Committee for Clinical Laboratory Standards) guidelines for susceptibility testing of yeasts (and proposed for hyphomycetes) are most important for standardization. Meanwhile, essential parts of this test procedure are accepted, but it should still be improved. The concept of using only one test medium for all drugs and test organisms is not realized so far. There are also some test situations that prevent the NCCLS standard from being applied. Based on our experience, this article describes the NCCLS methods and their modifications. It places emphasis on lipophilic drugs showing controversies despite standardization. Furthermore, the prediction of MICs on the clinical outcome is discussed. Since there are some pitfalls in testing antifungals, this should be done in experienced laboratories only. The MIC has to be regarded as only one, but an important, factor in the management of fungal diseases. Host-, drug-, and pathogen-specific data should be considered simultaneously.

Contents

Keywords

Antifungal susceptibility testing, standardization, hyphomycetes, yeasts, *in vitro-in vivo* correlation, lipophilic drugs.

Glossary of abbreviations

ATCC®, American type culture collection; AUC, area under the curve; CFU, colony forming units; CYG, Casiton Yeast Extract Glucose; DIN, Deutsche Industrie-Norm; DMSO, dimethyl sulfoxide; EMEM, Eagle's Minimal Essential Medium; EMTA, Endomethylene-tetrahydrophtalic acid; ESCMID, European Society of Clinical Microbiolgy and Infectious Diseases; EUCAST, European Committee for Antifungal Susceptibility Testing; FIC, fractional inhibitory concentration; HAART, highly active antiretroviral therapy; HR, Heath-Robinson or High Resolution; MEC, minimum effective concentration; MFC, minimal fungicidal concentration; MIC, minimal inhibitory concentration; MLC, minimal lethal concentration; MOPS, 3-(N-morpholino) propanesulfonic acid; MTT, [3-(4,5-dimethyl-2-thiazolyl)-2,5-diphenyl-2*H*-tetrazolium];

NCCLS, National Committee for Clinical Laboratory Standards; QC, quality control; RPMI, Roswell Park Memorial Institute; v/v, volume per volume; XTT, [(2,3bis(2-methoxy-4-nitro-5-sulfophenyl)-5-[(phenylamino) carbonyl]-2*H*-tetrazolium hydroxide)].

1 Introduction

1.1 Need for antifungal susceptibility testing

Because of the increasing number of life-threatening fungal infections with a high mortality rate in immunocompromised patients, information on the susceptibility of these etiological agents is of growing interest.

Further demand for information is given by a shift of fungal isolates to up to now less frequently isolated species [1–5]. This also includes emerging or re-emerging fungal pathogens. Particularly for uncommon agents, little information exists about their so far unpredictable susceptibility.

The development of resistance, especially under long-term therapy, makes susceptibility testing necessary. The widespread prescription of fluconazole was followed by an increase in the resistance of *Candida albicans* isolates [6–10]. A considerable amount of *Candida* spp. – up to one-third of all clinical isolates in HIV patients before HAART – showed resistance under standard therapy [11]. In *C. albicans* isolates of AIDS patients suffering from oropharyngeal candidosis, 46% had increased MICs for fluconazole [12].

Monitoring of susceptibility may give hints to the development of resistance. This is indicated whenever the clinical course of the fungal infection under therapy is not as effective as expected. Susceptibility testing of fungi is mainly of clinical interest.

In most clinically relevant fungal infections, however, primarily an empiric therapy is started. Antifungal testing is required to judge the likelihood of clinical response from a fungal agent to therapy. Decreased susceptibility under therapy, going along with delayed or refractory clinical response, raises the question of whether, e.g., to increase the dosage or to change the antifungal treatment. As in bacteriology, cross-resistance of antifungal agents in the same drug class is not uncommon [13].

In vitro testing is essential for the development of new drugs. The number of available antifungal drugs is limited. As already known, it is a long time between screening of substances for their antifungal properties to the development of new drugs. This article focuses mainly on *in vitro* testing of clinical interest; therefore, aspects of screening on antifungal activity of new substances are not considered further.

The *in vitro* susceptibility of fungi is of epidemiological interest. *In vitro* testing informs on the pattern of susceptibility in different populations, e.g., in hospitalized patients. It must be mentioned that nosocomial isolates with resistance are consistently reported. According to § 23 Abs.1 of the *Infektionsschutzgesetz* (IfSG), hospitals in Germany are obliged to observe fluconazole-resistant *Candida* spp. if a susceptibility test within clinical-microbiological diagnostics has been performed [14].

1.2 Clinical indications for antifungal susceptibility testing

Susceptibility testing should be based on a clear indication. Routine testing is not recommended. While resistance of *Candida* spp. to flucytosine was the most prevalent one in the 1980s and therefore the main indication for susceptibility testing, the dramatic development of resistance to azoles, especially to fluconazole, became the main cause for *in vitro* testing in the 1990s. Nowadays, the increasing number of life-threatening hyphomycoses in immunocompromised patients, often amphotericin B resistant (*Scedosporium* spp., *Aspergillus terreus*, and others), are a challenge for microbiologists for *in-vitro*-based therapeutical recommendations. The decision to perform testing requires not only trained and experienced lab staff but also good collaboration between the microbiologist and the clinician. First of all, the relevance of an isolate should be checked thoroughly. *In vitro* susceptibility testing might be performed before or in context with systemic antifungal treatment only. With rare exceptions neither a topic antimycotic treatment nor isolates from materials like feces are indications for susceptibility testing. The local concentration of topically applied antifungal agents might be not definable, but it will be so high that the MIC is of secondary relevance. Likewise, susceptibility testing is not indicated when the etiologic agent is known to show intrinsic resistance, e.g., for fluconazole and *C. krusei* isolates [15, 16].

One should consider that each *in vitro* test is time- and money-consuming and that there are many pitfalls on the way from isolation of the etiological agent to the interpretation of a MIC (see Section 6). Table 1 roughly summarizes the clinical relevance for susceptibility testing of yeasts and hyphomycetes (moulds).

Table 1.
Indications and test organisms for antifungal susceptibility testing

Fluconazole	
Yeasts:	- Blood stream/invasive infections due to *Candida* spp., especially when amphotericin B and flucytosine are not tolerated - No or delayed response to fluconazole therapy of an infection due to *Candida* spp. - Suspicion of emergence/spread of resistant strains (additional molecular studies on clonal identity are indicated)
Moulds:	- Not relevant
Itraconazole, Voriconazole	
Yeasts:	- Presence or suspicion of resistance to fluconazole
Moulds:	- *Aspergillus* spp., dematiaceous fungi
Flucytosine	
Yeasts:	- When combined with amphotericin B for therapy (for *Cr. neoformans* routinely not necessary); - *Candida* isolates, refractory to azole therapy
Moulds:	- *Aspergillus* spp., dematiaceous fungi
Amphotericin B	
Yeasts:	- Therapy with amphotericin B in infections due to *Candida* spp. with high risk of resistance (e.g., *C. lusitaniae, C. guillermondii*) - *Candida* infections refractory to azoles (optional)
Moulds:	- *Aspergillus* spp., *Fusarium* spp., *Pseudallescheria boydii* and any not yet identified mould
Caspofungin	
Yeasts:	- Not indicated for the basidiomyceteous yeasts *Cryptococcus* spp. and *Trichosporon* spp.
Moulds:	- Systemic mycosis refractory to amphotericin B or if not tolerated

Antifungal susceptibility testing for the management of patients with candidosis is recommended by the NIAID (National Institute of Allergy and Infectious Diseases) Mycosis Study Group. *Note*: For antifungal susceptibility testing of hyphomycetes, neither interpretive breakpoints nor data on interpretation of these MICs are available (except for MICs of itraconazole to *Aspergillus fumigatus*).

2 Resistance

2.1 Definitions of susceptibility and resistance

In the 1980s the resistance of *Candida* to azoles was compared to beauty, which "can lie very much in the eye of the beholder" [17]. A multiside study showed that the minimal inhibition concentration (MIC), i.e., the lowest concentration of a drug effective for growth inhibition (see below), might differ by a factor of 50,000 [18]. This variation led to a judgment from "highly susceptible" to "highly resistant" for the same isolate depending on the labs and their methods used. It was recognized that the MIC is more or less strongly influenced by the test parameters. The MIC determination of an antifungal is not a physical or chemical measurement. It is more of an approximation to a biological property that is comparable only when the test parameters are defined. Therefore, it would be correct to use the term "a MIC" instead of "the MIC".

The first standardization of antifungal testing was published for flucytosine by the French Society of Medical Mycology [19]. Because of the efforts of a standardizing committee, the National Committee for Clinical and Laboratory Standards (NCCLS) in the U.S., reproducible data on the MICs of yeasts were achievable [20]. Additionally, through publication of interpretative breakpoints for antifungal agents, a judgment of susceptible, resistant, or susceptible-dose-dependent (resp. intermediate) was given for single antifungal substances (fluconazole, itraconazole, and flucytosine), even if not for all. In the literature the terms "resistance testing" and "susceptibility testing" are used synonymously (see Section 6). In this article we prefer the term susceptility testing.

A fungal isolate is regarded as susceptible to an antifungal when its growth is inhibited or reduced by a defined drug-specific concentration. Correspondingly, resistance is defined as absence of growth inhibition or strongly reduced growth only under an antifungal drug. Growth inhibition may reflect fungistatic or fungicidal activity. If the latter is of interest, the ratio between killed and still culturable fungi has to be calculated. The time-dependent antifungal activity can be assessed by time-kill curves. Antifungal activity can be measured by parameters other than growth inhibition:

- The effect on the metabolism of fungi, e.g., the consumption of glucose in the test assay, the reduction of colored substrates in the medium, or the decrease of ATP within the cell or the ergosterol content of the cell. The measurement of the latter is adequate only for antifungal agents with this target.
- The efficacy of antifungal agents on the virulence factors of the cell, e.g., the adherence, the urease activity, or the transition from yeast cells to hyphae [21–23].
- Furthermore, antifungal substances can be measured *via* their effect on

growth morphology. Fluconazole-resistant *Candida albicans* isolates are known to differ from susceptible ones in pseudomycel formation. Testing caspofungin to *Aspergillus fumigatus*, the measurement of antifungal activity on the micromorphology of hyphae seems to be superior compared to traditional methods [24].

Other surrogate parameters of growth inhibition are theoretically possible; often they have been taken over by methods used in bacteriology. How far new criteria of antibacterial activity such as the mutant prevention concentration [25] could be adopted for antifungal susceptibility testing cannot yet be predicted. Measurement of growth inhibition (resp. reduction of cell yield), however, may be of limited value for rapid assays in fungi. In contrast to bacteria with short doubling times, even fast growing yeasts such as *Candida albicans* show a generation time of more than 1 hour under test conditions.

2.2 Types of resistance

Although this article does not focus on resistance mechanisms, which are partly analyzed – even at the molecular level – and described elsewhere in detail, the terms of different types of resistance have to be pointed out briefly.

2.2.1 Primary resistance

Fungi are considered to have primary resistance to an antifungal agent when it is ineffective or only slightly effective against the growth of the fungus and when this is genetically based. For example, this is proven for flucytosine and fluconazole in almost any zygomycete. Also, the ineffectiveness of fluconazole to *Candida krusei* and *Candida norvegensis* is due to this intrinsic (inherent) resistance [26–28].

Broadly accepted data exist on primary resistance of fungi. However, one should be aware of a too rash classification of fungal species as "primary resistant". This attribution sometimes derives from fungal infections, refractory to therapy. Occasionally, the so-called primary (as well as secondary) *in vitro* resistance is based on tests not standardized when the resistance was described. The number of strains that have proved to be primary resistant may vary within the same species. As already mentioned, *C. krusei* is inherently resistant to fluconazole, whereas the percentage of isolates with resistance to flucytosine on average is 43% [29]. Nearly all of the clinical relevant moulds, e.g., *Aspergillus* spp., *Fusarium* spp., or *Scedosporium* spp., are inherently resistant to fluconazole, and several genera are resistant to all azoles.

2.2.2 Secondary resistance

When an isolate previously found to be susceptible loses this feature under therapy, it is considered to be secondary resistant. The underlying mechanisms depend on the antifungal substance and the etiological agent. The reasons for this secondary or acquired resistance are mutation and selection. The mechanism of resistance to flucytosine was the first one described in detail. In this case many steps are involved in the interaction between the antifungal substance and the cell, and mutation can take place at different sites of interaction. Therefore, a resistance can arise quickly.

Repeated prophylactic therapy or a suboptimal dosage can result in resistance to the antifungal drug. This problem increased dramatically under fluconazole in HIV-infected patients. Concomitantly with the emergence of azole resistance in *Candida albicans*, the underlying mechanisms were intensively investigated and understanding about the interaction of the drug with the fungal cell could be obtained [27, 30–32].

2.2.3 Clinical resistance

Primary or secondary resistant isolates are expected to be refractory to antifungal treatment. But even *in vitro* susceptible isolates can be refractory to therapy. This so-called "clinical resistance" may depend on the drug, the fungus, the mode of infection, the underlying disease, and the immune status of the patient. It is obvious that suboptimal dosage or drug interaction can reduce the benefit of the antifungal drug. It has to be considered that colonization of indwelling catheters even in susceptible strains is often not to be cured by an antimycotic treatment. Further connections between the *in vitro* situation and the clinical outcome are discussed in Section 6.

3 Methods of susceptibility testing of yeasts

In Sections 3 and 4, the NCCLS standards are discussed thoroughly. These methods are performed in most antifungal susceptibility testing laboratories as a result of comprehensive experience for many years. Nevertheless, this method could be improved. In parallel to the NCCLS, efforts for standardizing were done in Europe and other countries, i.e., by the Committee for Laboratory Standards of the Japanese Society for Medical Mycology.

Non-standardized methods in antifungal susceptibility testing will produce largely different results. Not only the test format (agar dilution, disk diffusion, broth macro- and microdilution) can influence the MIC but also test parameters such as medium (composition, pH, buffering), inoculum size, time and temperature of incubation, etc. Their effects on *in vitro* susceptibility are summarized in Table 2. The following sections present methods that were established in order to obtain reproducible data on the susceptibility of fungi. Detailed reviews on standardization and methods of susceptibility testing are given in [33, 34].

3.1 The NCCLS M27-A method

1982 a committee was founded in the U.S. in order to set up a standard for the antifungal susceptibility testing of fungi. In 1997, the long-lasting efforts resulted in the NCCLS M27-A protocol entitled, "Reference Method for Broth Dilution Antifungal Susceptibility Testing of Yeasts; Approved Standard" [20]. The preceding protocols (M27-P, M27-T) focused on reproducibility, the most important prerequisite for any susceptibility testing. This is provided in the final standard. Although not perfect, the NCCLS method is widely accepted as a base for studies on correlation to other test methods and finally to *in vivo* outcome. To attain reproducible MICs, one must regard a series of regulations

Table 2.
Influence of test parameters on the MIC of antifungals to yeasts

	Amphotericin B (AMB)	Flucytosine (FCY)	Azoles
Medium	+ Possible antagonism with sterols or sterol-like substances. Spread of MIC range with Antibiotic Medium 3	+ Purines and pyrimidines of complex media act antagonistically with FCY! Differences of MIC even among fully defined media	–/+ Fluconazole testing little affected; MICs of very hydrophobic substances in complex media are lower (see Section 3.1)
Inoculum	–/(+)	+ High inocula raise MIC	+ High inocula raise MIC, may impede the reading and lead to false resistance (see Section 3.1)
Buffer, if not present	+ Raises MIC	+ Lowers MIC	+ Raises MIC (up to 1000-fold)
Temperature	+/– No uniform effects on MIC	+ MIC lower at 25 °C vs. 37 °C	+/(–) Lower temperature often resulting in lower MICs
Light	+ Prolonged exposure to light could degrade AMB	–	–
Incubation time	+/(–) MIC often raises with prolonged time	+ Raising of MIC with prolonged time	+ MIC raises with prolonged time, depending on substance and medium
Reading	– Mostly clear-cut endpoints, trailing uncommon	–/+ Less sharp endpoints for some species	+ Trailing endpoints not uncommon

+, effects evidently observed; +/(–), effect often present but sometimes absent; (+), less or no effect seen; –, effects not seen or very rarely; ±, effects may be present or not, depending on the substance and/or medium; –/(+), effects can differ from – to (+) but are considered marginally.

described in the document in detail. Because of the importance of the NCCLS standard, the main features are presented (Tab. 3). The procedure is commented upon critically, especially the problematic handling of highly lipophilic (hydrophobic) substances.

Table 3.
Parameters of the NCCLS M27-A method for testing yeasts

Test organisms	*Candida* species, *Cryptococcus neoformans*
Test format	Broth macrodilution or microdilution assay
Test medium	RPMI-1640 medium (with glutamine, without bicarbonate), buffered to pH 7.0 (25 °C) with 0.165 M MOPS
Drugs and test ranges	0.03–16 μg/ml for amphotericin B, itraconazole and ketoconazole; 0.12–64 μg/ml for flucytosine and fluconazole
Inoculum	0.5×10^3–2.5×10^3 CFU/ml (final concentration)
Preparation of inoculum	Standardization by spectrophotometric adjustment to a turbidity of McFarland 0.5
Incubation period/temperature	46–50 h for *Candida* spp., 70–74 h for *Cryptococcus neoformans*, 35 ± 1 °C
Reading	Visually, by mirror
Definition of inhibition	Endpoint for amphotericin B: 100% inhibition (score of 0) Endpoint for flucytosine and azoles: - macrodilution: ≈ 80 % reduction compared to growth control - microdilution: score of 2 (prominent decrease in turbidity, approx. equal to or greater than 50% reduction)
Quality control strains (established for broth macrodilution)	*C. krusei* ATCC® 6258 *C. parapsilosis* ATCC® 22019 (recommended limits for four reference strains: *C. albicans* ATCC® 90028 and ATCC® 24433, *C. parapsilosis* ATCC® 90018 and *C. tropicalis* ATCC® 750)
Interpretive breakpoints for *Candida* species	
Fluconazole (except for *C. krusei*)	- susceptible: ≤ 0.12–8 μg/ml - susceptible-dose dependent: 16–32 μg/ml - intermediate: not defined - resistant: ≥ 64 μg/ml
Itraconazole	- susceptible: ≤ 0.125 μg/ml - susceptible-dose dependent: 0.25–0.5 μg/ml - intermediate: not defined - resistant: ≥ 1 μg/ml
Flucytosine	- susceptible: ≤ 4 μg/ml - susceptible-dose dependent: not defined - intermediate: 8–16 μg/ml - resistant: ≥ 32 μg/ml

3.1.1 Test organisms

The suitability of this test method for yeasts is restricted to *Candida albicans* and partly to the clinical relevant non-*albicans Candida* species. This limitation must be seen in context with the test format as broth dilution test. The yeasts might sink to the bottom of the well (broth microdilution test) or test tube (broth macrodilution test) after inoculation, finding nearly anaerobic conditions. Diffusion of oxygen into the medium may be insufficient for non-, weak- or slow-fermenting yeasts like *Debaryomyces hansenii* (*C. famata*), *Rhodotorula* spp., *C. inconspicua, C. norvegensis* (*Pichia norvegensis*), or *C. valida* (*Pichia membranifaciens*). The restricted availability of oxygen also may be growth limiting for the non-fermenting, oxygen-requiring yeast *Cryptococcus neoformans* and *Trichosporon* spp. [33, 35, 36]. The agar dilution test (see Section 5.4) provides the non-fermenting organisms with sufficient oxygen. This test should be performed exceptionally, because the following problems have to be considered:

(1) Agars are not fully definable. The concentration of cations especially may influence the growth and the MICs.
(2) This alternative requires a technology not described in detail such as the NCCLS method.
(3) Agar plates once produced can be used for a limited time in contrast to microtiter plates, which can be stored frozen at –70 °C for a long time.

Modifications for testing of *Cr. neoformans* are mentioned but are not part of the formal M27-A method. The modification recommends Yeast Nitrogen Base medium, which may enhance the growth of *Cr. neoformans* and improve the clinical relevance of antifungal MICs [37–39].

3.1.2 Inoculum

It is widely accepted that the amount of the inoculum can influence the MICs (see Tab. 2). Too high inocula are reported to lead to resistance, especially when fungistatic substances are tested. In the opinion of the authors, this resistance can be fictitious only. Even under effective concentrations of a fungistatic antifungal, yeast cells can grow by dividing up to 10 times and more before growing is stopped completely (data not published). This results in an increase of up to 1000-fold for the inoculum. Thus, high inocula lead to false (fictitious) resistance when MICs are determined. In the case of the recommended inoculum of about 10^3 CFUs/ml, each well of the microtiter plate contains about 200 cells. It is self-evident that lower inocula lead to a variance of the cell number in each well and could impair the reproducibility of MICs. Inocula under 10^3 CFUs/ml will prolong the incubation time since the test can be read only if growth is visible. Results in our lab confirm that increasing the inoculum to 10^4 CFUs/ml might result in higher MIC mostly in the range of one to two dilution steps, depending on the isolate and antifungal tested. The tendency to false resistance rises markedly when the inocula are higher than 10^4 CFUs/ml. The recommended inoculum of the McFarland turbidity standard of 0.5 is prepared by photometrical adjustment or visually and has to be further diluted to give the final cell concentration. Alternative methods may be used, however, the correctness of these methods has to be ensured. For details on the preparation of the inoculum, see the NCCLS M27-A document.

3.1.3 Test medium

The demands on a test medium can be summarized as follows: reproducibility of MICs, no interference with test substances, good availability, and low cost. The NCCLS recommends MOPS-buffered RPMI-1640 medium (with glutamine, without bicarbonate, and with a pH indicator), which is then abbreviated as RPMI medium. This medium, already common for a long time as a cell culture medium, was used for the development of the NCCLS M27 standard [40, 41]. It was found to be suitable for antifungal susceptibility testing of yeasts, being at least as satisfactory as other synthetic media. The RPMI medium can be purchased as powder from different companies. The buffer MOPS [3-(N-morpholino) propanesulfonic acid] is not taken up by the cell and stabilizes within the neutral pH range optimally. The pH of the medium is set to pH 7.0 (±0.1) at room temperature (25 °C). The content of glucose and buffering of this medium are discussed below in detail. The concentration of glucose (2 g/L) resembles the *in vivo* situation (about 1 g/L). This relatively low amount leads to a limitation of growth after 24 hours for fast growing yeasts due to the consumption of glucose. The yield of cells is more or less dependent on the concentration of glucose in the medium. A higher content of glucose will be a better basis for the discrimination of susceptible or resistant isolates. It is known that isolates tested to fungistatic antifungal agents might show residual growth even under an effective drug concentration. There can be up to 10 or more cell divisions until their growth is stopped independently from the glucose concentration.

The growth control, i.e., the growth in drug-free medium, which is the basis for the calculation of the MIC, is set to 100% growth or 0% inhibition. It is clear that a decision on susceptibility may be difficult when the growth control is low in media with little glucose content and the tested isolate shows residual growth. Because of a better discrimination, many labs add 18 g glucose per liter without significant changes in the MIC [42–44]. The usefulness of phenol red as a pH indicator in the medium remains unclear since the medium is well buffered (see below).

Use of a buffer substance is obviously necessary because products of the yeast metabolism are excreted into the medium. Most of these products are acids that lower the pH of the test medium if not buffered. A decrease of the pH being species- or strain-specific leads to false *in vitro* resistance, especially in azoles. Buffering of the medium according to the NCCLS is done with 0.165 M MOPS. The high buffering capacity of 0.165 M MOPS might not be necessary, as the higher yield of growth given with 2% of glucose (the plain medium contains 0.2% of glucose) also holds the pH stable.

TRIS buffer was not considered by the NCCLS because of its interaction with flucytosine. Phosphate buffer was judged as inadequate since it will traverse the membrane of the fungal cell and therefore might interact with the antifungal and/or the metabolism of the cell. It is remarkable that the German standard (draft) using HR medium includes phosphate buffer. MOPS, on the other hand, is reported to be not as good as another zwitterion buffer, EMTA (endomethylene-tetrahydrophtalic acid [5 norbornene-2-endo, 3-endo-dicarbonic acid]), with regard to the growth of the yeasts [45]; unfortunately, EMTA is not cost-effective. But phosphate (see Sections 3.2 and 3.4) as well as other buffering substances are not well accepted.

3.1.4 Antifungal agents, solubilization

The NCCLS recommendations deal with water-soluble agents (flucytosine and fluconazole) and those requiring solvents other than water (amphotericin B, ketoconazole, and itraconazole). For the latter agents, there is no strict recommendation on the solvent. Most laboratories use dimethyl sulfoxide (DMSO) for solubilization of these antifungal agents. The use of other solvents, i.e., polyethylene glycol, could influence the MIC [46]. It is recommended to dissolve such drugs at least 100 times to the highest final concentration. The dilution series should be prepared in the same solvent. Each drug in intermediate concentrations has to be diluted to the final concentration. This is done by a first dilution step with medium to a 10-fold concentration, and a further 10-fold dilution gives the final solvent concentration of 1% (v/v). The macrodilution method gives the final concentration by adding 0.9 ml of inoculum to 0.1 ml of the 10-fold concentrated (water-insoluble) antifungal, whereas in the broth microdilution modification, the 10-fold concentration has to be diluted 1:5 with medium by a separate dilution step. This 1:5 dilution is further 1:2 diluted by adding the inoculum. This separate dilution step might influence the correlation between macro- and microdilution with extreme lipophilic substances due to a further "sticking effect" (see Section 3.1.5).

The final DMSO concentration of the solvent amounts to 1%. The drug-free growth control may be unaffected thereby, but the relatively high concentration of solvent might influence the permeability of the cell membrane and thus the MIC. The concentration of 1% DMSO is questionable since 3% may lead to a fungistatic effect. In azole testing with a casitone medium, such a high concentration of the solvent is not necessary. Even with ≤ 0.2% (v/v) DMSO, reliable results can be achieved [47].

Unfortunately, the influence of solvent on the MICs of lipophilic substances respective to their solubility in test media is not considered often enough. The precipitation of itraconazole at higher concentrations in the test medium was accepted as a problem only recently [48]. MICs of 16 µg/ml and higher are reported uncritically, although visible precipitations are seen above 2–4 µg/ml itraconazole. Highly itraconazole-resistant strains could not be detected with the NCCLS method because their MICs exceed the concentration where precipitation of itraconazole occurs. It is described that itraconazole dissolved in DMSO is soluble at no more than 0.7 µg/ml in the defined EMEM (Eagle's Minimal Essential Medium) medium as well as in the complex CYG (Casiton Yeast Extract Glucose) medium [49].

Antifungal agents not listed in the NCCLS M27-A recommendations must be handled according to the information provided by the drug manufacturer. Actually, the echinocandin caspofungin and newer triazoles like voriconazole and posaconazole are of interest for susceptibility testing. The need for testing these new substances is similar to those already introduced. Caspofungin is available as its acetate and can be solubilized directly with distilled water or with test medium. The lipophilic substances voriconazole

Table 4.
Effect of plastic- and glassware used for preparation of the dilution series and the test assay on the itraconazole MIC_{80} (µg/ml). Method: NCCLS M27-A, microdilution

Strains	Dilution series in:			
	Polypropylene		Glass tubes	
	Microtiter plates of			
	Polystyrene	Glass	Polystyrene	Glass
C. albicans ATCC®90028	0.500	0.250	0.062	0.016
C. albicans RKI 2594/95	1.000	0.125–0.250	0.250	0.062
C. krusei ATCC®6258	1.000	0.500	0.500	0.125
C. parapsilosis ATCC®22019	1.000	0.500	0.250	0.031–0.062

and posaconazole also have to be dissolved in DMSO and diluted in the same way as the water-insoluble substances described above.

3.1.5 Test format and test materials

All test procedures by NCCLS are performed in or with plastic material. For broth macrodilution, sterile 12 × 75 mm test plastic tubes are recommended. For the microdilution test sterile, disposable, 96-well microbilution plates (U-shaped wells/round-bottomed) are used. But the test material might influence the MICs [36, 47]. Itraconazole shows lower MICs when tested in glass material instead of in plastic microtiter plates (see Tab. 4). Additionally, the MICs proved to be more reproducible in glass compared to those performed in plastic material. This could be explained by "sticking" of extremely hydrophobic (lipophilic) substances to the plastic material and thus lowering the available drug concentration. This is evident not only for itraconazole but also for the lipophilic antifungal substance terbinafine, an agent used locally or systemically in infections from dermatophytes. Terbinafine is also prescribed for compassionate use since it is effective in some systemic mycoses [50, 51]. The "sticking effect" applies more or less to miconazole, ketoconazole, and posaconazole. Lower MICs and a high reproducibility of itraconazole MICs testing *Aspergillus* in glassware (with complex medium) is reported in [52], but a "sticking effect" is not discussed.

The NCCLS standard is based on the broth macrodilution method. Concordance to the broth microdilution is reported by several authors [53–57]. Because of the ease of performance, the microdilution proved to be more attractive. Microtiter plates can be stored at –70 °C or below for months without any loss of activity. The plates must be sealed and checked for correct activity of the components by quality control strains with defined MIC ranges.

The microdilution test requires 12 wells for each drug. The highest concentration (64 μg/ml for flucytosine or fluconazole, 16 μg/ml for the others) is followed by 9 1:2 dilutions each (prepared in separate dilution series). Number 11 will contain the growth control, and the remaining well is inoculated with medium for sterility control only.

3.1.6 Incubation time

The NCCLS standard was established on the basis of an incubation time of 48 hours for *Candida* species. Based on a better reproducibility of MICs, this prolonged incubation period was recommended [40]. In the meantime, MIC reading of *Candida* after 24 hours is more and more accepted, provided the growth control is positive. Only a few clinical *Candida* isolates show insufficient growth after 24 hours. MICs after 24 hours will not differ significantly from those of 48 hours for most isolates. It is hard to understand that a strain was stable in its susceptibility to fluconazole even after a prolonged incubation time but its susceptibility to itraconazole should have changed to resistance after this period of 48 hours [58]. Reading after 24 hours also is preferred because these MICs correlate more with the therapeutical outcome than do those after 48 hours [59–62]. Thus, isolates might be susceptible even when changing to higher MICs after prolonged incubation. The benefit of a shorter incubation period is of practical consequence: a decision on antifungal therapeutic regimen can be made earlier. The recommended incubation time for *Cryptococcus neoformans* is 70–74 hours since it grows slowly in RPMI medium. Substitution of RPMI medium with other media can shorten the incubation time to 48 hours. Some labs use a 10-fold higher inoculum than recommended so that the reading can be done earlier, but higher inocula might increase the MICs (see Section 3.1.2).

3.1.7 Incubation temperature

The incubation temperature of 35 °C is essential. Since most of the isolates being tested originate from human body sites, the growth of test organisms is not hampered by this temperature. Alteration of the incubation temperature may influence the MICs significantly, either increasing or decreasing depending on the species and antifungal used.

3.1.8 Incubation atmosphere

Ambient air is considered to be sufficient for growth of yeasts. Evaporation of medium has to be avoided, i.e., by a humid chamber. An atmosphere enriched with carbon dioxide (CO_2) is reported to influence the MICs in a different way. A more significant effect was observed for hyphomycetes than for yeasts [63]. In agar dilution tests (see Section 5.4) under CO_2-enriched atmosphere, no trailing endpoints (see Section 3.1.9) were observed [64].

3.1.9 Reading results

Endpoint reading

The MIC is the lowest concentration of an antifungal that shows substantial inhibition of growth of the test organism detectable visually. The growth control (drug-free) is compared to the tubes or wells containing different drug concentrations. Inhibition is defined differently depending on the test procedure and the test substance (see Table 3). In microdilution, growth is scored from 0 to 4. 0 is optically clear; 1, slightly hazy; 2, prominent decrease in turbidity; 3, slight reduction in turbidity; and 4, no reduction in turbidity. Sometimes isolates growing in clumps have to be resuspended to homogeneity. In the broth macrodilution as well as in the microdilution, the MIC for amphotericin B is defined as the lowest concentration of score 0. Flucytosine and azoles show less sharp endpoints and thus a 50% inhibition of growth by spectrophotometry (score 2) in the microdilution is considered as MIC. This best approximates the visual endpoint. In macrodilution, the 80% inhibition standard (identical to an allowable turbidity of 20%) can be estimated by diluting 0.2 ml of drug-free control growth with 0.8 ml of medium. Before the NCCLS method was established, the endpoint reading in fluconazole testing differed from 30% to 90% inhibition [15]. According to the recommendations of the NCCLS, scoring has to be done visually for macrodilution and with the help of a reading mirror in microdilution tests. This scoring seems to be one of the most problematic parameters of testing and might be the source of unsatisfactory interlaboratory reproducibility and thus is discussed in detail here. This problem is not seen when testing amphotericin B, which shows mostly clear-cut endpoints within a few dilutions for sensitive strains (see Fig. 1). Trailing endpoints – no clear-cut endpoints are detectable or drug concentrations within a large range allow trace growth – are seen in at least 5% of *Candida* isolates tested to azoles or flucytosine with RPMI medium. Here a decision on inhibition is rather subjective. Figure 1 shows the dose-response curve of amphotericin B, a fungicidal agent, and of fluconazole to a clinical *C. albicans* isolate. Amphotericin B shows a clear-cut endpoint at 0.5 μg/ml. Contrary to RPMI medium, the reading of the fluconazole MIC is easier in casitone medium (see Section 3.4) where endpoints are sharper and trailing is quite an exception. With RPMI medium the isolate shows trailing, and a MIC determination (defined as reduction of growth of at least 50% or 80 %) might be influenced by a subjective visual reading, especially when read without any agitation and/or subsequent spectrophotometrical reading (see below).

Collaborative studies have found a better reproducibility of MIC readings with small inocula [41, 54, 65] (see Section 3.1.2). Furthermore, it was noticed that trailing in antifungal susceptibility testing is pH dependent [61]. Until now the influence of pH on the trailing phenomenon has not been considered in any standard, since the practical consequences still have to be extended. The pH effect might be dependent on the antifungal agents and the medium used. The increasing fungicidal activity of a substance (e.g., voriconazole) generally decreases the trailing problem.

The growth of cells in the microtiter plate ranges from well-defined buttons or isles to more or less thick layers coating the wall of the wells. The NCCLS recommends dispersion of the yeast suspension by pipetting, vortexing, or other techniques if growth hinders the scoring. Undoubtedly, spectrophotometrical reading is the most objective way to calculate the antifungal effect. This method of antifungal susceptibility testing of yeasts was proposed as early as 1976 [66]. Endpoint reading of the microdilution test – either visually or spectrophotometrically – proved to be reliable and most objective when done after agitation immediately before reading [67, 68]. A

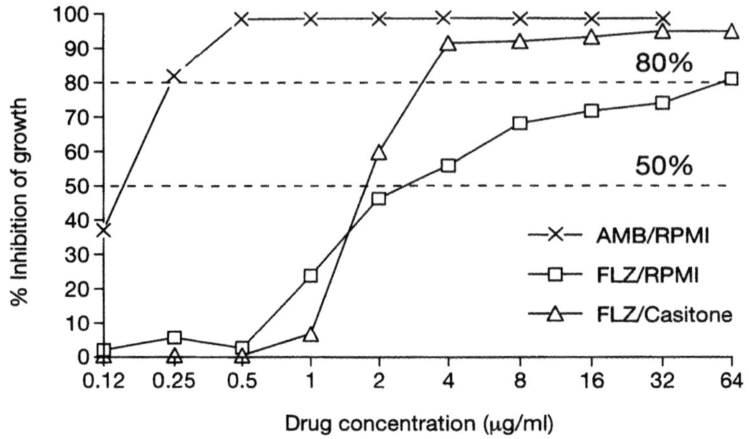

Fig. 1.
Curve (x) shows a rapid transition to the growth inhibition endpoint by AMB for *Candida albicans* RKI 1470/94. Curve (□) shows the inhibition of *Candida albicans* by fluconazole. A reduced but persistent growth in high concentrations of fluconazole is seen. Curve (△) shows clear-cut endpoints for fluconazole in casitone medium. All tests were done according to the NCCLS M27-A method except medium. Inhibition was determined spectrophotometrically at 630 nm. The growth control was set to 100% growth or 0% inhibition, respectively.

homogenous suspension of cells provides clearer endpoints than reading by eye. It may reduce false resistant readings, especially in isolates showing trailing [69]. Shaking with a microplate shaker as recommended by some authors often is not sufficient for dispersion. Resuspending by a multichannel pipette, starting with the wells containing the highest antifungal concentration, is easy to handle and is most effective.

3.1.10 Interpretation of results

The benefit of amphothericin B MICs for *Candida* spp. has to be doubted. A MIC of > 1 μg/ml is likely to be resistant to amphotericin B, but clinically resistant *Candida* spp. isolates do not consistently show MIC values above 1 μg/ml. The tight clustering of amphotericin B MICs between 0.25 and 1 μg/ml suggests low discrimination between resistance and susceptibility.

Some laboratories use Antibiotic Medium 3 to discriminate better between resistant and susceptible isolates [70]. But this medium must still be evaluated concerning reproducibility and correlation to the outcome of infection.

Using RPMI medium, interpretive breakpoints are given for flucytosine, fluconazole, and itraconazole in the appendix of the NCCLS M27-A document (see Tab. 3). These data are discussed in Section 6.

3.1.11 Quality control

This very important section of the NCCLS recommendations describes comprehensive procedures in quality control. The accepted MIC ranges for the quality-control strains are valid for the visual reading of the macrodilution test after 48 hours only. The two recommended control strains represent only a limited spectrum of susceptibility or resistance, respectively. In the meantime, quality-control ranges were expanded for the broth microdilution test of newer azoles and echinocandins for 24 and 48 hours of incubation [71]. Further quality-control strains should be defined, especially those showing resistance to azoles.

3.1.12 *In vitro* susceptibility testing of *Cryptococcus neoformans*

In susceptibility testing of *Cryptococcus neoformans*, the following factors have to be considered: (1) The growth of this organism in RPMI medium is not sufficient; substituting Yeast Nitrogen Base (YNB) medium for RPMI medium might improve growth (see Section 3.1.6) as well as the clinical relevance of MICs [37, 38]. (2) The established *Candida* interpretive breakpoints are not valid for *Cryptococcus neoformans*.

3.2 The German standard of susceptibility testing of fungi against antifungal agents (DIN standard, draft version 08/1999)

As mentioned above, the NCCLS standard has not found general acceptance. The standard of the German Institute for Standardization, the Deutsche

Industrie Norm (DIN), is based on the HR medium (originally Heath-Robinson, now High Resolution medium) which has been recommended for *in vitro* testing of fluconazole by Pfizer. Special requirements for susceptibility testing of fungi against antifungal agents are described in the draft version of DIN 58940-84 (edited August 1999). This document is based on DIN 58940-8, which deals with general method-specific requirements for the microdilution. The main features are listed in Table 5.

The proposed DIN standard differs from the NCCLS method mainly in the medium (HR medium) and buffer. HR medium is more common in Europe [11, 72–78]. This medium, as well as the RPMI medium, is a synthetic medium, but HR medium is phosphate-buffered and contains more glucose (2%), ammonium salts, and trace elements than the RPMI medium. This altered composition of the HR medium leads to fluconazole MICs similar to those in RPMI medium [77, 79]. Other azoles also do not differ markedly when comparing the two media [80, 81]. The type of microtiter plates (flat-bottomed or U-shaped wells in the DIN standard vs. round-bottomed in the NCCLS method) and their reading (without agitation in the DIN standard) might also influence the concordance of MICs by these two methods. We observed differences in MICs when the DIN standard was performed either in flat-bottomed microtiter plates or round-bottomed microtiter plates in individual cases (not published). Unfortunately, reading with previous agitation (see Section 3.1.9), which results in more reliable MICs, is not considered in the DIN standard.

Identical to the NCCLS method, the DIN standard requires that hydrophobic drugs have to be dissolved with organic solvents, which has not been pointed out in detail. Both methods describe the preparation of 100-fold concentrated dilution series in the solvent. Thus, there might be problems in reproducibility preparing, e.g., itraconazole with polyethylene glycol (PEG) or DMSO as already mentioned in Section 3.1.4.

"Sticking" of hydrophobic test substances to the wells of the plastic microtiter plates (see Section 3.1.5) could also be shown in evaluation of the German standard by the authors. Further questions are: What's the difference of early *versus* late reading? Will the criteria of endpoint reading be defined more precisely? Does the supplementation of HR medium with methylene blue (optional) reduce any trailing without influencing the MICs? Last but not least, the *in vivo-in vitro* correlation is most important. A study on this subject is running presently.

Table 5.
Antifungal susceptibility testing according to the proposed DIN standard

Test organisms	Yeasts
Test format	Broth microdilution assay
Test material	Microtiter plates (flat-bottomed or U-shaped)
Test medium	HR (high resolution) medium supplemented with glucose and asparagine, phosphate buffered (0.1 M) to pH 7.0 ± 0.2
Antifungals/solvents	Identical to the NCCLS method, voriconazole listed additionally
Inoculum	5×10^3 CFU/ml
Incubation temperature	36 ± 1 °C (if no growth: 30 ± 2 °C)
Incubation time	18 h (reading when growth control is positive) or 24 h Second reading after 48 h
Reading	Visually (without agitation) or by spectrophotometer (530–620 nm)
Endpoint	Prominent decrease in turbidity (amphotericin B not further specified)
Quality-control strains	Preliminary ranges for 11 strains (strains clearly resistant to azoles not provided)
Interpretive breakpoints	In study

3.3 The EUCAST method

In 1999 the European Committee for Antifungal Susceptibility Testing (EUCAST) of the ESCMID (European Society of Clinical Microbiology and Infectious Diseases) presented a preliminary document on the susceptibility testing of yeasts for discussion. The "Method for Determination of Minimum Inhibitory Concentration (MIC) by Broth Dilution of Fermentative Species of Yeasts" deals with the NCCLS method but differs markedly (see Tab. 6).

The EUCAST method uses inocula distinctly higher (100-fold) than other test standards, possibly leading to false resistant MICs. This will be re-checked with a lower inoculum by the EUCAST. The endpoint definition corresponds to the NCCLS M27-A for azoles and flucytosine. Surprisingly, the endpoint of 80% inhibition is proposed for amphotericin B, although amphotericin B acts as a fungicidal and therefore a 100% inhibition is asked for. Practically speaking, the calculation of 100% inhibition is achievable only with high-quality spectrophotometers; thus, a 95% inhibition would be more practical. The dilution of antifungal agents in the microtiter plate is actually recommended. This simplified method as well as other parameters might be changed before final recommendation (publication announced for the middle of 2002). Since we emphasize the problem of handling hydrophobic substances, we cannot accept this dilution procedure that provokes the "sticking effect" (see Section 3.1.5).

Table 6.
Parameters of the European Committee for Antifungal Susceptibility Testing (EUCAST) method (draft version) of antifungal susceptibility testing of yeasts

Test organisms	Fermenting yeasts
Test format	Microdilution assay with flat-bottomed microtiter plates
Test medium	RPMI-1640 medium according to the NCCLS method modified to 2% glucose (final concentration) Antibiotic Medium 3 for amphotericin B
Antifungals/solvents	According to the NCCLS standard but dilution of antifungals is done by log_2-dilutions in the microtiter plate
Inoculum	$0.5–2.5 \times 10^5$ CFU/ml (100× higher than NCCLS method)
Incubation time	24 and 48 hours
Reading	By spectrophotometer (previously agitated)
Endpoints	Inhibition of 80% (compared to growth control) for amphotericin B Inhibition of 50% for flucytosine and azoles
Interpretive breakpoints for flucytosine	≤ 4 µg/ml susceptible 8–16 µg/ml intermediate ≥ 32 µg/ml resistant

The concept of the EUCAST method clearly recognizes the weak point in reading results in the NCCLS standard. Objective reading done by spectrophotometer of resuspended cells is therefore compulsory. Furthermore, testing of *Cryptococcus neoformans* is not included and has to be done by a different test procedure for non- or weak-fermenting yeasts, e.g., *Candida valida* (*Pichia membranifaciens*), *C. inconspicua*, and non-*Candida* species, e.g., *Trichosporon asahii*. These organisms show no or insufficient growth when tested with the microdilution method. Finally, in the EUCAST method amphotericin B MICs are considered to be more relevant when given with Antibiotic Medium 3.

3.4 Use of complex media for antifungal susceptibility testing

Several synthetic media were investigated for suitability as a universal test medium (see Section 3.1.3). It was the concept of the NCCLS to use only one medium for antifungal susceptibility testing. Because of the insufficient growth of *Cryptococcus neoformans* in RPMI medium, a further medium was proposed: the synthetic Yeast Nitrogen Base medium, buffered and supplemented with glucose. For amphotericin B testing, the use of complex media is still under discussion, and the RPMI medium will possibly be replaced by the complex medium Antibiotic Medium 3 (see Section 3.1.10).

Complex media were not considered because of their antagonism with flucytosine [82]. This observation is widely accepted. Antagonism of Sabouraud bouillon and brain-heart infusion bouillon as complex media with clotrimazole and fluconazole also has been reported to result in elevated MICs of azoles [82, 83]. But the criticism on complex media in azole susceptibility testing has to be discussed. Our *in vitro* data demonstrate that antagonism does not apply for casitone. Fluconazole MICs in casitone medium correlate well with those in synthetic media such as RPMI medium or HR medium.

Apart from interaction of some substances in complex media with antifungal agents, a possible lot-to-lot variation of compounds was the reason for not considering complex media for susceptibility testing. Differences in media not fully definable were considered to be responsible for the decrease of the reproducibility of MICs. A variablity of amphotericin B MICs due to lot-to-lot differences of Antibiotic Medium 3 was reported during testing of *Candida* species [84]. No other reports discuss the influence of varying composition of the same medium on the MIC in detail. Antibiotic Medium 3 contains three complex components: beef extract, yeast extract, and peptone. But a constant quality of the commercial products used for this medium is guaranteed by the manufacturers. Although there are some variations in composition of complex media, these should not influence any MIC. Several laboratories use media with casitone or similar ingredients for azole susceptibility testing of yeasts (e.g., [52, 85–87]), as do we. When testing dermatophytes (not mentioned in this article), such media are essential. Complex ingredients such as peptone, casitone, tryptone etc. are components of media used for standardized susceptibility testing also of bacteria, e.g., Mueller-Hinton medium. Even complex media are standardized, not with respect to each molecule but to a defined property, e.g., the absence of substances interfering with the agent tested. The use of casitone agar was recommended for the Etest (see Section 5.6.1) in testing azoles for many years. Etest with casitone was in better agreement with the NCCLS method than Etest with RPMI medium for all the azoles [87]. In our experience, Etest MICs of azoles with casitone were highly reproducible, easier to read than with RPMI medium, and well correlated to the clinical outcome [88, 89].

3.4.1 The in-house method of antifungal susceptibility testing of yeasts to azoles at the Robert Koch-Institut Berlin, Germany

The reported interaction of fluconazole with complex media (see above) is not evident when using a modified casitone medium (see below). In the late 1980s, before standardization with synthetic media was established, we looked for a test medium enabling fast growth of yeasts. A modified casitone medium was evaluated; supplemented with vitamins, trace elements, and other components; and buffered to pH 7.2 with 0.1M phosphate [47]. This medium proved to be superior to synthetic and non-modified casitone medium and is used for testing yeasts and hyphomycetes to azoles in the microdilution test in our lab. Fluconazole MICs obtained with this medium are more or less identical to those in synthetic media. Unfortunately, there are no studies available for the use of casitone medium in amphotericin B testing. Casitone media could possibly be just as beneficial for amphotericin B testing as Antibiotic Medium 3. The test parameters of our method are shown in Table 7.

The advantages of our own method, which is extensively studied for testing of *Candida* spp. to azoles, are (1) the fast growth of yeasts so that the incubation period can be shortened, (2) a high reproducibility even for hydrophobic test substances, and (3) a satisfactory correlation to the clinical outcome [90]. Generally, MICs are beneficial only if there is no doubt about their interpretation. Intralaboratory results obtained in our lab show that MICs differ within 3 $\log_2$ dilution steps with RPMI medium, which is in the allowed range of the NCCLS guidelines. But when testing the identical strains with casitone medium, these variations are significantly lower. Three $\log_2$ dilution steps are equivalent to a 4-fold difference in MIC. It is evident that isolates with MICs in the "intermediate" range could be categorized falsely when their MICs will vary. Note: The MICs of itraconazole are lower with casitone medium than with RPMI medium. This has already been described for other complex media like brain-heart-infusion broth, Sabouraud broth [91], or similar media [52].

Any modification of a method could lead to discordant results, as seen, e.g., in susceptibility testing of itraconazole in casitone medium showing significantly lower MICs compared to the NCCLS method. The precondition for modifying a method has to be the evaluation of correlation with MICs of quality-control strains and with clinical outcome. It has to be considered that the breakpoints could be different from the original method.

Table 7.
Test parameters of antifungal susceptibility testing of *Candida* species to azoles at the Robert Koch-Institut

Test format	Microdilution assay
Test material	Plastic microtiter plates for testing hydrophilic substances (U-shaped). Glass microtiter plates* for testing hydrophobic substances
Test substances	Azoles
Inoculum	~1×10^3 CFU/ml
Incubation temperature	35 ± 1 °C
Incubation time/reading	When showing turbidity of 0.2–0.6 spectrophotometrically at 630 nm (log-phase of growth, for most *Candida* species after ~ 18 h)
Endpoints	IC_{80} for azoles
Quality-control strains	*C. krusei* ATCC®6258, internal QC strains of *C. albicans*, responding, delayed responding or refractory to azole therapy

*When the assay was established, only flat-bottomed microtiter plates were available (Firma Hellma, Germany)

3.5 Early standardization of antifungal susceptibility testing of yeasts in Europe

In 1981 the French Society of Medical Mycology [19] presented a paper on the standardization of antifungal susceptibility testing. A further recommendation for susceptibility testing of flucytosine and amphotericin B was published by the German *Paul Ehrlich Gesellschaft* in 1987 [92]. But the synthetic medium used was not further examined for other test substances. In flucytosine testing for the first time there was a clear correlation between the results of *in vitro* testing and the clinical outcome [93]. The interpretation of MICs is handled in Section 6 in detail.

4 Antifungal susceptibility testing of hyphomycetes

4.1 The NCCLS M38-P standard

Based on the achievements of yeast susceptibility testing, the NCCLS subcommittee started working out a reference method for antifungal susceptibility testing of conidium-forming fungi (moulds). Two collaborative studies resulted in the establishment of the following test conditions for a reproducible test method (see Tab. 8): preparation and size of inoculum, time and temperature of incubation, medium, and the MIC determination [94, 95]. The procedure is described in the document NCCLS M38-P: Reference Method for Broth Dilution Antifungal Susceptibility Testing of Conidium-Forming Filamentous Fungi; Proposed Standard [96].

Critical comments

Because the method for testing hyphomycetes is closely related to the one for yeasts (NCCLS M27-A), the substantial criticism of the latter also applies for the NCCLS M38-P method. The test parameters influencing the MICs of moulds have not yet been evaluated to such an extent as for yeasts. The M38-P method encompasses three sporulating genera of hyphomycetes (*Aspergillus, Rhizopus, Fusarium*) and the two species *Pseudallescheria boydii* and *Sporothrix schenckii* only.

4.1.1 Test format

The proposed standard recommends the microdilution method. The macrodilution method may be used as a modification, since some labs might prefer this common method for safety reasons. But the correlation of macrodilution with microdilution is described controversially [94, 97]. When testing clinically itraconazole-resistant *A. fumigatus* isolates, the macrodilution test proved to be better correlating than other tests [98].

4.1.2 Itraconazole testing

Section 3.1.4 describes that the lipophilic character of itraconazole is not considered enough in the NCCLS standard for yeasts. In the proposed testing method for hyphomycetes, the final concentration of itraconazole is done by one dilution step, whereas in the microdilution test for yeasts, the final concentration is given by a second dilution step. In the NCCLS M38-P method, the dilution of the 100-fold concentrated itraconazole solution by one dilution step only reduces the "sticking effect" of itraconazole to plastic material but is still present, especially when plastic tubes are used for the dilution series and microdilution is performed in plastic microtiter plates. The

Table 8.
Parameters of the NCCLS M38-P method for susceptibility testing of hyphomycetes

Test organisms	Conidia of conidium-forming fungi of the genera: *Aspergillus*, *Fusarium*, *Rhizopus* and of *Pseudallescheria boydii*, *Sporothrix schenckii*
Test format	Microdilution assay (macrodilution modification)
Medium	RPMI-1640 medium (identical with NCCLS M27-A method)
Drugs and test ranges	0.03–16 μg/ml for amphotericin B, ketoconazole and itraconazole, 0.125–64 μg/ml for flucytosine and fluconazole
Inoculum size	0.4×10^4–5×10^4 CFU/ml (final concentration) (spectrophotometrically standardized); *P. boydii* two times higher
Incubation period	21–26 h for *Rhizopus* species 46–50 h for *Fusarium* and *Aspergillus* species and *Sporothrix schenckii* 70–74 h for *Pseudallescheria boydii*
Reading	Visually (by a reading mirror) scoring from 0 (optically clear) to 4 (no reduction in growth)
Endpoints	Amphotericin B: score of 0 Azoles and flucytosine: prominent growth reduction (score of 2, approx. 50 % inhibition compared to growth control)
Quality-control strains	2 ATCC® strains of *Aspergillus*, not named
Interpretive breakpoints	Not established at present

loss of itraconazole activity, when exposed to plastic material, applies also to susceptibility testing of hyphomycetes (data not shown).

4.1.3 Endpoint reading

The definition and reading of the endpoint makes any standardization difficult (see Section 3). Improvement in determination of MICs is described in detail for yeasts (see Section 3.1.9), focusing on agitation before reading and/or spectrophotometric measurement of growth. This is generally not applicable for moulds. Resuspension of a layer hardly can be done in this case. Spectrophotometric reading is not allowed because fructified moulds would contaminate the instrument. The endpoint for azoles and flucytosine determined visually as score 2 (in microdilution) might be of practical benefit when standardizing a method. But it gives little evidence on the effectiveness to inhibit the fungus substantially. For detection of azole resistance in *Aspergillus*, it is possible to use an optically clear endpoint (score 0) instead of a score 2 [99]. Comprehensive studies on azole activity are based on the endpoint reading of ≥ 50% inhibition compared to the growth control [100, 101]. Reports on reading the IC_{80} or IC_{75} (growth inhibition of ≥80 % or 75%, respectively) are published too [102–104]. Better reading might be achievable by a colorimetric indicator, which will be described as a modification in the final NCCLS M38-P standard. This indicator, a dye, is a modified resazurin, but there is no detailed information. Clear-cut endpoints in a different colorimetric assay for antifungal susceptibility testing of *Aspergillus* species are based on the reduction of a tetrazolium salt (XTT) in the presence of menadione [105]. The use of colorimetric markers is further commented in Section 5.1.1.

4.1.4 Inoculum

As for yeasts, the inoculum of hyphomycetes is an important parameter of antifungal susceptibility testing. A significant effect from the size of the inoculum on the MICs of flucytosine and itraconazole was reported [106]. A 10-fold higher inoculum than for yeasts (0.5×10^4 to 5×10^4 CFU/ml) was found to be suitable for hyphomycetes [94, 95]. The NCCLS method provides correct inocula by ranges of optical density of conidia for each organism being adjusted photometrically. Hyphae are the target of antifungal agents *in vivo*. Nevertheless, the inoculum is prepared with conidia since it is obvious that an inoculum of conidia is easier to handle and can be standardized better. Little is known about any differences in the susceptibility of conidia *versus* hyphae. Dermatophytes are reported to show a different suseptibility of conidia and hyphae [33], but these organisms are not the focus of this article. When comparing the *in vitro* antifungal susceptibilities of conidia and hyphae of *Aspergillus* species, there is little published on higher MICs of hyphae [107], whereas others did not find any differences [108–110]. For non-*Aspergillus* species, higher MICs and MFCs (for the latter, see Section 5.1.2) of hyphal *versus* conidial inocula were reported [111]. Testing of non-sporulating moulds is not the subject of the NCCLS M38-P method. For testing these organisms, see Section 4.2.

4.1.5 MICs of quality-control strains

Until recently, hyphomycetes for quality control have not been specified. Therefore, the yeast quality-control strains (NCCLS M27-A) should be used for checking the dilution series. For the reference isolate *Paecilomyces variotii* (ATCC®22319), MIC ranges were described [94, 100]. But for itraconazole, the (tentative) QC limit ranging from 0.03 to 1 μg/ml indicates the problematic handling of this substance. For purposes of comparison, our own standard shows itraconazole MICs from 0.016 to 0.031 μg/ml for this strain.

4.1.6 Detection of amphotericin B resistance

Contrary to susceptibility testing in yeasts, amphotericin B testing in moulds is more important due to the high frequency of resistance in non-*Aspergillus fumigatus* isolates. Studies have to demonstrate the benefit of replacing RPMI medium with Antibiotic Medium 3. How far a reported lot-to-lot variation of this medium influences not only the amphotericin B MICs of yeasts but also those of moulds has yet to be shown. Maybe the MFC determination (see Section 5.1.2) of amphotericin B is more suitable for detecting resistance to this drug, as is shown for yeasts [112].

4.2 The in-house standard at the Robert-Koch Institut

Based on the long experience of testing yeasts by microdilution (see Section 3.4.1) in our lab, we adopted this technique for susceptibility testing of hyphomycetes (see Tab. 9).

Contrary to the NCCLS method, we harvest the conidia when their formation is obvious, but not later than after 5 days of incubation at 35 ± 1 °C. This allows earlier *in vitro* results but is in contrast to the instructions of the standard method: preculturing for 7 days at 35 °C, with the exception of *Fusarium* spp., which first have to be incubated at 35 °C (2–3 days) and later at 25–28 °C (until day 7). As recommended by the NCCLS method, we use potato dextrose agar for preculturing. We emphasize an isolate-specific incubation time in our test. When reading too late, i.e., the growth control is grown to a thick layer and/or the fungus has heavily sporu226lated, the MIC result is questionable since growth in the other wells is difficult to compare (semi-)quantitatively with this drug-free growth. As with yeasts, the most noticeable difference between the NCCLS standard and our method is docu-

Table 9.
Test parameters of antifungal susceptibility testing in hyphomycetes at the Robert Koch-Institut

Test organisms	Hyphomycetes growing well under the test conditions (if not, see Section 5.4), precultured on potato-dextrose-agar
Test format	Microdilution assay
Test material	Microtiter plates (U-shaped) Glass ware for hydrophobic test substances
Medium	Modified casitone medium (as used for yeasts)
Inoculum	Conidia when produced (otherwise mycelia), final concentration: 1×10^4 CFU/ml (counted by a modified hemocytometer)
Incubation temperature	35 ± 1 °C
Incubation time	Until growth control is positive, i.e. for *Rhizopus* ~ 18–24 h, *Aspergillus* ~ 30–48 h, *P. boydii* 60–72 h
Reading	Visually by reading mirror
Endpoints	Amphotericin B: 100% inhibition Azoles and flucytosine: 80% inhibition (compared to growth control)
Quality-control strains	*Paecilomyces variotii* ATCC® 22319 and yeast quality control strains

mented in testing hyphomycetes with extremely hydrophobic drugs: these show generally higher MICs in the NCCLS M38-P method compared to the RKI standard, because the NCCLS method does not consider the chemophysical properties of extreme lipophilic substances (see Sections 3.1.4 and 3.1.5). As shown for yeasts, highly reproducable MICs even of lipophilic substances are given with the RKI standard (data not shown).

Preparing an inoculum of non-sporulating moulds can be a problem. Absence of sporulation is found in pathogens not mentioned in the NCCLS method, especially in basidiomycetes and in rare *Aspergillus* and *Pseudallescheria* isolates. Probably because of a long-lasting adaptation to the human body, the latter have lost or reduced their ability to produce conidia. Subculturing on potato dextrose agar or cultivation on oatmeal agar might induce sporulation. Moulds sporulating insufficiently can be tested by an agar dilution method [78] (see Section 5.4). This is done simply by placing a block of agar of the precultured fungus on the drug-containing plate. Some labs use sonified mycelium as inoculum independently of any sporulation of the test organism. In our method the conidial inoculum is calculated by a counting chamber (a modified hemocytometer) followed by cultivation of the diluted suspension on Sabouraud glucose agar for determination of CFUs.

5 Modifications and alternatives of the NCCLS standards M27-A and M38-P

The standards (see Sections 3.1 and 4.1) can hardly be used as a routine method in laboratories performing antifungal susceptibility testing. Because of the time-consuming and cumbersome handling of the NCCLS method and because of the non-applicability for several organisms, modifications exist. These might be justified, e.g., by resulting in a higher reproducibility of MICs, as we see with itraconazole and casitone medium. Thus, MICs may differ from the ones of the NCCLS method, but they should not considered to be false. Any alterations have to be done while checking for concordance to the NCCLS method, and correlation of MICs to clinical outcome has to be evaluated as far as possible. A panel of quality-control strains and isolates with known clinical outcome for comparative studies generally is recommended. This should encompass sensitive, as well as resistant, isolates.

5.1 Modifications of the standard methods

As pointed out in Section 3.1.1, modifications are done in order to make the standard method easier and more objective. The following modifications for testing yeasts are commonly used: glucose supplementation with 18 g/L, reading after 24 hours photometrically with previous agitation. Testing hyphomycetes supplementation of RPMI medium with glucose is not favourable. By using a spectrophotometer, the MICs of yeasts can be calculated in a simple way. The microdilution assay has become widely accepted. The microdilution plates can be prefabricated and stored and are easier to handle, to read and are more cost-effective. Sometimes test organisms require the use of another method (e.g., non-fermenting yeasts or moulds not able to form conidia). Alternatives are described in Sections 5.3 and 5.4.

5.1.1 Use of colorimetric markers

Colorimetric markers are used to make a decision on inhibition more distinctly.

Since the growth of cells is associated with a change of the redox potential of the culture medium, colored redox indicators can serve as a surrogate parameter of growth or inhibition. The best evaluated substance is Alamar Blue™ (Alamar Biosciences, Inc., Sacramento, CA, also known as Resazurin). Growth is indicated by a color change from blue (no growth) to red that is detectable visually. Alamar Blue™ is used in commercial tests like the ASTY Colorimetric Microdilution Panel (see Section 5.6.1) and Fungitest® (see Section 5.6.2). The correlation between MICs with medium containing Alamar Blue™ and those with the reference method (NCCLS) was excellent in one study of yeasts [113], showing concordance of 95% for amphotericin B, fluconazole, and flucytosine after 24 hours and of 84%–98% after 48 hours. In a further multisite study, a most satisfactory interlaboratory reproducibility was found [114]. Furthermore, Alamar Blue™ can be handled more easily than other possibly harmful substrates that indicate the growth of cells (see below). Spectrophotometrical measurement at 570 nm and 600 nm allows an earlier reading. A high correlation of an 8-hour rapid assay for fluconazole susceptibility of *Candida albicans* was shown with the reference method (NCCLS M27-A; unpublished data). It should be considered that Alamar Blue™ does not generally improve a given method. When used in combination with Antibiotic Medium 3, the discrimination between susceptible and resistant isolates decreased [115].

Incorporation of MTT [3-(4,5-dimethyl-2-thiazolyl)-2,5-diphenyl-2*H*-tetrazolium] or XTT [(2,3bis(2-methoxy-4-nitro-5-sulfophenyl)-5-[(phenylamino) carbonyl]-2*H*-tetrazolium hydroxide)] as a colorimetric marker for redox potential (oxidation-reduction indicator) is described for yeasts and moulds [116–119]. XTT is preferred due to an easier handling, but both substances show good correlation to the reference methods.

5.1.2 Determination of the MFC (syn. MLC)

In severely immunocompromised patients, it cannot be assumed that the antifungal drug and the host act additively or synergistically. At body sites without any defense mechanisms, the fungicidal potency is of more importance than the fungistatic effect. The MFC thus can give more information on the power of the substance. Interestingly enough, itraconazole and voriconazole were found to be fungicidal to *Aspergillus* species but were fungistatic only to *Candida* species [102]. The time-kill curves give the maximum information [120]. The determination of the MFC is quite simple: an amount (mostly 10 μl) out of the optically clear wells of the microtiter plate is given onto the culture medium (Sabouraud glucose medium), and after incubation (2 day for yeasts, 2–7 days for hyphomycetes) growth is documented. The MFC represents the lowest concentration of the antifungal drug that killed at least 99% of the inoculum [100]. We prefer this definition. Since there are no official recommendations, the MFC calculation is also set to 95% killing [103]. MFCs are considered neither in the NCCLS M38-P method nor in any other standard method. The evaluation of the clinical value of MFCs *versus* MICs is addressed to standardizing committees. An insight into this problem is provided in [121, 122]. Determination of the MFC seems to be especially useful for the detecting of amphotericin B resistance. It has to be considered that high drug levels in serum corresponding to the MFC often are not achieved.

5.2 Testing of new azoles and echinocandins

Antifungal susceptibility testing of voriconazole is not mentioned in the NCCLS guidelines, but, meanwhile, many reports exist without any evidence of *in vitro* test problems. Less is known about the new triazole SCH 56592 and the echinocandin MK-0991 (caspofungin). Because of the high lipophilic character of SCH 56592, problems may arise as described for itraconazole in this article. In caspofungin testing of *Aspergillus* isolates, an until-now unconsidered parameter, the minimum effective concentration (MEC), was described to be more adequate compared to the MIC of the NCCLS microdilution method [24].

5.3 The agar diffusion test

This alternative technique is the method most often used. A tray with the test substance is put on the agar plate, which is inoculated with the test organism. The antifungal tray is usually a disk; thus it is called a disk (diffusion) test. Diffusion of the test substance into the agar leads to inhibition of growth around the disk if the test organism is susceptible. The diameter of growth inhibition reflects the susceptibility of the fungus. The use of this method strongly depends on the chemophysical property of the test substance. Diffusion is poor with water-insoluble substances such as amphotericin B and itraconazole but is excellent with flucytosine and fluconazole. Furthermore, clinically relevant (tentative) interpretive breakpoints are not mentioned, with the exception of the water-soluble substances flucytosine [93] and fluconazole [123]. Flucytosine showed a good correlation between MICs and the *in vivo* outcome of a systemic candidosis model [93]. The suitability of the disk diffusion test depends on the concentration of the test substance. The flucytosine disk is loaded with 1 μg. When testing fluconazole, the use of the 25-μg fluconazole disk – compared to a lower loading – improves reading and correlation. Good intralaboratory reproducibility was reported with this 25-μg fluconazole disk and HR medium, but interlaboratory agreement of only 58% was reported [124].

5.4 The agar dilution test

The NCCLS standards do not claim to be suitable for all fungi. The oxygen availability in broth cultures is growth-limiting for weak-fermenting or non-fermenting organisms (see Section 3.1.1). For example, a filamentous basidiomycete causing an ocular infection did not grow in the broth microdilution test, but testing with the agar dilution method was successful [125]. Even if no interpretive breakpoints exist for such organisms (except for *Cr. neoformans*, which are under study), there is some information on the *in vitro* susceptibility.

In the agar dilution method (also referred to as agar incorporating method), the test substance has to be dissolved before incorporating it into the solidified (usually with 1.5% agar) medium. Producing these plates is enormously time-consuming, and the plates can be stored for a limited time only. With the help of a multipoint inoculator, more than 20 isolates can be tested for comparative studies on one agar plate simultaneously. When evaluating seven methods of testing *in vitro* susceptibility of clinical isolates to fluconazole, the agar dilution test showed the best correlation (>95% concordance) with microdilution [76].

5.5 Other methods

There are several other methods for testing antifungal susceptibility [34]. This publication describes routine methods commonly used. The efforts and expenses of other methods impede their broad acceptance, although they may show good correlation to standard methods. An example is the flow cytometry being beneficial due to its extreme time saving [126].

5.6 Commercial susceptibility tests

For commercial tests it is a precondition that they are concordant to existing standards. Apart from the test quality, the concordance depends on the experience of a test lab, the selected strains, and the antifungal agents. There are hardly any problems testing *C. albicans* to fluconazole. But concordance of species like *C. tropicalis*, *C. glabrata*, and *C. krusei* might be insufficient especially when lipophilic drugs like itraconazole are tested.

5.6.1 Tests covering the full range of antifungal concentrations

The Etest

The commercial test evaluated best of all, the Etest (AB Biodisk, Solna, Sweden), is a mixture of the agar diffusion and agar dilution tests. Test strips generate stable gradients of antifungal concentrations in the solidified medium, and inhibition is shown by an elliptical zone. At its intersection with the strip, the MIC can be read. There are numerous publications on the correlation of Etest MICs to the NCCLS method and to other tests which state that the correlation is species and substance dependent. Correlation of the Etest with the reference method is shown to vary from 34% to 97% [57, 127]. It is reported that the Etest is superior to the NCCLS method in detecting amphotericin B resistance [128]. Testing fluconazole in 42 *Candida* isolates, 32 of them from HIV-infected patients, showed in 41/42 (97.6%) a correlation to the clinical outcome [89].

The Etest may be beneficial if only an orientation on the susceptibility is needed. Most isolates will be clearly susceptible or resistant. To what extent the Etest will detect any development of resistance has to be checked by further studies. As far as we know, quality-control strains have mostly been elaborated for the Etest. Ranges have been proposed for fluconazole, itraconazole, ketoconazole, amphotericin B, and flucytosine for the same strains as in the NCCLS method. Recently, the Etest was evaluated for susceptibility testing of hyphomycetes to amphotericin B and itraconazole [129]. The results were encouraging with respect to correlation with the M38-P method. Nevertheless, some experience is necessary for handling of hyphomycetes and reading the results. The risk of contamination by release of conidia is probably higher in the Etest compared to the NCCLS method. In many labs the Etest is preferred since it is an easy-to-handle method showing high reproducibility.

Other tests

Other full-range tests are less evaluated than the Etest. The broth-based ASTY (Kyokuto Pharmaceutical Industrial Co., Ltd., Tokyo, Japan) gives an excellent correlation (90%–99%) with the NCCLS standard [130]. The quality of this commercial system is similar to a different colorimetric liquid panel, the "Sensititre Yeast One Colorimetric Antifungal Panel", produced by Trec Diagnostic Systems, Ohio [131].

5.6.2 Breakpoint tests

Most commercially available tests are breakpoint tests. They provide a number of drug concentrations selected as critical breakpoints only. Data on correlation with the NCCLS method are published on a limited scale. A possible development of resistance can hardly be detected, and thus the benefit of these tests is limited. Since breakpoint tests give qualitative results (susceptible, intermediate, or resistant), their correlation to the reference method (NCCLS M27-A) will be better than for a full range test. This was shown for amphotericin B and flucytosine susceptibility testing (100% and 99% correlation, respectively) with the Fungitest® (BIO-RAD SDP, Paris, France). On the other hand, the concordance of this test with the reference method for itraconazole (86%) was lower [132].

5.7 Susceptibility testing of drug combinations

Combination therapy in bacterial infections is well established. Monotherapy often is regarded to be insufficient for fungal infections, especially by hyphomycetes because of the high mortality rate of these infections (see Chapter 4, by A. Polak). The efficacy of combination therapy is checked by a special *in vitro* testing technique, the checkerboard titration of antifungal agents. One therefore can judge the *in vitro* effects of one antifungal combined with another one or a non-antifungal drug as antagonistic, indifferent, additive, or synergistic in its effect. The test format commonly is the microdilution assay, since it is more standardized than any agar-based technique. The checkerboard titration in microtiter plates requires quite an effort: two dilution series have to be prepared and checked against each other. In the plate, the different concentrations for each substance are applied in the checkerboard manner. Each well has to be filled with 50 μl of the four-fold (final) concentration of the antifungal substance for a final test volume of 200 μl. The combination effect is calculated by the FIC (fractional inhibitory concentration) index, which is defined as FIC = A/MICA + B/MICB. A is the lowest concentration of the drug inhibiting in the presence of the second drug; MIC is the MIC of the drug alone. The FIC index is interpreted as synergy (FICs ≤ 0.50), additivism (FICs > 0.50 to 1.0), indifference (FICs > 1.0 to ≤ 2.0), and antagonism (FICs > 2.0). Especially for testing hyphomycetes, this method is limited by the problem of reading endpoints, as discussed already. Therefore, a modified checkerboard microdilution method employing the dye MTT was proposed. This alternative technique, the response surface modeling, seems quite promising [133].

6 Interpretation of the MICs

In vitro susceptibility testing gives hints about the activity of a drug but does not guarantee reliable evidence for the clinical outcome. Numerous reports on the correlation of MICs with the clinical outcome of mycoses in animal experiments (see Chapter 4, by A. Polak) are quite important. The best *in vivo-in vitro* correlation was found for flucytosine. In antifungal agents for which there is no consensus on how to determine their MICs (e.g., itraconazole, caspofungin), this correlation is more difficult.

Studies on *in vivo-in vitro* correlation mainly concern yeast isolates from patients with oral candidosis. For hyphomycetal infections in animal experiments, comprehensive data exist for the classical antifungal agents. In humans correlation is documented mostly in case reports; for selected agents, see, e.g., [134, 135]. A correlation with a NCCLS M38-P-like method could be established for itraconazole and *Aspergillus fumigatus* [98].

The most comprehensive study for correlation of fluconazole and itraconazole MICs of *Candida* isolates to the clinical outcome was initiated by the NCCLS committee. It was concluded that a MIC defined as susceptible does not uniformly predict therapeutic success, and *in vitro* resistance correlates often, but not generally, with therapeutic failure [136]. Because a MIC interpreted as resistant is considered to be more predictive for the clinical outcome (therapeutical failure highly probable) than a MIC interpreted as susceptible (no guarantee for therapeutical success), one might use the term resistance instead of susceptibility testing. Data from the NCCLS study are of limited value only. Most of the patients were suffering from oropharyngeal candidosis (due to HIV infection), and the results are based on the original version of the NCCLS methodology (macrodilution method, incubation period of 48 hours, plain RPMI medium), which meanwhile had been changed (see Sections 3.1.1 and 5.1) in order to get data that were more reproducible and that correlated better with the clinical outcome. In other studies a good, high or excellent *in vivo-in vitro* correlation is documented [77, 86, 90, 137–140].

Rare Amphotericin B-resistant *Candida* isolates were readily identified with Antibiotic Medium 3 as test medium [70]. Reports on correlation testing of hyphomycetes seem to be promising [98, 141, 142].

The following observations support a further correlation of MICs with the clinical outcome:

(1) *Candida albicans* isolates from patients never having been exposed to azoles will show up to > 90% low MICs of fluconazole interpreted as susceptible. If one of these "azole-naive" patients has to be treated with fluconazole, a therapeutic success rate of over 90% can be stated.
(2) Clinical failures correlate well with higher MICs. Infections due to *Aspergillus terreus* generally are known to be refractory to amphotericin B therapy. This correlates well with the MICs. The species *Aspergillus fumigatus* usually is *in vitro* susceptible to itraconzole. But *Aspergillus fumigatus* isolates under therapy refractory to itraconazole showed MICs of > 16 μg/ml [98]. This correlation could be confirmed in murine systemic aspergillosis [137]. Further therapeutic failure is found in other fungi with high MICs, e.g., infections due to *Fusarium* spp. and *Scedosporium* spp. treated with

amphotericin B. Experimental *Fusarium solani* infections not responding to amphotericin B therapy correlated with MICs > 1 μg/ml [143].

The duration an etiological agent is detectable culturally often correlates well with its MIC. So *Candida albicans* isolates susceptible to fluconazole under therapy in AIDS patients usually will be eliminated within a relative short time, whereas the *in vitro* less susceptible species *Cryptococcus neoformans* is eliminated within a longer period.

An absolute *in vitro-in vivo* correlation might be limited for the following reasons:

1) The test conditions never will reflect real life.
- The doubling time of fungal cells in the human body is far less than that of the test assay. One can calculate that cells of *Candida albicans* double within about 90 minutes in the microdilution test. Presuming this growth rate in an infection, the amount of yeasts grown within 3 days would exceed the body weight of the patient.
- The glucose content is 0.08–0.12% *in vivo* instead of 2% *in vitro* (modified RPMI medium for testing of yeasts), which declines to 0% in the test assay. The ratio of fermentation of cells (provided that they can grow anaerobically) decreases during the incubation time, while the respiration increases when glucose is lowered. In the test assay, the fermentation-to-respiration ratio of yeasts is uncontrolled. In an infection this ratio might be influenced not only by strain specifity but also by the availibility of oxygen at the site of the infection.
- The inoculum of ~ 10^3 cells/ml for yeasts and ~ 10^4 conidia/ml for hyphomycetes, respectively, was arbitrarily chosen for reasons of better test performance as well as the endpoints of reading (50% inhibition). Infections cannot be calculated quantitatively, e.g., an abscess will have a higher quantity of yeast cells.
- The availability of oxygen and the presence of carbon dioxide, respectively, possibly influencing the susceptibility is not yet studied enough.
- The test procedure is a batch assay constantly buffered to pH 7.0, different from the situation in the infected patient.
- It is not yet understood why the addition of serum to the test assay for *in vivo* simulation influences the MICs in such a way that they will be contrary to those without any serum.

- Immune cells cannot be incorporated into the test assay.
- The reproducibility of some test methods is not satisfactory. MICs often range between three 2-fold dilutions for the same isolate, even in quality control strains. Other isolates often show a higher variability in their MICs. Isolates with MICs between susceptible and resistant (so-called "intermediate" MICs) can be categorized as susceptible as well as resistant if their MICs are allowed to vary within three 2-fold dilutions.
- The conclusions from different MICs obtained with round- or flat-bottomed microtiter plates testing yeasts (data from our lab, not published) are not drawn yet.

2) The etiological agent.
Some open questions concerning the test organisms are rarely considered in the test assay.

- Blastoconidia of yeasts and conidia of hyphomycetes are used as inoculum, whereas *in vivo* different morphological structures (e.g., pseudomycelium, hyphae) are seen.
- Patients might harbor different clones of the same species with varying susceptibility [144, 145]. Our findings agree with these authors. In 62% of AIDS patients with oropharyngeal candidosis undergoing azole therapy, more than one DNA subtype could be isolated [146]. Molecular typing only might allow one to discriminate between the replacement of one strain with another or the change of the resistance pattern. There is no guarantee that resistant clones will be detected among susceptible colonies in clinical specimens unless culture media containing different antifungal concentrations are used.
- In antifungal susceptibility testing, it is generally implied that *in vivo* resistance is stable *in vitro*. Only limited data exist on this.
- The virulence of the etiological agents is not checked by the test system. Susceptible isolates with high virulence could be more resistant to therapy compared to those with lower virulence.

3) The antifungal substances.
Without understanding pharmacodynamic data, a correlation of MICs with clinical outcome is difficult to establish. The MIC should not be seen absolutely. The peak serum (the c_{max}/MIC ratio) and trough levels, the tissue

concentrations, the duration of exceeding the antifungal concentration in serum or tissue, and the MIC and the AUC (area under the curve)/MIC ratio are essential for judgment on therapeutic outcome.

Most test systems hardly consider the chemophysical property, e.g., the lipophilic (hydrophobic) character, of itraconazole or posaconazole. Itraconazole is about 100,000-fold less hydrophilic compared to fluconazole (see also Section 3.1.4). Good correlations are expected for antimycotic drugs, for which determination of their antifungal activity *in vitro* is easy and which have calculable pharmacokinetic data. Therefore, correlation for itraconazole might be not as good as that for fluconazole [136, 147].

Serum levels usually are the basis for such a prediction, although the main site of infection is not the blood. A fictitious discrepancy between *in vivo* and *in vitro* results is seen, e.g., if itraconazole was poorly absorbed. Such situations will be detected by determination of the serum level.

4) The patient.

Some patient-related factors will contribute to the predictive value of a MIC:

- The immunological status of the patient undoubtedly influences the outcome of an infection. This status has to be seen not only in the context of the patient's underlying disease but also on the site and/or severity of the fungal infection and on the local defense mechanism, e.g., varying in different organs or in an abscess.
- Yeast isolates from colonized catheters might be *in vitro* susceptible but are refractory to therapy. This does not contradict any correlation because "biofilms", a complex entity, might be an explanation [148].
- Drug interactions have to be considered. Data on correlation are not valid when drug interactions with the antifungal are suspected.
- Pharmacokinetic parameters on the correlation must be considered. For example, itraconazole is highly bound to plasma proteins and blood cells and generates individual levels of this substance in serum (and tissue). Its active metabolic product, hydroxy-itraconazole, does not directly correlate to the serum level. Fluconazole serum levels of patients with leukemia are reported to be significantly lower than in other patient groups. Furthermore, fluconazole shows other pharmacokinetics for children than for adults. These few drug-specific examples are representative only of the complexity of the in the *in vivo-in vitro* correlation.

Acknowledgements

The authors are grateful to Annemarie Polak and Birgit Willinger for helpful comments and critical reading of the manuscript.

References

1 M. Borg-von Zepelin, H. Eiffert, M. Kann and R. Rüchel: Mycoses *35* (Suppl.). 21–25 (1992).
2 F. Ancarani: Clinician *11*, 6–9 (1993).
3 K. Tintelnot: Tätigkeitsbericht des Robert Koch-Instituts RKI, MMV Medizin Verlag GmbH, München 1995, 54–55.
4 J. Berenguer, V. Fernández-Baca, R. Sánchez and E. Bouza: Eur. J. Clin. Microbiol. Infect. Dis. *14*, 362–365 (1995).
5 M. Knoke, K. Schulz and H. Bernhardt: Mycoses *40*, 105–110 (1997).
6 J.R. Maenza, W.G. Merz, M.J. Romagnoli, J.C. Keruly, R.D. Moore and J.E. Gallant: Clin. Infect. Dis. *24*, 28–34 (1997).
7 B. Dupont: 4th Congress ECMM, Glasgow, U.K., Abstract (1998).
8 L.A. Joseph, C.B. Moore, D. Law, D.M. Thornton, B.J.M. Bowles and D.W. Denning: 4th Congress ECMM, Glasgow, U.K., Abstract (1998).
9 K.A. Marr, R.A. Bowden and T.C. White: 38th Annual ICAAC (Abstr. J-32), San Diego, CA (1998).
10 F.M. Müller and T.J. Walsh: 50. Kongress DGHM u. 25. Jahrestg. DGI, Berlin, Abstract (1998).
11 D. Law, C.B. Moore, H.M. Wardle, L.A. Ganguli, M.G. Keaney and D.W. Denning: J. Antimicrob. Chemother. *34*, 659–668 (1994).
12 C. Waskow, M. Seibold, K. Tintelnot and F. Bergmann: 30. Wissensch. Tagung DMykG Kiel, Abstract (1996).
13 J.D. Cartledge, J. Midgley and B.G. Gazzard: AIDS *11*, 1839–1844 (1997).
14 Bundesgesundheitsbl. – Gesundheitsforsch. – Gesundheitsschutz *43*, 887–890, Springer-Verlag, Berlin/Heidelberg 2000.
15 D.W. Denning, G.G. Baily and S.V. Hood: Eur. J. Clin. Microbiol. Infect. Dis. *16*, 261–280 (1997).
16 K. Venkateswarlu, D.W. Denning and S.L. Kelly: J. Med. Vet. Mycol. *35*, 19–25 (1997).
17 F.C. Odds, in: *Candida* and Candidosis, 2nd ed., Baillière Tindall, London-Philadelphia-Toronto-Sydney-Tokyo 1988, 279–313.
18 J.N. Galgiani, J. Reiser, C. Brass, A. Espinel-Ingroff, M.A. Gordon and T.M. Kerkering: Antimicrob. Agents. Chemother. *31*, 1343–1347 (1987).
19 Groupe d'études de la Société Française de Mycologie Medicale: Bull. Soc. Fr. Mycol. Med. *10*, 131–134 (1981).
20 National Committee for Clinical Laboratory Standards. NCCLS Document M27-A: NCCLS, Wayne, PA (1997).
21 M. Borg-von Zepelin, T. Niederhaus, U. Gross, M. Seibold, M. Monod and K. Tintelnot: AIDS *16*, 1237–1244 (2002).

22 Y. Nakamura, R. Kano, S. Watanabe, H. Takahashi and A. Hasegawa: Mycoses *41*, 41–44 (1998).

23 K.C. Ha and T.C. White: Antimicrob. Agents Chemother. *43*, 763–768 (1999).

24 S. Arikan, M. Lozano–Chiu, V. Paetznick and J.H. Rex: Antimicrob. Agents Chemother. *45*, 327–330 (2001).

25 J.M. Blondeau, X. Zhao, G. Hansen and K. Drlica: Antimicrob. Agents Chemother. *45*, 433–438 (2001).

26 P. Marichal, J. Gorrens, M.C. Coene, L. Le Jeune and H. Vanden Bossche: Mycoses *38*, 111–117 (1995).

27 J.H. Rex, M.G. Rinaldi and M.A. Pfaller: Antimicrob. Agents Chemother. *39*, 1–8 (1995).

28 P. Sandven, K. Nilsen, A. Digranes, T. Tjade and J. Lassen: Antimicrob. Agents Chemother. *41*, 1375–1376 (1997).

29 A. Polak: Ancotil Flucytosin: Status Quo and Perspektiven, ed. ICN Pharmaceuticals, Herbert Utz Verlag, München 1999.

30 D. Sanglard, F. Ischer, M. Monod and J. Bille: Antimicrob. Agents Chemother. *40*, 2300–2305 (1996).

31 T.C. White, K.A. Marr and R.A. Bowden: Clin. Microbiol. Rev. *11*, 382–402 (1998).

32 M.A. Ghannoum and L.B. Rice: Clin. Microbiol. Rev. *12*, 501–517 (1999).

33 A. Espinel-Ingroff, F. Barchiesi, K.C. Hazen, J.V. Martinez-Suarez and G. Scalise: Med. Mycology *36* (Suppl. I), 68–78 (1998).

34 J.H. Rex, M.A. Pfaller, T.J. Walsh, V. Chaturvedi, A. Espinel-Ingroff, M.A. Ghannoum, L.L. Gosey, F.C. Odds, M.G. Rinaldi, D.J. Sheehan et al.: Clin. Microbiol. Rev. *14*, 643–658 (2001).

35 F.C. Odds, T. DeBacker, G. Dams, L. Vranckx and F. Woestenborghs: J. Clin. Microbiol. *33*, 995–997 (1995).

36 K. Tintelnot and M. Seibold: Mycoses *39* (Suppl. 2), 22–26 (1996).

37 M.A. Ghannoum, A.S. Ibrahim, Y. Fu, M.C. Shafiq, J.E. Edwards and R.S. Criddle: J. Clin. Microbiol. *30*, 2881–2886 (1992).

38 M.D. Witt, R.J. Lewis, R.A. Larsen, E.N. Milefchik, M.A.E. Leal, R.H. Haubrich, J.A. Richie, J.E. Edwards Jr. and M.A. Ghannoum: Clin. Infect. Dis. *22*, 322–328 (1996).

39 H. Sanati, S.A. Messer, M. Pfaller, M. Witt, R. Larsen, A. Espinel-Ingroff and M. Ghannoum: J.Clin. Microbiol. *34*, 1280–1282 (1996).

40 M.A. Pfaller, M.G. Rinaldi, J.N. Galgiani, M.S. Bartlett, B.A. Bodey, A. Espinel-Ingroff, R.A. Fromtling, G.S. Hall, C.E. Hughes, F.C. Odds et al.: Antimicrob. Agents Chemother. *34*, 1648–1654 (1990).

41 R.A. Fromtling, J.N. Galgiani, M.A. Pfaller, A. Espinel-Ingroff, K.F. Bartizal, M.S. Bartlett, B.A. Bodey, C. Frey, G. Hall, G.D. Roberts et al.: Antimicrob. Agents Chemother. *37*, 39–45 (1993).

42 J.L. Rodríguez-Tudela and J.V. Martinez-Suarez: Antimicrob. Agents Chemother. *38*, 45–48 (1994).

43 J.L. Rodríguez-Tudela and J.V. Martinez-Suarez: J. Antimicrob. Chemother. *35*, 739–749 (1995).

44 A. Espinel-Ingroff, J.L. Rodríguez-Tudela and J.V. Martinez-Suarez: J. Clin. Microbiol. *33*, 3154–3158 (1995).

45 E. Werner, M. Seibold and E. Antweiler: Mycoses *36*, 125–130 (1993).

46 J.N. Galgiani and M.L. Lewis: Antimicrob. Agents Chemother. *41*, 180–183 (1997).

47 M. Seibold and E. Werner: Mycoses *38*, 443–448 (1995).

48 C.B. Moore, N. Sayers, J. Mosquera, J. Slaven and D.W. Denning: J. Infect. *41*, 203–240 (2000).

49 M. Borgers and M.A. van de Ven: Rev. Inf. Dis. *9* (Suppl. 1), 33–42 (1987).

50 N.S. Ryder: Mycoses *42* (Suppl.), 2, 115–119 (1999).

51 C.J. Jessup, N.S. Ryder and M.A. Ghannoum: Med. Mycol. *38*, 155–159 (2000).

52 H. Yamada, S. Kohno, S. Maesaki, H. Koga, M. Kaku, K. Hara and H. Tanaka: J. Clin. Microbiol. *31*, 1009–1012 (1993).

53 A. Espinel-Ingroff, T.M. Kerkering, P.R. Goldson and S. Shadomy: J. Clin. Microbiol. *29*, 1089–1094 (1991)

54 A.Espinel-Ingroff, C.W. Kish, T.M. Kerkering, R.A. Fromtling, K. Bartizal, J.N. Galgiani, K. Villareal, M. Pfaller, T. Gerarden, M.G. Rinaldi et al.: J. Clin. Microbiol. *30*, 3138–3145 (1992).

55 F. Barchiesi, A.L. Colombo, D.A. McGough and M.G. Rinaldi: J. Clin. Microbiol. *32*, 2494–2500 (1994).

56 M.A. Pfaller, C. Grant, V. Morthland and J. Rhine-Chalberg: J. Clin. Microbiol. *32*, 506–509 (1994).

57 D.L. Sewell, M.A. Pfaller and A.L. Barry: J. Clin.Microbiol. *32*, 2099–2102 (1994).

58 A.W. Fothergill: Focus on fungal infections 6, New Orleans, Louisiana 1996, 31–33.

59 S.G. Revankar, W.R. Kirkpatrick, R.K. McAtee, A.W. Fothergill, S.W. Redding, M.G. Rinaldi and T.F. Patterson: J. Clin. Microbiol. *36*, 153–156 (1998).

60 J.H. Rex, P.W. Nelson, V.L. Paetznick, M. Lozano-Chiu, A. Espinel-Ingroff and E.J. Anaissie: Antimicrob. Agents Chemother. *42*, 129–134 (1998).

61 K.A. Marr, T.R. Rustad, J.H. Rex and T.C. White: Antimicrob. Agents Chemother. *43*, 1383–1386 (1999).

62 O. Uzun, S. Arikan, S. Kocagöz, B. Sancak and S. Unal: Diagnost. Microbiol. Infect. Dis. *38*, 101–107 (2000).

63 B. Rambali, J.A. Fernandez, L. van Nuffel, F. Woestenborghs, L. Baert, D.L. Massart and F.C. Odds: J. Antimicrob. Chemother. *48*, 163–177 (2001).

64 T. Yoshida, K. Jono and K. Okonogi: Antimicrob. Agents Chemother. *41*, 1349–1351 (1997).

65 R.A. Cook, K.A. McIntyre and J.N. Galgiani: Antimicrob. Agents Chemother. *34*, 1542–1545 (1990).

66 J.N. Galgiani and D.A. Stevens: Antimicrob. Agents Chemother. *10*, 721–726 (1976).

67 E.J. Anaissie, V.L. Paetznick and G.P. Bodey: Antimicrob. Agents Chemother. *35*, 1641–1646 (1991).

68 M.A. Pfaller, S.A. Messer and S. Coffmann: J. Clin. Microbiol. *33*, 1094–1097 (1995).

69 E.J. Anaissie, V.L. Paetznick, L.G. Ensign, A. Espinel-Ingroff, J.N. Galgiani, C.A. Hitchcock, M. LaRocco, T. Patterson, M.A. Pfaller, J.H. Rex et al.: Antimicrob. Agents Chemother. *40*, 2387–2391 (1996).

70 J.H. Rex, C.R. Cooper, W.G. Merz, J.N. Galgiani and E.J. Anaissie: Antimicrob. Agents Chemother. *39*, 906–909 (1995).

71 A.L. Barry, M.A. Pfaller, S.D. Brown, A. Espinel-Ingroff, M.A. Ghannoum, C. Knapp, R.P. Rennie, J.H. Rex and M.G. Rinaldi: J. Clin. Microbiol. *38*, 3457–3459 (2000).

72 P. Sandven, A. Bjorneklett, A. Maeland and the Norwegian Yeast Study Group: Antimicrob. Agents Chemother. *37*, 2443–2448 (1993).

73 C. Imbert-Bernard, A. Valentin, J. Reynes, M. Mallie and J.M. Bastide: Europ. J. Clin. Microbiol. Infect. Dis. 13, 711–716 (1994).

74 M. Ruhnke, E. Engelmann, B. Geiseler and M. Trautmann: Infection *22*, 132–136 (1994).
75 M. Ruhnke, A. Schmidt-Westhausen, E. Engelmann and M. Trautmann: J. Clin. Microbiol. *34*, 3208–3211 (1996).
76 A.F. Schmalreck, I. Kottmann, A. Reiser, U. Ruffer, E. Scharr and E. Vanca: Mycoses *38*, 359–368 (1995).
77 S. Metzger and H. Hofmann: Mycoses *40* (Suppl. 1), 56–63 (1997).
78 S.A. Radford, E.M. Johnson and S.W. Warnock: Antimicrob. Agents Chemother. *41*, 841–843 (1997).
79 M. Ruhnke, A. Schmidt-Westhausen and M. Trautmann: Antimicrob. Agents Chemother. *41*, 575–577 (1997).
80 A.F. Schmalreck, I. Kottmann, A.Reiser, P.Tränkle and E. Vanca: Mycoses *43*, 208–209 (1999).
81 W. Fegeler, A. Schmalreck and Working Group of the German Speaking Mycological Society: Rev. Iberoam. Micol. *17*, P9-008 abstr (2000).
82 P.D. Hoeprich and P.D. Finn: J. Infect. Dis. *126*, 353–361 (1972).
83 M.S. Marriott and K. Richardson, in: R.A. Fromtling and J.R. Prous (eds.): The discovery and mode of action of fluconazole. Prous Science, Barcelona 1987, 81–92.
84 M. Lozano-Chiu, P.W. Nelson, M. Lancaster, M.A. Pfaller and J.H. Rex: J. Clin. Microbiol. *35*, 270–272 (1997).
85 P. Chavanet, J. Lopez, M. Grappin, A. Bonnin, M. Duong, A. Waldner, M. Buisson, P. Camerlynck and H. Portier: AIDS *8*, 945–950 (1994).
86 C. Quereda, A.M. Polanco, C. Giner, A. Sánchez-Sousa, E. Pereira, E. Navas, J. Fortún, A. Guerrero and F. Baquero: Europ. J. Clin. Microbiol. & Infect. Dis. *15*, 30–37 (1996).
87 A.M. Tortorano, M.A. Viviani, F. Barchiesi, D. Arzeni, A.L. Rigoni, M. Cogliati, P. Compagnucci and G. Scalise: J. Clin. Microbiol. *36*, 1578–1583 (1998).
88 M. Seibold: Antiinfect. Drugs Chemother. *14*, 61 Abstract (1996).
89 M. Seibold, E. Engelmann, F. Esdorn, B. Graf and R. Schiller: 3rd Meeting of the European Confederation of Medical Mycology, Lisboa, Abstract (1996).
90 K. Tintelnot, G. Just-Nübling und M. Seibold: 28. Wissensch. Tagung der DMykG Montreux, Schweiz, Abstract (1994).
91 J. Van Cutsem, F. van Gerven and P.A.J. Janssen: Rev. Infect. Dis. *9* (Suppl. 1), 15–32 (1987).
92 A.Polak: Mykosen *30*, 306–314 (1987).
93 R.L. Stiller, J.E. Bennett, H.J. Scholer, M. Wall, A. Polak and D.A. Stevens: Antimicrob. Agents Chemother. *22*, 482–487 (1982).
94 A. Espinel-Ingroff, K. Dawson, M. Pfaller, E. Anaissie, B. Breslin, D. Dixon, A. Fothergill, V. Paetznick, J. Peter, M. Rinaldi et al.: Antimicrob. Agents Chemother. *39*, 314–319 (1995).
95 A. Espinel-Ingroff, M. Bartlett, R. Bowden, N.X. Chin, C. Cooper, jr, A. Fothergill, M.R. McGinnis, P. Menezes, S. A. Messer, P.W. Nelson et al.: J. Clin. Microbiol. *35*, 139–143 (1997).
96 National Committee for Clinical Laboratory Standards. NCCLS document M38-P: NCCLS, Wayne, PA (1998).
97 K.L. Oakley, C.B. Moore and D.W. Denning: J. Antimicrob. Chemother. *42*, 91–94 (1998).
98 D.W. Denning, S.A. Radford, K.L. Oakley, L. Hall, E.M. Johnson and D.W. Warnock: J. Antimicrob. Chemother. *40*, 401–414 (1997).
99 A. Espinel-Ingroff: 39th ICAAC, San Francisco, 544, Abstract (1999).

100 A. Espinel-Ingroff: J. Clin. Microbiol. *36*, 2950–2956 (1998).
101 S. Arikan, M. Lozano-Chiu, V. Paetznick, S. Nangia and J.R. Rex: J. Clin. Microbiol. *37*, 3946–3951 (1999).
102 E.K. Manavathu, J.L. Cutright and P.H. Chandrasekar: Antimicrob. Agents Chemother. *42*, 3018–3021 (1998).
103 E.M. Johnson, A. Szekely and D.W. Warnock: J. Antimicrob. Chemother. *42*, 741–745 (1998).
104 J. Meletiadis, J.F.G.M. Meis, J.W. Mouton, J.L.Rodriquez-Tudela, J.P. Donnelly, P.E. Verweij and the EUROFUNG Network: Antimicrob. Agents Chemother. *46*, 62–68 (2002).
105 J. Meletiadis, J.W. Mouton, J.F.G.M. Meis, B.A. Bouman, J.P. Donnelly, P.E. Verweij and Eurofung Network: J. Clin. Microbiol. *39*, 3402–3408 (2001).
106 A. Gehrt, J. Peter, P.A. Pizzo and T.J. Walsh: J. Clin. Microbiol. *33*, 1302–1307 (1995).
107 C. Lass-Flörl, M. Nagl, E. Gunsilius, C. Speth, H. Ulmer and R. Würzner: Mycoses *45*, 166–169 (2002).
108 V. Bezjak: J. Clin. Microbiol. *21*, 509–512 (1985).
109 E.K. Manavathu, J.L. Cutright and P.H. Chandrasekar: J. Clin. Microbiol. *37*, 858–861 (1999).
110 A. Espinel-Ingroff: Antimicrob. Agents Chemother. *45*, 605–607 (2001).
111 J. Guarro, C. Llop, C. Aguilar and I. Pujol: Antimicrob. Agents Chemother. *41*, 2760–2762 (1997).
112 M.H. Nguyen, C.J. Clancy, V.L. Yu, Y.C. Yu, A.J. Morris, D.R. Snydman, D.A. Sutton and M.G.Rinaldi: J. Infect. Dis. *177*, 425–430 (1998).
113 M.A. Pfaller and A.L. Barry: J. Clin. Microbiol. *32*, 1992–1996 (1994).
114 M.A. Pfaller, Q. Vu, M. Lancaster, A. Espinel-Ingroff, A. Fothergill, C. Grant, M.R. McGinnis, L. Pasarell, M.G. Rinaldi and L.Steele-Moore: J. Clin. Microbiol. *32*, 1625–1628 (1994).
115 M. Lozano-Chiu, M.V. Lancaster and J.H. Rex: Diagn. Microbiol. Infect. Dis. *31*, 417–424 (1998).
116 B. Jahn, A. Stuben and S. Bhakdi: J. Clin. Microbiol. *34*, 2039–2041 (1996).
117 C.J. Clancy and M.H. Nguyen: J. Clin. Microbiol. *35*, 2878–2882 (1997).
118 S.P. Hawser, H. Norris, C.J. Jessup and M.A. Ghannoum: J. Clin. Microbiol. *36*, 1450–1452 (1998).
119 J. Meletiadis, J. Meis, J.W. Mouton, J.P. Donnelly and P.E. Verweij: J. Clin. Microbiol. *38*, 2949–2954 (2000).
120 M.E. Klepser, E.J. Ernst, R.E. Lewis, M.E. Ernst and M.A. Pfaller: Antimicrob. Agents Chemother. *42*, 1207–1212 (1998).
121 I. Pujol, C. Aguilar, J. Fernández-Ballart and J. Guarro: Med. Mycology *38*, 23–26 (2000).
122 A. Espinel-Ingroff: J. Clin. Microbiol. *39*, 954–958 (2001).
123 W.R. Kirkpatrick, T.M. Turner, A.W. Fothergill, D.I. McCarthy, S.W. Redding, M.G. Rinaldi and F. Patterson: J. Clin. Microbiol. *36*, 3429–3432 (1998).
124 M.A. Pfaller, B. Dupont, G.S. Kobayashi, J. Müller, M.G. Rinaldi, A. Espinel-Ingroff, S. Shadomy, P.F. Troke, T.J. Walsh and D.J. Warnock: Antimicrob. Agents Chemother. *36*, 1805–1809 (1992).
125 K.U. Bartz-Schmidt, K. Tintelnot, M. Steffen, M. Özel, B. Kirchhof and K. Heimann: Clin. Exp. Ophthalmol. *234*, 591–593 (1996).
126 C. Wenisch, K.F. Linnau, B. Parschalk, K. Zedtwitz–Liebenstein and A. Georgopoulos: J. Clin. Microbiol. *35*, 5–10 (1997).

127 M.A. Pfaller, S.A. Messer, A. Bolmström, F.C. Odds and J.H. Rex: J. Clin. Microbiol. *34*, 1691–1693 (1996).
128 A. Wanger, K. Mills, P.W. Nelson and J.H. Rex: Antimicrob. Agents Chemother. *39*, 2520–2522 (1995).
129 A. Espinel-Ingroff: J. Clin. Microbiol. *39*, 1360–1367 (2001).
130 M.A. Pfaller, S. Arikan, M Lozano-Chiu, Y.-S. Chen, S. Coffman, S.A. Messer, R. Rennie, C. Sand, T. Heffner, J.H. Rex et al.: J. Clin. Microbiol. *36*, 2609–2612 (1998).
131 A. Espinel-Ingroff, M. Pfaller, S.A. Messer, C.C. Knapp, S. Killian, H.A. Norris and M.A. Ghannoum: J. Clin. Microbiol. *37*, 591–595 (1999).
132 B. Willinger, P. Apfalter, A.M. Hirschl, A. Makristathis, M. Rotter and M. Seibold: Diag. Microbiol. Infect. Dis. *38*, 11–15 (2000).
133 D.T.A. Te Dorsthorst, P.E. Verweij, J.F.G.M. Meis, N.C. Punt and J.W. Mouton: Antimicrob. Agents Chemother. *46*, 702–707 (2002).
134 O. Cornely, J. Chemnitz, H.G. Broichhagen, K. Lemmer, H. Schütt, D. Söhngen, P. Staib, C. Wickenhauser, V. Diehl and K. Tintelnot: Emerg. Infect. Dis. *7*, 149–152 (2001).
135 I. Sobottka, H. Albrecht, D. Mack, H.-J. Stellbrink, J. van Lunzen, K. Tintelnot and R. Laufs: Eur. J. Clin. Microbiol. Inf. Dis. *15*, 256–259 (1996).
136 J.H. Rex, M.A. Pfaller, J.N. Galgiani, M.S. Bartlett, A. Espinel-Ingroff, M.A. Ghannoum, M. Lancaster, F.C. Odds, M.G. Rinaldi, T.J. Walsh et al. for the Subcommittee on Antifungal Susceptibility Testing of the National Committee for Clinical Laboratory Standards: Clin. Infect. Dis. *24*, 235–247 (1997).
137 E. Dannaoui, E. Borel, F. Persat, M.F. Monier and M.A. Piens: J. Med. Microbiol. *48*, 1087–1093 (1999).
138 S.-C. Lee, C.-P. Fung, J.-S. Huang, C.-J. Tsai, K.-S. Chen, H.-Y. Chen, N. Lee, L.-C. See and W.-B. Shieh: Antimicrob. Agents Chemother. *44*, 2715–2718 (2000).
139 F. Lacassin, F. Damond, C. Chochillon, P. Longuet, J. Lebras, J.-L. Vildea and C. Leport: Antimicrob. Agents Chemother. *40*, 1961–1963 (1996).
140 J.L. Rodríguez-Tudela, J.V. Martinez-Suarez, F. Dronda, F. Chaves and E. Valencia: J. Antimicrob. Chemother. *35*, 793–804 (1995).
141 C. Lass-Flör, G. Kofler, G. Kropshofer, J. Hermans, A. Kreczy, M.P. Dierich and D. Niederwieser: J. Antimicrob. Chemother. *42*, 497–502 (1998).
142 F.C. Odds, F. van Gerven, A. Espinel-Ingroff, M.S. Bartlett, M.A. Ghannoum, M.V. Lancaster, M.A. Pfaller, J.H. Rex, M.G. Rinaldi and T.J. Walsh: Antimicrob. Agents Chemother. *42*, 282–288 (1998).
143 J. Guarro, I. Pujol and E. Mayayo: Antimicrob. Agents Chemother. *43*, 1256–1257 (1999).
144 A. Schoofs, F.C. Odds, R. Colebunders, M. Ieven, L. Wouters and H. Goossens: Antimicrob. Agents Chemother. *41*, 1625–1635 (1997).
145 E. Dannaoui, V. Lacoste, C. Prat and M.A. Piens: Mycoses *40*, 279–282 (1996).
146 M.A. Pfaller, J. Rhine-Chalberg, S.W. Redding, J. Smith, G. Farinacci, A.W. Fothergill and M.G. Rinaldi: J. Clin. Microbiol. *32*, 59–64 (1994).
147 P. Phillips, J. Zemcov, W. Mahmood, J.S.G. Montaner, K. Craib and A.M. Clarke: AIDS *10*, 1369–1376 (1996).
148 J. Chandra, D.M. Kuhn, P.K. Mukherjee, L.L. Hoyer, T. McCormick and M.A. Ghannoum: J. Bacteriol. *183*, 5385–5394 (2001).

Index